HOME BIRTH

HOME BIRTH

HOME BIRTH

ANNA-MARIE MADELEY
Registered Midwife, BSc(Hons)
Midwifery, MSc (Oxon), PGCertTHE, FHEA
Doctoral Researcher
School of Health, Wellbeing & Social Care,
Faculty of Wellbeing Education & Language Studies
Open University, Milton Keynes
United Kingdom

ELSEVIER

ISBN: 978-0-323-93501-2

Content Strategist: Andrae Akeh
Content Project Manager: Shivani Pal
Design: Ryan Cook

Printed in India

Last digit is the print number: 9   8   7   6   5   4   3   2   1

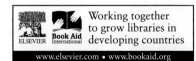

Working together
to grow libraries in
developing countries

www.elsevier.com • www.bookaid.org

CONTENTS

PREFACE

At the time of writing, homebirth rates in the UK remain low, representing 2.4% of births in 2020, rising from 2.1% in 2019 (ONS, 2020). Despite this rise, attributed in part to the effects of the coronavirus (COVID-19) pandemic, the rate of homebirth has remained relatively stable over the last decade, declining from a rate of approximately 2.5% in 2010. What influences decisions for place of birth has been explored both in general terms and specifically for homebirth (Coxon *et al.*, 2017; Naylor Smith *et al.*, 2018) with factors such as availability and clarity of information supporting all options to inform choices, confidence in and reliability of maternity services, views of families, friends and health care professionals, and personal beliefs around risk and safety. The National Maternity Review in England (NHS England, 2016) and National Institute for Health and Care Excellence in the UK (NICE, 2017) suggest women should be provided with clear, unbiased, evidence-based information to support their decision about their preferred place of birth which includes offering home as an option for healthy women and birthing people at lower risk of complications. For many, the choice to labour and birth at home will be something that perhaps they have never considered and for some, this may have been their preference for some time. In either case the key to safe and respectful care is acknowledging the needs, wants, and preferences of each woman and birthing person as an individual, ensuring discussions and recommendations related to *any* place of birth be grounded in a personalised approach to care planning, considering individual biopsychosocial influences, motivations, and clinical presentation informed by the best available evidence.

The aim of this book is not to convince anyone to choose one place or mode of birth over another but to explore, discuss, and describe what it means to safely facilitate homebirth in the UK. This book also does not aim to be a definitive guide; this would be impossible given the scope of service provision across the UK. Facilitating safe birth at home requires a particular set of skills, knowledge, resources, and confidence to safely support antenatal, intrapartum, and postnatal care whilst remaining alert to identifying deviations from expected physiology and escalate this in a safe and timely manner. This book therefore aims to provide a starting point to consider how national and local policies, guidelines, and governance arrangements can support women and birthing people's choice to birth at home, touching on key practice points for reflection at an individual and institutional level as well a practical consideration for resources and equipment.

For some midwives, perhaps new to the profession or even those with extensive experience of intrapartum care within a hospital environment, attending and facilitating birth at home might be a daunting prospect as there exists a wide variety of exposure to experiences of home birth for clinicians and students alike. The sociodemographic profile of women and birthing people who access homebirth services and the range of geographical challenges presented by many areas in the UK, whether these be inner city or remote and rural locations, all influence how planning for homebirth is conducted as a strategic and individual level. Threaded throughout this book are themes of safety, ongoing risk assessment, personalised care planning, best available evidence, working with the wider multidisciplinary team, pathways for escalation, management of emergencies, and clinical self-efficacy, all informed by national reports and reviews.

By drawing upon the expertise of midwives leading and working in models supporting homebirth, neonatal clinicians, doulas, educators and academics, consultant midwives, and lead clinical paramedics, this book hopes to inspire and develop confidence in discussing, planning, and facilitating birth evidence-based care at home with reference to local and national guidelines. The book begins with an exploration of the evidence for homebirth which provides a foundation for the following chapters, which cover subjects such as homebirth in education, service, and antenatal planning, managing labour at home, postnatal care, water birth at home, emergency birth including breech birth at home, working alongside paramedics during transfer and emergencies, the neonatal perspective, freebirth, and planning for women with complex needs. Alongside the chapters the book presents a collection of reflective vignettes from a consultant midwife, doula, homebirth midwife, and service user on what it means to them to have experience in homebirth from their own unique perspectives.

Planning and facilitating safe homebirth has been a passion for me since I first embarked on my own midwifery career, having been exposed and involved early in my student journey to respectful, safe, and skilful care by inspiring midwives and role models. Both in my clinical practice as a senior midwife leading a homebirth team and subsequently as a midwifery educator, when asked to signpost to contemporary books that addressed safe homebirth, existing texts were few and far between. This began a chain of events that led to the development of this book and subsequent connections with like-minded contributors who, like me, are committed to the development and dissemination of safe care practices alongside supporting women in their choices. I hope that by bringing together the expertise of the contributors of this book it will go some way to developing the knowledge and supporting ongoing safe practice of student midwives, midwives, and the wider maternity community and multidisciplinary team.

Anna-Marie Madeley

REFERENCES

Coxon, K. *et al.* (2017) 'What influences birth place preferences, choices and decision-making amongst healthy women with straightforward pregnancies in the UK? A qualitative evidence synthesis using a "best fit" framework approach', *BMC Pregnancy and Childbirth*, 17(1), p. 103. Available at: https://doi.org/10.1186/s12884-017-1279-7.

Naylor Smith, J. *et al.* (2018) '"I didn't think you were allowed that, they didn't mention that." A qualitative study exploring women's perceptions of home birth', *BMC Pregnancy and Childbirth*, 18(1), p. 105. Available at: https://doi.org/10.1186/s12884-018-1733-1.

NHS England (2016) 'National Maternity Review. Better Births'. NHS England.

NICE (2017) 'Intrapartum care for healthy women and babies.' National Institute for Health and Care Excellence. Available at: https://www.nice.org.uk/guidance/cg190/chapter/recommendations#pain-relief-in- labour-nonregional.

ONS, (2020) 'Births in England and Wales: 2019 Live births, stillbirths and the intensity of childbearing, measured by the total fertility rate. ' Office for National Statistics. Available at: https://www.ons.gov.uk/peoplepopulationandcommunity/birthsdeathsandmarriages/livebirths/bulletins/birthsummarytablesenglandandwales/2019.

LIST OF CONTRIBUTORS

Carla Jayne Avery, BsC (Hons) Midwifery, PGCTHE, MA Medical Education
Associate Professor in Midwifery
School of Nursing, Midwifery and Allied Health
Buckinghamshire New University, Aylesbury
United Kingdom

Ethel Burns, PhD
Faculty of Health and Life Sciences
Oxford brookes University, Oxford
United Kingdom

Claire Feeley, RM, BSc (Hons), MSc, PhD
Lecturer
Nursing, Midwifery & Palliative Care
King's College London, Milton keynes
United Kingdom

Mari Greenfield, PhD, PGCHE, MA, MA, MPA, BA
Postdoctoral Fellow
Women and Children's Health
King's College, London, London
United Kingdom

Lesley Kilby, RGN, PGCAP, PGDip ME, FHEA, BSc Neonatal Studies
ANNP/Senior Lecturer Neonatal Care
Milton Keynes University Hospital
University of Bedfordshire

Amy Meadowcroft, BSc Hons
Midwife
Maternity Services
Northern Care Alliance NHS Foundation Trust, Oldham
United Kingdom

Lydia Naomi Miller, BSc Hons, MCPara
Learning Development Officer
Learning and Development
SWAST, Bristol
United Kingdom

John Pendleton, BA (Hons), BSc (Hons), MSc, RM, FHEA
Senior Lecturer
Faculty of Health, Education & Society
University of Northampton, Northampton
United Kingdom

Katy Powis, BN
Senior Lecturer in Neonatal Care
School of Nursing, Midwifery and Health Education
University for Bedfordshire, Luton
United Kingdom

Carolyn Rooth, MSc, MA, BSc(Hons) RM
School of Nursing, Midwifery & Health Education
University of Bedfordshire, Luton
LU1 3JU
United Kingdom

Emma Spillane BSc (Hons), MSc
Consultant Midwife
St Georges NHS Foundation Trust

Samuel Todd, Registered Midwife, BSc (Hons), Professional Midwifery Advocate
Midwifery Lecturer
Midwifery
Birmingham City University, Birmingham
United Kingdom

Shawn Walker, RM, PhD
Senior Research Fellow
Women and Children's Health
King's College London, London
United Kingdom
Researcher in Residence
Midwifery
Imperial College London, London
United Kingdom

Becky Louise Westbury, BMid, MSc
Community Midwife Team Leader
Maternity
Hywel Dda University Health Board, Aberystwyth
United Kingdom

Aimee Yarrington, FCPara, MSc, BSc (hons)
Midwife and Paramedic
College of Paramedics
College of Paramedics, West Midlands
United Kingdom

ACKNOWLEDGEMENTS

A heartfelt thank you to all contributors to this book, including those who shared their reflections on homebirth as service users, clinicians, and birth workers. Each one of you has been working in intensely challenging circumstances in the 3 years running up to the production of this book and it is a testament to your commitment to safe clinical care and education that you have dedicated your time to producing such valuable words. Thank you to Mhairi McLellan for your wisdom around facilitating birth in remote and rural locations, Chriss Doyle for your unique perspective, and Belle for being my voice of reason. Thank you to the Elsevier team and Claire for your support and advice in navigating this process. A massive thank you to Christine Cooper, who not only introduced me to safe and respectful homebirth and began a journey that I will forever be grateful for but also role-modelled midwifery advocacy and instilled in me the skills, knowledge, and confidence necessary to support women and birthing people to labour birth safely at home. Finally, I wish to express my thanks to every family who has allowed me to provide support and care in your home. You inspire me every day to be a better advocate and clinician.

CHAPTER 1

HOMEBIRTH – THE EVIDENCE

Samuel Todd

The Nursing and Midwifery Council (2018) and General Medical Council (2020) are clear and unanimous regarding the importance of and need for women to receive clear, accurate, and up-to-date information which is based on the best available evidence. It is important to acknowledge both professional bodies as although most women will have contact with a midwife there will be occasions where women receive care from obstetricians and general practitioners. However, when it comes to discussing homebirth as a place of birth option with women it is clear they do not always receive clear, accurate, up-to-date information from their healthcare professionals. This can be supported by reviewing the uptake of homebirth in the UK. The rates of homebirth in England and Wales remain consistently low, with only 2.4% of all births in 2020 occurring at home, compared with 2.9% in 2007 and 2008 (the greatest percentage of women giving birth at home over the last three decades) (Office for National Statistics, 2022). The COVID-19 pandemic had the potential to increase rates of homebirth due to women and their families wanting to avoid the virus and to have birth partners of their choosing present at the birth. However, multiple NHS Trusts scaled back midwifery-led birth options including homebirths and both freestanding and alongside midwifery-led units (Moore, 2021). In doing this NHS Trusts potentially increased the exposure of mothers and babies to COVID-19, whereas homebirth could have offered protection against contracting the virus. Research by Selma-Royo et al. (2020) identified that being born at home is beneficial to a baby's immune system and results in a stronger epithelial barrier function and maturation. Furthermore, there appears to be a higher immunological response in babies born at home. Outside of the COVID-19 pandemic there are numerous factors that may contribute to the continued low uptake of homebirth. Factors may include unreliable homebirth services (e.g. midwives escalated to work in inpatient maternity services) and homebirth not being actively promoted as a viable birthplace option (e.g. due to low confidence in facilitating homebirth by midwives offering the service), both of which can lead to reduced confidence in women considering this as an option. However, arguably the biggest factor that impacts informed decision making is healthcare professionals ignoring the evidence regarding the place of birth and therefore not providing accurate information. More often, myths and misinformation are often verbalised by healthcare professionals when faced with questions from women regarding the possibility of a homebirth or suitability for homebirth, including primiparous women not being 'suitable' or women with identified complexities (regardless of what they are) being told that they are 'high risk' and will need to birth on an obstetric unit.

Midwives and obstetricians are viewed as trustworthy by those accessing maternity services and, as such, have a duty to ensure that women receive the correct information based on evidence to make decisions regarding place of birth choices. Cook and Loomis (2012) identified that women rely on their healthcare professionals for them to make birth-related decisions during the birth planning phase. Furthermore, they recommend that all members of the woman's birthing team need to support women in making informed choices and negotiating decisions during the birth process. The National Maternity Review (2016) recommends that care is personalised, centred on the woman and her family, and based on the woman's needs and her decisions, where they have genuine choice that has been informed by unbiased information. A systematic review undertaken by Henshall et al. (2016) identified that during place of birth discussions some midwives assumed decision-making responsibility for women when deciding birthplace options. This was done by stereotyping women according to their social background, age, and literacy levels or because midwives felt they should not be granted access to information which might sway their decision making. In these situations, midwives were reported to either omit place of birth options or present them in such a way that women would be unlikely to disagree with their suggestions. Choosing the place to give birth is arguably the biggest decision a woman may make when planning her birth options and women should be able to choose to birth at home, in a midwifery unit, or in an obstetric unit and their choice should be supported (National Institute for Health and Care Excellence, 2017). Information about midwifery-led units and obstetric led-units may be more readily available and health professionals may feel more confident discussing these place of birth options; however, it has been identified that women often seek information regarding homebirth from sources outside of contact with health professionals including the internet and the opinions of friends and family (Naylor-Smith et al., 2018; Yuill et al., 2020). This could suggest that women do not receive comprehensive and consistent information about homebirth from trusted healthcare professionals.

Ideally women would receive information about all of their birth options from their named midwife during pregnancy. However, pressures such as increased case loads may impact on the ability of the midwife to have these conversations due to reduced time for a well-rounded conversation to take place which includes the risks and benefits of all place of birth options. Instead, at a booking appointment following a risk assessment a recommended place of birth option may be discussed and documented. In many NHS Trusts the pathways of care usually follow an opt-out model for women who are 'low-risk', with their default place of birth option being a midwifery unit. For women who are deemed 'high-risk' will be placed on a pathway where they will birth in an obstetric unit. Midwives should discuss and offer homebirth as a place of birth option; however, as exposure to homebirths is low midwives may have reduced confidence to talk about home as a place of birth option. Drip-feeding information may be a beneficial approach to take when planning the place of birth with women. At each antenatal contact providing small quantities of information regarding birthplace options may allow the woman to ask questions and engage with the process. This would avoid a decision needing to be made at the booking appointment which may have taken place at or before 10 weeks (Green, 2016), supporting flexibility in decision making later in the pregnancy. Ideally the decision to birth at home should be finalised by 34-36 weeks gestation, however the woman should be made aware that they can change their mind at any point leading up to labour and birth. Furthermore, it could be argued that place of birth should not be chosen until the woman goes into labour. This could be supported by the offer of a home assessment in labour by a midwife. Janssen et al. (2003) identified that home assessments in labour are associated with reduced opioid analgesia use, reduced neonatal intensive care unit admissions, and increased rates of established labour on admission to the hospital. If this was widely offered to all women there is the potential that more women may choose to continue to labour and birth at home; however, further research is required in this area to understand the implications of this (including maternal and neonatal outcomes and experiences).

Historically 'home' was the 'normal' birthplace, and most readers of this book are likely to be descended from one or two generations away from a homebirth. However, it is important to note that although this was the usual place of birth this would not have been without certain challenges. Prior to modern maternity care there would have been a lack of national standardised risk assessments, guidelines, and resources. For example, in extremely rural areas there may have been no appropriate transport to the hospital if the need arose (obstetric flying squads were only introduced in the 1930s), and for some these delays would most certainly have been a contributing factor to morbidity and mortality for either/both mother and newborn. Most women who had homebirths during this time would have been cared for primarily by a midwife and if further support was needed (e.g. if there was a delay in the second stage of labour) the woman's general practitioner would attend. The Peel Report (Standing Maternity and Midwifery Advisory Committee, 1970) was a major turning point for place of birth as it stated, 'sufficient facilities should be provided to allow for 100% hospital delivery'. It could be argued that it was the publication of this report that led numerous healthcare professionals and our wider society to believe that homebirth was not as 'safe' as a hospital birth and may have been the beginning of many myths surrounding the safety of homebirth. Beech (2012) identified that when undertaking the Peel Report no women were asked if they wanted to birth in a hospital and no evidence was found to suggest that increasing hospital-based births would reduce adverse outcomes. The Peel Report was a major turning point for how the public perceives homebirth and more importantly the perceived 'danger' of giving birth at home. Anecdotally, even today many would openly question the safety of homebirth based on misconceptions arising from this period and women who have birthed at home may face comments such as 'did you plan to birth at home?' or 'you are brave'. However, the same cannot be said for women who birth in a hospital and the potential for iatrogenic harm.

Evidence suggests that this move towards hospital-based births has resulted in increased rates of interventionist births. It would be remiss not to acknowledge that for some women intervention can be lifesaving (either for the mother and/or baby), for example, in cases of severe pre-eclampsia, fetal hypoxia, and postpartum haemorrhage. However, intervention during childbirth (such as episiotomy or instrumental births) is an identified risk factor for perinatal mental health problems (PMHPs). It is reported that one in five women is affected by PMHPs including anxiety, depression, and postpartum psychosis (NHS England, 2020). This is significant as if the PMHPs are directly related to the woman's experience of childbirth then this can be classified as morbidity. Furthermore, women may experience PMHPs any time from conception and up to a year following the birth (Mind, 2020). The impact of this can be devastating, as when left untreated PMHPs can lead to loss of resources, exacerbation of existing medical conditions, substance abuse, and suicide (Kendig et al., 2017). Ertan et al. (2021) identified that women who experienced childbirth as distressing and those who had unplanned caesarean births were more vulnerable to developing post-traumatic stress disorder. Conversely research by Bland (2009) identified that women who had a homebirth had lower rates of postnatal depression, felt more control over their birth experience, and were more satisfied with their birth experience. Therefore, it is essential that professionals working in maternity services are aware of our changing birth statistics and the impact of this on the short- and long-term health outcomes of women and babies. In England in the period 2020–2021, only 47.3% of all births commenced spontaneously (34.4% of all births were induced and the caesarean birth rate was 18.3%), compared to the period 2005–2006, in which 68.8% of all births commenced spontaneously (20.5% of all births were induced and the caesarean birth rate was 10.7%) (Michas, 2022).

The appetite for change regarding the perception and promotion of homebirth has only occurred relatively recently: the publication of the Birthplace in England Cohort Study (Birthplace in England Collaborative Group, 2011) provided the impetus for NHS hospitals and clinical commissioning groups to reevaluate the provision and promotion of homebirth services (Todd, 2021). The study identified that for 'low-risk' multiparous women, home was as safe as the hospital, with added benefits such as significantly and substantially reduced rates of unplanned caesarean birth, instrumental birth, or episiotomy. Although this research was positively received, it suggested that for nulliparous women there was a slight increase in adverse neonatal outcomes. For some NHS Trusts this would have given credence to the pervasive myth that homebirth is unsafe, especially for primiparous women, and therefore should not be promoted as a place of birth option. The Birthplace in England Cohort Study (Birthplace in England Collaborative Group, 2011) highlighted that the cost of a planned birth in an obstetric-led unit was approximately £1631 compared to a cost of £1067 for a planned homebirth. The findings of this study, including potential financial benefits, provided the impetus for NHS Trusts to review their current homebirth service provision and review how services were delivered; some trusts demonstrated forward thinking by creating dedicated homebirth teams (National Institute for Health and Care Excellence, 2014; Cross-Sudworth et al., 2018; Foley and Olusile, 2021). This model appears to have become increasingly popular with the development of increased numbers of dedicated homebirth teams nationally. The Royal College of Midwives (2017) has acknowledged that demands on maternity services are rising due to increased birth rates, increased complexity, a shortage of midwives, and an aging midwifery profession. Since 2010 the entire growth of the midwifery workforce has been among the oldest midwives, closest to their retirement date. The impact of this is the loss of typically more experienced midwives, who are replaced by newly qualified, less experienced midwives. With only a small population of women choosing to birth at home, combined with the loss of older midwives experienced in homebirths (due to retirement), the overall impact or likely outcome is that confidence in this area of midwifery practice will reduce compared with hospital-based care (Todd, 2020). Furthermore, due to lack of opportunity for student midwives and early-career midwives to learn from these experienced midwives who facilitate homebirth there is the potential for homebirth rates to decrease further. Common (2015) identified that it was difficult for midwives who work exclusively in community with low homebirth rates to maintain their intrapartum skills. This is of particular concern, with newly qualified midwives being allocated core community posts early in their careers. It is essential that midwives consolidate their knowledge and skills in observing and supporting physiological birth so that they can manage and avert complications that may arise. Without these skills midwives may have lower thresholds for transferring women from homebirths, whereas more experienced midwives may feel confident to continue intrapartum care at home (e.g. when there is an occipito-posterior labour with slower than expected progress). With the changing midwifery workforce, this gap in midwifery expertise will further impact women who choose to birth 'outside the system' as they are less likely to be listened to when expressing birth preferences that do not conform to 'normal' expectations.

Feeley et al. (2020) have expressed their concern at the lack of equitable services meeting the needs of women seeking a normal physiological birth. Women who are 'higher-risk' may feel their only option to achieve a normal physiological birth is to birth 'outside the system'. Jackson et al. (2012) identified that women who choose to pursue a 'higher-risk' homebirth feel that birthing 'outside the system' is a choice that protects them and their babies from the risks associated with birthing in a hospital and thus provides the best and safest birthing option. The Birthplace in England 'follow-on' study (Li et al., 2015) identified that 18–23% of 'higher-risk' multiparous women required transfer in labour compared to 12% of 'low-risk' multiparous women. Interestingly, in 'higher-risk' women, compared with planned obstetric-led unit births, planned homebirth was associated with a significantly reduced risk of an adverse perinatal outcome. Planned homebirth was associated with a reduced risk of maternal intervention or adverse outcome requiring obstetric care and an increased probability of a physiological vaginal birth compared with the obstetric-led unit. Home might appeal as the most appropriate place of birth for 'higher-risk' women or women who feel that they are given real choices rather than perceived choices, giving them feelings of empowerment, as identified by Bernhard et al. (2014). There has been increased media coverage regarding the mortality rates of women of colour in the UK during pregnancy and childbirth (McKenzie, 2019) following the publication of the *Saving Lives, Improving Mothers' Care* report (Knight et al., 2019) which reported that non-white women are more likely to die than white women in childbirth. In the most recent *Saving Lives, Improving Mothers' Care* report (Knight et al., 2021) these harrowing statistics have improved slightly (Table 1.1); however, they suggest and support the prevalence of racism in maternity care. Henderson et al. (2013) identified that women from minority ethnic groups were less likely to receive pain relief in labour and Black African women, in particular, were more likely to have an unplanned caesarean birth. Furthermore, they report that women from minority ethnic groups were less likely to feel spoken to in a way that they could understand and be treated with kindness and were less likely to be sufficiently involved in decisions, which impacted their confidence and trust in the staff. Holten et al. (2018) suggest that if healthcare professionals want fewer women to 'birth outside the system', then hospitals need to be perceived as safe again. This can only be accomplished by establishing a reputation of respect, trustworthiness, and equality between women and professionals.

For higher-risk women a combination of continuity of carer, meaningful place of birth discussions, and options that include homebirth and individualised care planning may offer a protective factor against adverse outcomes for both mother and baby. The Royal College of Midwives (2018) reports that women who received midwifery-led continuity models of care, compared to standard care, are more likely to know the midwife who cares for them in labour, feel satisfied with their experience of maternity care, and have a normal physiological birth. Furthermore, they are less likely to experience a fetal loss, premature birth, and instrumental birth or receive unnecessary intervention.

Table 1.1 Maternal Mortality Rates by Ethnicity (Knight et al, 2021)

MATERNAL MORTALITY RATIO 2015–2017		MATERNAL MORTALITY RATIO	
White women	7/100,000	White women	7/100,000
Asian women (2×)	13/100,000	Asian women (2×)	12/100,000
Mixed ethnicity women (3×)	23/100,000	Mixed ethnicity women (2×)	15/100,000
Black women (5×)	38/100,000	Black women (4×)	32/100,000

Dunkley-Bent (2018) reports that continuity of carer enables women to build a trusting relationship with their midwife and is the best way to help women have a safe, positive, and empowering experience of pregnancy, birth, and parenthood. In addition, continuity of carer ensures that women are physically and psychologically well so that they can develop a responsive and nurturing relationship with their children. Hunter (2006) identified that women want and need both a healthy baby and a satisfying childbirth experience. For women with 'higher-risk' pregnancies, in order to facilitate the woman's preference for a homebirth a care plan should be created. The purpose of this is to ensure the woman's safety; outline parameters for transfer; and take into account her wishes for labour and birth. According to Schwartz (2010) care plans act as a voice for women to be heard by healthcare professionals and include informed decision making, care planning, advocacy, and patient satisfaction. The care plan should be personalised to the woman and include the woman's medical and obstetric history. The clinical concern should be highlighted and state that the woman is planning a homebirth outside of guidance; a summary of why this would be a homebirth against advice should be sensitively documented. The anticipated time of transfer to the hospital should be estimated (which includes the time it would take for an ambulance to attend the home and the time it would take to transfer from the home) and documented in the care plan so that the woman is aware and comprehends that there may be a delay in commencing potentially lifesaving treatment should this be required. For women who are considered as having a 'higher-risk' pregnancy it is the recommendation of the author that two midwives be present during labour and birth. Lothian (2008) identified that autonomy of women during childbirth is necessary to tap into personal and authoritative knowledge, to develop confidence, and to make decisions. Otherwise, women are manipulated and swayed, and they give up control. The midwife creating the care plan should ensure that the woman is respected, valued, and honoured for her personal knowledge and can demonstrate this by documenting the woman's wishes, thoughts, and preferences in the care plan. The care plan should be agreed upon by the woman and her birthing team (the named midwife, a senior midwife such as a consultant midwife, and a consultant obstetrician). By involving the woman in the development of the care plan she may experience feelings of choice and control. The woman should receive a copy of the care plan for her own records and a second copy should be made available in her notes. This type of care planning can ensure that women who historically may not have been offered homebirth as an option have physically, psychologically, and culturally safe outcomes and experiences. Furthermore, it may readdress the disproportionate rates of mortality experienced by BAME women, in particular Black women. By individualising care that falls outside of guidance women may feel more involved in their care and empowered rather than disempowered by a medically managed maternity system and environment.

The vast majority will feel that their home is a safe space that is restful. Zielinski et al. (2015) suggest that labouring at home is linked to greater control over events and is more satisfying. Flint (2020) suggests that labour pain is more easily managed at home, with most labours only lasting a few hours; if a woman requires further analgesia or assistance then transfer to the hospital can be facilitated. There appears to be a power shift that occurs during home-births; when a woman attends a hospital in labour, she may feel that she is a 'guest' in the 'home' of the midwife. However, when a midwife attends a homebirth she becomes a 'professional guest' and this power shift can be empowering for women. Brailey et al. (2015) identified that women may be influenced to birth at home as they feel that they will have more autonomy and less medical intervention and will be in a more relaxing environment to give birth. Meredith and Hugill (2017) report that women deciding on a homebirth are essentially seeking places of emotional and physical safety for birth. The benefits of giving birth at home extend to fathers; Sweeney and O'Connell (2015) identified that homebirth gives fathers greater involvement in, and ownership of, the birth experience and fathers can be positively impacted emotionally as a result. When homebirth services are suspended or when the offer of homebirth is withdrawn the impact of this on women planning to birth at home should not be ignored. It is apparent that midwife-led birth options such as homebirth and midwifery-led units are seen as 'nice' extras that only lead to enhanced experience rather than the physical benefits of giving birth at home. In order to sustain homebirth provision NHS Trusts need to examine how best to plan for a workforce that can accommodate this place of birth option, giving it equal attention and importance as workforce planning for obstetric-led units.

The usual model for homebirths in the UK is for women to be attended by two midwives, who are usually based within the community. The responsibility to maintain a 24/7 on-call homebirth service for women often lies with the community teams. However, during high activity and short staffing within the hospital those community midwives are often escalated to support services. It has been reported that midwives are significantly more likely to want to work in a continuity-based model, which included intrapartum care for homebirths only, compared with intrapartum care across all settings (Taylor et al., 2019). A potential solution to improving homebirth provision would be for NHS hospitals to develop new dedicated homebirth teams and continue to support existing ones. Moreover, when designing dedicated homebirth teams, consideration should be made about the inclusion of midwifery support workers (MSWs) as the second birth attendant for low-risk births only. It has been identified that with appropriate training, such as the completion of a maternity pathway foundation degree, MSWs could be used as second birth attendants, freeing up midwifery time and providing a reliable homebirth service (Taylor et al., 2019). For this model to be safe and effective, it is essential that the MSWs are part of the team and not escalated from their usual place of work to attend homebirths to avoid familiarity with setting, location and working practices. By working in a dedicated homebirth team, MSWs can provide care during the antenatal, intrapartum, and postnatal period, contributing to the woman receiving continuity of carer. Furthermore, it could be argued that the potential for adverse outcomes in low-risk births is further reduced because there is no confusion over who is the lead at the birth. The midwife is responsible for maintaining safety and recognising any deviations, while the MSW is there to primarily support the midwife in their role (Taylor et al, 2018).

Table 1.2 Key Benefits of Birth at Home According to Contemporary Systematic Review	
Hutton et al. (2019): perinatal or neonatal mortality among women who intend at the onset of labour to give birth at home.	Reitsma et al. (2020): maternal outcomes and birth interventions among women who begin labour intending to give birth at home.
• There was no significant difference by intended place of birth in adverse neonatal outcomes regardless of parity. • An Apgar score of <7 at 5 minutes occurred less frequently among intended homebirths in multiparas women.	• >40% less likely to give birth by caesarean • >50% less likely to have an instrumental birth • 70% less likely to use epidural analgesia • 5% less likely to have an episiotomy • >40% less likely to experience a third- or fourth-degree perineal tear • >60% less likely to receive oxytocin augmentation of labour • >75% fewer reported maternal infections • >30% fewer reported postpartum haemorrhages

For midwives providing homebirth services the most recent evidence should confirm and enhance existing learnt knowledge about the benefits. However, for healthcare professionals who may not have experience with homebirth or who may be unsure of what the evidence suggests it would be remiss not to update knowledge in this area which may contribute to dispelling myths. As such, there has never been a better time for those providing and commissioning maternity services to re-evaluate guidelines and provide women with up-to-date evidence. Dahlen (2019) suggests that evidence is now very convincing for homebirth in both primiparous and multiparous women. Table 1.2 highlights the key benefits of homebirth, and these findings were derived from the largest systematic reviews and meta-analyses of 500,000 planned homebirths.

Regan (2020) suggests that a randomised control trial of homebirth is not possible and that these meta-analyses represent our best current knowledge about the safety of homebirth for low-risk women. With the publication of recent evidence supporting the safety and benefits of homebirth, there has never been a better time to feel optimistic about changing the place of birth culture. There is real potential to increase the uptake of homebirth nationally and this will benefit from the creation of more dedicated homebirth teams, alongside women receiving continuity of carer.

REFERENCES

Beech, B. (2012) The benefits of homebirth: Evidence of safety, effectiveness and women's experience. Available at: https://www.aims.org.uk/assets/media/3/benefits-of-home-birth.pdf

Bernhard, C., Zielinksi, R., Ackerson, K. and English, J. (2014) Homebirth after hospital birth: Women's choices and reflections, Journal of Midwifery & Women's Health; 59(2): 160–166.

Birthplace in England Collaborative Group, Brocklehurst, P., Hardy, P., Hollowell, J. et al. (2011) Perinatal and maternal outcomes by planned place of birth for healthy women with low-risk pregnancies: The Birthplace in England national prospective cohort study, BMJ; 23(343): d7400.

Bland, M. (2009) The influence of birth experience on postpartum depression, Midwifery Today; 89: 65–66.

Brailey, S., Jarrett, P., Luyben, A. and Poat, A. (2015) Swimming against the tide: Women's experience of choosing a homebirth in Switzerland, British Journal of Midwifery; 23(11). Available at: https://doi.org/10.12968/bjom.2015.23.11.780

Common, L. (2015) Homebirth in England: Factors that impact on job satisfaction for community midwives, British Journal of Midwifery; 23(10): 716–722.

Cook, K. and Loomis, C. (2012) The impact of choice and control on women's childbirth experiences, The Journal of Perinatal Education; 21(3): 158–168.

Cross-Sudworth, F., Hindley, J., Cheatham, C., Clarke, P. and McAree, T. (2018) Creating a dedicated homebirth service: Results of a 3-year pilot, British Journal of Midwifery; 26(3). Available at: https://www.britishjournalofmidwifery.com/content/research/creating-a-dedicated-homebirth-service-results-of-a-3-year-pilot

Dahlen, H. (2019) Is it time to ask whether facility based birth is safe for low-risk women and their babies? The Lancet; 14: 9–10.

Dunkley-Bent, J. (2018) The importance of continuity of carer in maternity services. Available at: https://www.england.nhs.uk/blog/the-importance-of-continuity-of-carer-in-maternity-services/

Ertan, D., Hingray, C., Burlacu, E., Sterlé, A. and El-Hage, W. (2021) Post-traumatic stress disorder following childbirth, BMC Psychiatry; 21. Available at: https://doi.org/10.1186/s12888-021-03158-6

Feeley, C., Byrom, A., Byrom, S. and Tizard, H. (2020) Normal birth, The Practising Midwife; 23(1): 34.

Flint, C. (2020) Reasons to be joyful. Available at: https://www.midwifery.org.uk/blog/midwifery-skills/reasons-to-be-joyful-by-caroline-flint/?fbclid=IwAR0y2A5C150B-x_Sy3eC1zGcxJS6F_H8xA_4qootl1hbmYiPd8aSYIN7jjY

Foley, C. and Olusile, M. (2021) A dedicated homebirth team, two years on, The Practising Midwife; 24(3). Available at: https://www.all4maternity.com/a-dedicated-home-birth-team-two-years-on/

General Medical Council. (2020) Guidance on professional standards and ethics for doctors: Decision making and consent. Available at: https://www.gmc-uk.org/-/media/documents/gmc-guidance-for-doctors—-decision-making-and-consent-english_pdf-84191055.pdf

Green, C. (2016) Preparing women for homebirth, The International Journal of Birth and Parent Education; 3(4): 7–10.

Henderson, J., Gao, H. and Redshaw, M. (2013) Experiencing maternity care: The care received and perceptions of women from different ethnic groups, BMC Pregnancy and Childbirth; 13(196). https://doi.org/10.1186/1471-2393-13-196

Henshall, C., Taylor, B. and Kenyon, S. (2016). A systematic review to examine the evidence regarding discussions by midwives, with women, around their options for where to give birth, BMC Pregnancy and Childbirth; 16(53). https://doi.org/10.1186/s12884-016-0832-0

Holten, L., Hollander, M. and de Miranda, E. (2018) When the hospital is no longer an option: A multiple case study of defining moments for women choosing homebirth in high-risk pregnancies in the Netherlands, Qualitative Health Research; 28(12): 1883–1896.

Hunter, L.P. (2006) Women give birth and pizzas are delivered: Language and Western childbirth paradigms, Journal of Midwifery & Women's Health; 51(2): 119–124.

Hutton, E., Reitsma, A., Simioni, J., Brunton, G. and Kaufman K. (2019) Perinatal or neonatal mortality among women who intend at the onset of labour to give birth at home compared to women of low obstetrical risk who intend to give birth in hospital: A systematic review and meta-analyses, The Lancet; 14: 59–70.

Jackson, M., Dahlen, H. and Schmied, V. (2012) Birthing outside the system: Perceptions of risk amongst Australian women who have freebirths and high risk homebirths, Midwifery; 28(5): 561–567.

Janssen, P.A., Iker, C.E. and Carty, E.A. (2003) Early labour assessment and support at home: A randomized controlled trial, Journal of Obstetrics and Gynaecology Canada; 25(9): 734–741.

Kendig, S., Keats, J.P., Hoffman, C.M., Kay, L.B., Miller, E.S., Moore Simas, T.A., Frieder, A., Hackley, B., Indman, P., Raines, C., Semenuk, K., Wisner, K.L. and Lemieux, L.A. (2017) Consensus bundle on maternal mental health: Perinatal depression and anxiety, Journal of Midwifery & Women's Health; 62(2): 232–239. Available at: https://doi.org/10.1111/jmwh.12603

Knight, M., Bunch, K., Tuffnell, D., Patel, R., Shakespeare, J., Kotnis, R., Kenyon, S. and Kurinczuk, J.J. (Eds.) on behalf of MBRRACE-UK. Saving Lives, Improving Mothers' Care (2021) Lessons learned to inform maternity care from the UK and Ireland Confidential Enquiries into Maternal Deaths and Morbidity 2017–19. Oxford: National Perinatal Epidemiology Unit, University of Oxford.

Knight, M., Bunch, K., Tuffnell, D., Shakespeare, J., Kotnis, R., Kenyon, S. and Kurinczuk J.J. (Eds.) on behalf of MBRRACE-UK. Saving Lives, Improving Mothers' Care (2019) Lessons learned to inform maternity care from the UK and Ireland Confidential Enquiries into Maternal Deaths and Morbidity 2015–17. Oxford: National Perinatal Epidemiology Unit, University of Oxford.

Li, Y., Townend, J., Rowe, R., Brocklehurst, P., Knight, M., Linsell, L., Macfarlane, A., McCourt, C., Newburn, M., Marlow, N., Pasupathy, D., Redshaw, M., Sandall, J., Silverton, L. and Hollowell, J. (2015) Perinatal and maternal outcomes in planned home and obstetric unit births in women at 'higher risk' of complications: Secondary analysis of the Birthplace national prospective cohort study, BJOG: An International Journal of Obstetrics and Gynaecology; 122(5): 741–753.

Lothian, J.A. (2008) Choice, autonomy, and childbirth education, The Journal of Perinatal Education; 17(1): 35–38.

McKenzie, G. (2019) MBRRACE and the disproportionate number of BAME deaths, AIMS Journal; 31(2): 18–23.

Meredith, D. and Hugill, K. (2017) Motivations and influences acting on women choosing a homebirth: Seeking a 'cwtch' birth setting, British Journal of Midwifery; 25(1). Available at: https://doi.org/10.12968/bjom.2017.25.1.10

Michas, F. (2022) Distribution of child deliveries in National Health Service (NHS) hospitals in England from 2005/06 to 2020/21, by type of labor onset. Available at: https://www.statista.com/statistics/936564/method-of-labor-onset-in-england/

Mind. (2020) Postnatal depression and perinatal mental health. Available at: https://www.mind.org.uk/information-support/types-of-mental-health-problems/postnatal-depression-and-perinatal-mental-health/about-maternal-mental-health-problems/

Moore, A. (2021) Covid crisis forces suspension of maternity services. Available at: https://www.hsj.co.uk/coronavirus/covid-crisis-forces-suspension-of-maternity-services/7029261.article

National Institute for Health and Care Excellence. (2014) Birmingham's dedicated homebirth service. Available at: https://www.nice.org.uk/sharedlearning/birmingham-s-dedicated-homebirth-service

National Institute for Health and Care Excellence. (2017) Intrapartum care for healthy women and babies. Available at: https://www.nice.org.uk/guidance/cg190/resources/intrapartum-care-for-healthy-women-and-babies-pdf-35109866447557

National Maternity Review. (2016) Better births: Improving outcomes of maternity services in England – A five year forward view for maternity care. Available at: https://www.england.nhs.uk/wp-content/uploads/2016/02/national-maternity-review-report.pdf

Naylor-Smith, J., Taylor. B., Shaw, K., Hewison, A. and Kenyon, S. (2018) 'I didn't think you were allowed that, they didn't mention that'. A qualitative study exploring women's perceptions of homebirth, BMC Pregnancy and Childbirth; 18. Available at: https://doi.org/10.1186/s12884-018-1733-1

NHS England. (2020) Better Births Four Years On: A review of progress. Available at: https://www.england.nhs.uk/wp-content/uploads/2020/03/better-births-four-years-on-progress-report.pdf

Nursing and Midwifery Council. (2018) The Code: Professional standards of practice and behaviour for nurses, midwives and nursing associates. Available at: https://www.nmc.org.uk/globalassets/sitedocuments/nmc-publications/nmc-code.pdf

Office for National Statistics. (2022) Birth characteristics in England and Wales: 2020. Available at: https://www.ons.gov.uk/peoplepopulationandcommunity/birthsdeathsandmarriages/livebirths/bulletins/birthcharacteristicsinenglandandwales/latest

Regan, M. (2020) Homebirth meta-analyses across two reviews: Hutton et al., 2019 and Reitsma et al., 2020, The Practising Midwife; 24(3).

Reitsma, A., Simioni, J., Brunton, G., Kaufman, K. and Hutton E. (2020) Maternal outcomes and birth interventions among women who begin labour intending to give birth at home compared to women of low obstetrical risk who intend to give birth in hospital: A systematic review and meta-analyses, The Lancet; 21: 1–10.

Royal College of Midwives. (2017) The gathering storm: England's midwifery workforce challenges. Available at: https://www.rcm.org.uk/media/2374/the-gathering-storm-england-s-midwifery-workforce-challenges.pdf

Royal College of Midwives. (2018) Position statement: midwifery continuity of carer (MCOC). London: RCM. Available at: https://www.rcm.org.uk/media/2946/midwifery-continuity-of-carer-mcoc.pdf

Selma-Royo, M., Calatayud Arroyo, M., García-Mantrana, I., Parra-Llorca, A., Escuriet, R. Martínez-Costa, C. and Collado, M.C. (2020) Perinatal environment shapes microbiota colonization and infant growth: impact on host response and intestinal function, Microbiome; 167(8). https://doi.org/10.1186/s40168-020-00940-8

Schwartz, J. (2010) Birth plans: Why pay attention? International Journal of Childbirth Education; 25(1): 5–9.

Standing Maternity and Midwifery Advisory Committee. (1970) Domiciliary midwifery and maternity bed needs. Report of the sub-committee. Chairman: Sir John Peel. London: HMSO; 1970.

Sweeney, S. and O'Connell, R. (2015) Puts the magic back into life: Fathers' experience of planned homebirth, Women and Birth; 28(2): 148–153.

Taylor, R., Cross-Sudworth, F., Goodwin, L., Kenyon, S. and MacArthur, C. (2019) 'Midwives' perspectives of continuity-based working in the UK: A cross-sectional survey, Midwifery; 75: 127–137.

Taylor, B., Hensall, C., Goodwin, L. and Kenyon, S. (2018) Task shifting Midwifery Support Workers as the second health worker at a homebirth in the UK: A qualitative study, Midwifery; 62: 109–115.

Todd S. (2020) Am I eligible for a homebirth? Supporting women with a raised body mass index, MIDIRS Midwifery Digest; 30(4): 503–508.

Todd, S. (2021) Bringing birth home, The Practising Midwife; 24(3): 16–22.

Yuill, C., McCourt, C., Cheyne, H. and Leister, N. (2020) Women's experiences of decision-making and informed choice about pregnancy and birth care: A systematic review and meta-synthesis of qualitative research, BMC Pregnancy and Childbirth; 20. https://doi.org/10.1186/s12884-020-03023-6

Zielinski, R., Ackerson, K. and Kane Low, L. (2015) Planned homebirth: Benefits, risks and opportunities, International Journal of Womens Health; 7: 361–366.

CHAPTER 2

HOMEBIRTH IN UNDERGRADUATE, POSTGRADUATE, AND CLINICAL EDUCATION

Anna Madeley and Carolyn Rooth

INTRODUCTION

Professional education for homebirth has several focuses, pre-registration at undergraduate level, post-registration at either undergraduate or postgraduate level, and the provision of education for those who wish to explore home as an option for their place of birth. This involves being creative and focused on the provision of education, which aims to facilitate a positive and informative culture which ultimately empowers both healthcare professionals and service users alike. The aim of this chapter is to introduce some fundamental concepts of learning which apply to adult learning in the context of professional education and development whilst giving practical ideas for how this might be applied to services supporting homebirth and pre-hospital care.

DEVELOPING AND SUSTAINING THE LEARNING ORGANISATION

The movement of midwifery care to the hospital setting in the later part of the 20th century and the increase in the use of medical technology has undoubtedly influenced clinical practice. This has led to a focus on the acquisition of clinical competencies, which may not accurately reflect the needs of healthcare professionals and support staff working in women's homes and community-based settings. As financial considerations such as the need for cost-saving initiatives and the necessity to maintain safe staffing levels have also impacted, there has never been a greater need to develop and sustain a proactive learning culture where personal and organisational commitment to learning is seen as a core value rather than an optional extra.

A positive learning culture is much more than a tick box exercise which focuses on the meeting of mandatory training requirements or the development of skills and competencies. It is one which embraces the principles of a shared vision and team learning and provides the key to providing safe and effective care. Importantly a positive educational ethos not only develops and empowers the organisation through the development and empowerment of employees at all levels but in turn also ultimately empowers the women and the families who use maternity services (Hermansson and Mårtensson, 2010).

Skilful facilitation and leadership are required to achieve a positive learning culture which emphasises core values of providing safe and effective care, improving service user experience, and using the best available evidence to inform learning. This requires the application of adult learning theory (andragogy) and applies the following principles:

- Recognition of the need to develop, improve, and adapt at individual and organisational levels
- Valuing the sharing of knowledge
- Proactive use of acquired knowledge and skills
- Staff engagement with self-directed learning opportunities
- Access to tools and resources and the use of a variety of educational approaches to meet individual learning preferences
- Providing value for money

Senge's (1994) concept (Fig. 2.1) of a learning organisation can be applied to the development and need to sustain a positive learning culture. This concept embraces the principles of shared vision and team learning with an emphasis on five core elements of building a shared vision, systems thinking, mental models, team learning, and personal mastery.

The principles of shared vision, team learning, and personal mastery are perhaps self-explanatory whilst others require a little more explanation. Systems thinking relates to the whole picture and how each of the other elements interacts to achieve a shared goal. The concept of mental models considers how we as individuals perceive the world (or practice) through experiences which form our individual perceptions and assumptions. The knowledge and philosophies which underpin midwifery practice and maternity care are formed and informed through these concepts and are embedded in our experience of professional education. There is a recognition that education and practice are inextricably linked. When applied to the development and sustainability of positive and effective learning culture for homebirth education, the following considerations may be useful:

Shared vision:
- Maintaining/promoting/facilitating a culture that supports learning for all levels of staff
- Commitment to learning about homebirth in undergraduate and postgraduate theory and clinical practice experience

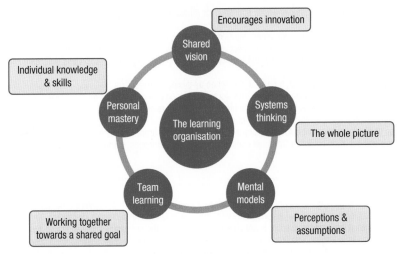

Fig. 2.1 Senge's (1994) concept.

- Empowerment healthcare professionals, women, and their families to use evidence to support informed choice
- Avoidance of a disconnect between what is being seen in practice and learnt in theory

Personal mastery:
- Recognition of learning as a lifelong process
- Revalidation and personal development and growth
- Developing confidence and the competencies needed to care for women in the family home

Team learning:
- Facilitation and provision of access to multi-professional education
- Working with non-healthcare professionals who may be called upon to attend a homebirth
- Seeking service user feedback to develop understanding of their views and experiences

Mental models:
- Using reflection to explore experiences
- Building trust and confidence in midwives and other healthcare professionals
- Acknowledgement of students' experience and view of homebirth
- Seeking feedback from service users
- Challenging unfounded assumptions

Systems thinking:
- Transformational leadership to ensure effective delivery of homebirth education and service provision
- Evaluation of both education and service provision through audit and feedback
- Ensuring that resources are available to support education and service provision

Other factors for consideration:
- Use of strategies to meet differing learning styles rather than a one-size-fits-all approach
- Providing resources for online and face-to-face education using a mix of interactive and non-interactive approaches
- Considering how to engage and motivate
- Ensuring that education is financially sustainable

PRACTICALITIES AND CONTENT

The content of face-to-face teaching activities for healthcare professionals in relation to homebirth will inevitably be influenced by local variations and focus on the management and required escalation of emergency situations. Educational activities aimed at service users are likely to focus on the practicalities of homebirth and again will be influenced by local variation. However, there is room for a more innovative approach which combines face-to-face activities and online educational packages related to homebirth, which can be worked through at the learner's own pace. Here the core principles of midwifery practice published in the *Lancet* series (Renfrew et al., 2014) may be useful in informing the content. These cover the following:
- Focusing on the needs of women, infants, and families
- Examination of care across the continuum from pregnancy to the early weeks after birth

- Employment of a human rights-based approach for all women and babies, regardless of context or circumstances
- Consideration of all relevant outcomes (mortality, morbidity, health, and well-being)
- Examination of personalised needs in all social settings (low, middle, and high-income)
- Taking a long-term view to achieve and maintain quality care and services (recognising that there are no quick fixes)
- Distinguishing between what, how, and who when analysing interventions
- Consideration of interdisciplinary and cross-sectoral working in the context of the healthcare system
- Consideration of a diverse workforce to achieve an appropriate skill mix
- Examination of the specific contribution of midwives
- Use of diverse sources of evidence using a rigorous and transparent approach
- Development of an evidence-informed consensus to inform guidelines, standard operational procedures, and policy

ADULT LEARNING

The development of adult learning theory (andragogy) was influenced by the work of Knowles (1984) (Fig. 2.2), who recognised that adults learn differently when compared with the way in which children learn (pedagogy). Knowles proposed that in adult learning the teacher is not considered to hold all the necessary knowledge and that adults are active participants in the educational process as individuals with unique life experiences adults were considered to have greater motivation to learn and to view the gaining of knowledge through a problem-solving perspective rather than being subject focused. This assumes that adults have an aim for their learning rather than this being imposed as it would be for a child. However, when applied to professional education, this view could be considered somewhat simplistic given that the content and outcomes for curricula are imposed by the governing bodies of each profession (Health & Care Professions Council, 2014; General Medical Council, 2018; Nursing and Midwifery Council (NMC), 2019). Additionally, it cannot be assumed that all adults are the same. Recognition that learning exists on a wide spectrum which will be influenced by multiple complex factors is important. Despite these considerations, the four adult learning principles of involvement, experience, motivation, and a need to problem solve suggested by Knowles remain relevant.

LEARNING STYLES

Although there are similarities in the way individuals learn, assimilate knowledge, and develop understanding, individual preferences will influence engagement with the learning that is offered. A preference for learning in a group setting or in a more solitary environment may also have influence on individual learning. Although there are a variety of theories

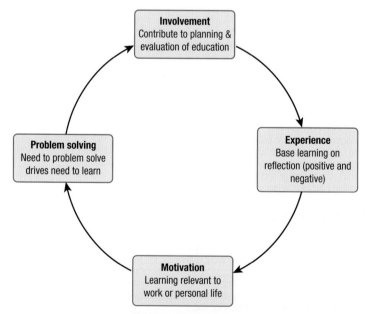

Fig. 2.2 The work of Knowles.

Table 2.1 Examples of Learning Styles Methods

VISUAL	AUDITORY	READING/WRITING	KINESTHETIC
Pictures	Lectures (Face to face & recorded)	Handouts	Hands-on practice
Posters		PowerPoints	Clinical experience
Video clips	Discussion groups	Books	Use of examples
Graphs	Podcasts	Guidance/policy documents	Role play
Diagrams	Audio recordings	Use of headings, notes, writing tasks/ reading tasks	Reflection
Use of colour/symbols	1:1 Tutorial		Visits
Body language	Use of mnemonics	Use of mnemonics	

which relate to learning styles, these are broadly described as being visual or auditory, preferring reading/writing, or being kinaesthetic, but there are other factors which less commonly influence learning style preferences (Pritchard, 2009). It may be somewhat simplistic to attribute one approach as the most appropriate in all circumstances and some learning will be gained through the adoption of all approaches to the presentation of information.

There is little research which focuses on learning styles in healthcare education, but a small study by Prithishkumar and Michael (2014) examined the experiences of undergraduate medical students with the use of a multiple-choice questionnaire designed to identify learning preferences. This found that the majority of students preferred more than one approach to learning (multimodal) and that only 13.8% were unimodal with a definitively identified preference. Auditory and kinaesthetic preferences were identified as the most common in this study. It is therefore important for facilitators of education to recognise that although there may be individual preferences, there is a necessity to devise a variety of ways with which to engage learners.

A variety of online tools can be used to determine which learning style an individual might wish to adopt but to maintain an effective learning environment, it is recommended that interactive student-centred approaches to facilitating learning are adopted. These could include the suggestions laid out in Table 2.1 above.

RESOURCES

The availability and use of resources such as visual aids, anatomical models, literature, and access to video resources need to be considered when planning educational activities. Funding may come from Trust educational budgets, but this may be a competitive process. It may therefore be necessary to bid from funding from other sources and the support of maternity managers will be required to facilitate this process.

UNDERGRADUATE MIDWIFERY EDUCATION

> *Skilled, knowledgeable, and compassionate midwifery care has a huge impact on outcomes and experiences for women and babies and is fundamental to quality maternity care.*
> —Renfrew et al., 2014

It is therefore essential that the woman or birthing person remain central to the provision of pre-registration midwifery education based on a 50% theory and 50% clinical practice split.

Whilst the higher education sector is responsible for delivery of theory components of pre-registration midwifery education, student midwife exposure in clinical placements to maternity care in the changing contexts of where and how current maternity services are provided is important. This includes the family home as a viable birthplace option. As a result, a workforce fit for purpose to care for women who opt for physiological birth either in a hospital or home setting needs to be central to every midwifery curriculum.

Within the UK, attainment of professional registration is guided by the NMC. The standards of proficiency for midwives and standards framework for midwifery education provide the core elements of curricula to ensure that midwives are both competent and confident to provide both universal and enhanced midwifery care at the point of registration (NMC, 2018, 2019). These standards align with the World Health Organization's (WHO) framework for action in strengthening midwifery education for universal health coverage (WHO, 2019) and the International Confederation of Midwives' (ICM) essential competencies for midwifery practice and global standards for midwifery education (ICM, 2018). Additionally, the UK-based standards and competencies were developed based on the *Lancet Midwifery* series, which adopted the following definition of midwifery:

> *...skilled, knowledgeable, and compassionate care for childbearing women, newborn infants, and families across the continuum throughout pre-pregnancy, pregnancy, birth, postpartum and the early weeks of life.*
> *Core characteristics include optimising normal biological, psychological, social and cultural processes of reproduction and early life; timely prevention and management of complications; consultation with and referral toother services, respect for women's individual circumstances and views; and working in partnership with women to strengthen women's own capabilities to care for themselves and their families.*
> —Renfrew et al., 2014, p. 1129

A robust curriculum therefore needs to ensure inclusion of all of these elements if student midwives are to be fully aware of the evidence-based knowledge that underpins midwifery practice and are able to provide care in all clinical settings. In addition, a pre-registration curriculum that is organised systematically and provides exposure to real-life experience of homebirth is essential if students are to be enabled to acquire the skills, knowledge, and behaviours essential to become autonomous practitioners who can facilitate physiological birth processes in both institutional and community settings, including women's homes (ICM, 2018). However, facilitating birth in community settings can be challenging, particularly where there are staffing and financial constraints. How student experience can be facilitated will inevitably be impacted by these factors as well as being influenced by local service provision and local design of any associated maternity care pathways.

> **Practice Point:**
> The implementation of a curriculum into clinical practice will be influenced by local variations such as geography, sociodemographic factors, the degree of implementation of continuity of care/carer, and the uptake of the option to birth at home. When developing a midwifery curriculum, consider how homebirth and pre-hospital care can be incorporated to meet local needs either through direct clinical practice or through simulation. This should be audited regularly during curriculum review cycles to maintain its fidelity.

Incorporation of the NMC standards of proficiency and ICM guidance for essential competencies for midwifery practice involves the promotion of strong links between theory and practice experience (ICM, 2018; NMC, 2019). In both spheres role modelling by teaching staff, practice supervisors, and assessors is needed to ensure that both theoretical and practice teaching is closely correlated and based on current evidence (ICM, 2018). For example, the Birthplace study (Brocklehurst et al., 2011) evidences the safety of planned homebirth in most circumstances where women chose to exercise their right to this birth option (Walton, 2012). Whilst place of birth can be explored from a theoretical perspective in a classroom setting, it is the exposure in clinical practice placements to homebirths which enables the student to apply this to her practice experience and thus integrate theory and practice more effectively. The introduction of homebirth teams and continuity models of care as part of the implementation of the recommendations of the Better Births report (NHS England, 2016) also provide unique opportunities for students to experience the planning, design, and delivery of safe, evidence-based homebirth (Moncrieff et al., 2020).

Pre-registration curricula therefore require core themes of:
- How midwives facilitate physiological birth processes in all clinical settings, including homebirth as part of physiological birth teaching.
- Recognition of complications and deviations from the expected norm and the importance of escalation to an appropriate healthcare professional.
- How to manage and act on complications and emergency situations using recognised referral pathways and appropriate escalation.
- Exploration of maternity care pathways which include homebirth.
- Promotion of informed choice based on best available evidence.
- Skill development to include management of a physiological third stage, examination of the newborn, perineal suturing, and cannulation.
- Delivery of antenatal education which meets the learning needs of the service user (including consideration of some educational theory and how to promote active birth).
- Simulation experiences (not simply simulation of how to deal with emergency situations).
- Reflective experiences which explore the realities of the student experience of physiological birth at home.
- Practice experience to ensure alignment of theory and practice experiences.

In addition, curricula would benefit from:
- Exploration of multidisciplinary perceptions and experiences of homebirth (including practice and education experience).
- Consideration of the available practice experience including how students can experience homebirth in a continuity model.
- Developing insight into alternative therapies.

> **Practice Point:**
> Higher education institutes and practice partners should maintain a relationship which maintains an oversight of the NMC standards for pre-registration and work together to achieve these.

> **Practice Point:**
> As a component of modules that deal with physiological labour and birth and obstetric emergencies, consider inclusion of these events occurring outside of a hospital environment. This should include simulation, discussion, reflection, and, where possible, multidisciplinary working and cross-over lectures/simulation.

Practice Point:
Taking into account the number of women who may opt for homebirth, all students should be given the opportunity to gain real-life clinical practice experience of homebirth. Consider how, using the standards for student supervision and assessment (SSSA) model (NMC, 2018), this might be achieved. In the absence of the opportunity to attend a homebirth in clinical practice, consider also how the curriculum might support the development of not just physical skills but decision making and care planning outside of the hospital environment.

Practice Point:
When creating simulation scenarios, consider how these might reflect a family home. Assess the equipment that you have available with practice partners to ensure that this equipment replicates that which might be carried by community-based midwives. Where possible, use opportunities to conduct training in available accommodation that could be used to mimic a domestic environment and discuss the logistics that might be encountered in the family home, for example, a front room, bedroom, toilet, ambulance, or stairs.

Practice Point:
As part of simulation for pre-hospital and homebirth care, use live simulation of handover or decision making over the phone. This might reflect a call to the emergency services or update and escalation to the maternity unit.

POSTGRADUATE MIDWIFERY EDUCATION: COMMITMENT TO LIFELONG LEARNING

The principle of lifelong learning is an important aspect of professional life which is supported by all professional bodies governing the healthcare professions. Continuing education for Registered Midwives is enshrined in NMC revalidation requirements (NMC, 2021), meaning that it is essential to keep both theoretical knowledge and practice skills up to date. However, inevitably updating focuses on employer requirements for statutory mandatory training, is influenced by actions which are implemented by NHS Trusts after critical incidents, and will unsurprisingly be driven by the specific interests of individual midwives. These competing priorities create a challenge for facilitators of education who by necessity must recognise the need to create an educational culture which is proactive rather than punitive and one which is promoted across healthcare disciplines. However, individual and organisational objectives are not exclusive and need to be complementary in nature, aiming to develop and maintain knowledge and clinical competency, as well as promote safety and improve service user experience. The development of a training needs analysis which centres on continuing professional development as well as the setting of an agenda to maintain clinical skills is essential.

The introduction of continuity models following publication of the Better Birth report (NHS England, 2016) set out a vision for the planning, design, and safe delivery of maternity services in both hospital and community settings. The report sets out how women, babies, and families will be able to get the type of care they want and how staff will be supported to deliver such care, particularly in those situations where the midwife is the lead professional and lacks easy access to obstetric expertise. Therefore education to achieve the aims of Better Births will in turn need to focus on how staff will maintain confidence and competence in providing care in community-based settings. This involves consideration of how midwives maintain and promote a culture of physiologically informed birth linked to the NMC standards of proficiency for midwives (NMC, 2018) as well as the recognition and escalation of complications and the management of emergency situations.

Practice Point:
All organisations providing homebirth services should ensure that mechanisms are in place to audit and monitor the acquisition and maintenance of skills (Ledger, 2021). These should be implemented to support homebirth and pre-hospital care and include hard skills such as facilitating a birth at home, cannulation, suturing, and management of obstetric and neonatal emergencies (BAPM, 2022). Additionally, the inclusion of skills such as clinical decision making, escalation, communication, managing conflict, and human factors and how these apply to homebirth is recommended.

Practice Point:
It is implicit within the NMC Code (2018) that midwives are required to ensure that knowledge, skills, and competencies remain up to date. This requires a good relationship between employer and employee to ensure that midwives can raise issues around deficits in knowledge and skills and be supported to develop required knowledge and skill.

The development of community-based continuity teams may have the effect of exposing some midwives to the need to provide care in the unfamiliar surroundings of the homes of service users. Whilst competence in providing the essential labour care is unlikely to be an issue, not all midwives will feel confident in providing midwifery care in a setting outside of a hospital. In addition, there may be clinical skills which require development, for example, cannulation, suturing, managing a physiological third stage of labour, and the management of emergency situations in a community setting. Development and maintenance of a skilled and responsive midwifery workforce which is both competent and confident requires an innovative and adaptive approach to practice development which meets the needs of the employing organisation, midwifery teams, and individual midwives alike. Teaching could be incorporated into topic-related study days or be combined into discrete education sessions either as online packages or as part of in-service training programmes. Suggested educational topics could include:

- Providing personalised care in partnership with women, birthing people, and their families.
- Promoting informed choice.
- Focus on physiological rather than pathological processes.
- Recognising and acting on complications.
- Managing emergency situations in the community setting, including neonatal resuscitation.
- Clinical skills, for example, cannulation, suturing, physiological third stage.
- Planning care for the expected and unexpected situation.
- Processes involved in escalation to secondary care.
- Caring for service users who opt for care outside of excepted guidelines.

> **Practice Point:**
> As a practice education team, facilitators should consider how to provide training and skills which reflect pre-hospital care and homebirth. You may wish to take study days outside of a clinical environment into a home space.

> **Practice Point:**
> When considering methods of continuous professional development and training, there are a variety of ways this can be achieved, for example, a mix of face-to-face, self-directed and online learning, workbooks, discussion forums etc.

> **Practice Point:**
> Births which are planned to take place in community settings have similar outcomes when compared to those which take place within obstetric units (British Association of Perinatal Medicine, 2022). However, the need for neonatal resuscitation cannot be predicted and the Resuscitation Council UK recommend that at least one person attending a birth in a community setting should successfully have completed an accredited neonatal course where competency has been formally assessed (Resuscitation Council UK, 2021). National Institute for Health and Care Excellence (NICE) (2017) intrapartum guidelines also suggest that all those providing intrapartum care should attend an annual course in neonatal resuscitation aligned with Resuscitation Council United Kingdom (RCUK) guidelines. Attendance should not only be facilitated by maternity service managers but feature as part of mandatory training to ensure that midwives attending homebirths are able to achieve the required level of skill acquisition and are assessed as competent.

MULTIDISCIPLINARY EDUCATION

The Better Births: Improving Outcomes of Maternity Services in England report (2016) highlights the need for multi-professional working to break down barriers between midwives, obstetricians, and other health professionals to enable the delivery of world-class, safe, personalised care for women and their babies. Education is crucial to the success of working in partnership with all members of multidisciplinary teams who may be involved in the management and care of women who opt to birth their babies at home. The evidence supporting multi-professional education and training, particularly in relation to obstetric emergencies, is well established, with charities such as PROMPT and Baby Lifeline providing evidence-based training packages actively aimed at standardising approaches to learning and simulation (Winter, 2018; Baby Lifeline 2020; Renwick et al., 2021). The overarching objective is to reduce harm and adverse outcomes through the development of knowledge, skills, and competency whilst providing appreciation of human factors and application of evidence-based information.

Whilst initially focussed on institution-based scenarios, recognition of the need for pre-hospital, community, and midwife-led settings, focussed training has come to the fore in recent years, along with the development of specific packages of training and scenario-based training (Renwick et al., 2021). As local guidelines and protocols for management of care, transfer to an institution, emergency care, and escalation, it is imperative that these all-form part of locally agreed approaches to facilitating the learning environment. It is essential that midwives practising within a home environment are involved in the development and review of guidance and policy.

> **Practice Point:**
> When developing guidelines and standard operating procedures and policy, efforts should be made to include local ambulance services and other stakeholders. This ensures that these documents remain fit for purpose and relevant to each professional group.

Structured simulation has become a core element of undergraduate and postgraduate education of all healthcare professionals, particularly for emergency scenarios (Miller, 2015). This offers the opportunity to facilitate the application of knowledge to practice-based scenarios and develop both individual and team working skills (Norris, 2008; Black, 2018). However, although clinical staff will be familiar with this educational activity, it may be as part of a discrete professional group rather than through a multidisciplinary or multi-agency approach. *Safe Birth: Everybody's Business* (Kings Fund, 2008) established the need for teams that work together to also train/learn together as a core activity rather than an optional extra. This was suggested as a hospital-based activity with regular multidisciplinary learning facilitated in a labour ward, but simulation, particularly of those situations which involve complications, is equally necessary to facilitate safety, competency, and confidence for practitioners involved in caring for women or birthing people who opt for homebirth.

A pilot study exploring fidelity for midwives engaging with simulated obstetric emergencies at home was undertaken by Komorowski et al. (2017), with a view to identifying whether a modified set of scenarios designed for institution skills and drills could maximise fidelity for those engaging with homebirth scenarios. They found that hospital-based scenarios could indeed be effective in being adapted for home-based scenarios whilst hypothesising that this might increase both confidence and effectiveness in skills. This approach has been supported by evidence from Australia, where Kumar et al. (2019) evaluated a homebirth–based simulation approach to skills development and its impact on and benefit to midwives and paramedics for birth-related emergencies in homebirth and found that applying simulation-based learning developed a breadth to their learning experiences and changed their clinical practice approach. Black (2018) cited the use of fidelity simulation within a UK NHS Trust as a method of training and assessing the competence of staff and showed that feedback from participants suggested that an increase in confidence and communication resulted and that participants valued this as a learning opportunity.

Taking into account the community-based nature of homebirth, it is recommended that educational activities (emergency and standard care) take place in an environment which can replicate a service user's home and wherever possible take place in a local community-based environment engaging not only with midwives but also with all healthcare professionals who might be called upon to attend a homebirth. Standardised education facilitates the adoption of a universal approach to the management of care for women and birthing people and is important in advancing safety in maternity care. The advantage that locally based community education adds to this approach is the potential to replicate the homebirth environment, to consider the needs of local populations, and to take into account human factors which may impact the provision of care in the family home. Additionally, there is an opportunity for healthcare professionals who may be called to attend homebirths but do not work together as a multidisciplinary team on a regular basis to get to know each other and develop mutual understanding of the underpinning principles of each other's profession.

It is recognised that it is optimal for teams who work together to train together but this may present challenges for maternity services. The competing priorities of busy clinical workloads and the unpredictable nature of maternity care impact the ability for staff to be released to attend educational activities. Additionally, in community settings, particularly those which are more rural and cover wide geographical areas ensuring staff availability and locating suitable venues may be problematic. However, whilst it is recognised that these factors can impact the provision of educational opportunities, it is important to highlight that healthcare professionals do not work in isolation and that wherever possible, opportunities for multi-professional education should be exploited. A report commissioned and undertaken by the charity Baby Lifeline (Ledger et al. 2018) identified that training based on emergency skills and drills in the community was lacking, with as few as 25% of NHS Trusts not providing community-specific training. The report recognised the need for organisations to be supported in providing ongoing education and training for all maternity staff, particularly during difficult times, and to decrease the incidence of avoidable harm and recommended the implementation of nationally agreed standards for ongoing evidence-based education and training competencies. Facilitators of education need therefore to work with the managers of maternity and related services to balance the acuity required for safe staffing with the need to ensure that staff from multidisciplinary teams can attend training sessions. The adoption of innovative approaches may be required to provide a balance between face-to-face and online educational activities but will ultimately ensure that the right staff, with the right skills, are deployed to the right place at the right time (Ledger et al. 2021). Organisations who have adopted these approaches have found that they not only enhance the skills development and safety of the service but also improve homebirth rates to some degree (Brown et al., 2012; Pauley and Dale, 2016).

Practice Point:
Organisations providing homebirth services should ensure that interprofessional and interagency education can be accessed and delivered. This requires coordination between all professions and agencies at both a local and a strategic level.

Increases in the use of technology have seen a move towards online rather than interactive education, and consequently, opportunities to engage in interactive learning need to be optimised with a blend of face-to-face and online multidisciplinary education (Ledger et al., 2021). However, the management of emergency situations will undoubtedly remain an important aspect of planning educational activities for the multi-professional team, but all aspects of birth at home should be a central focus of all education pertaining to homebirth. Simulation-based training for emergency situations, which assesses clinical, communication, and team skills within discrete exercises involving all maternity staff, paramedic, and ambulance services, should be facilitated to take into account the factor that healthcare professionals attending a woman or birthing person at home may not have previously met. This provides an opportunity to break down professional boundaries and build trust, respect, and collaboration (Pauley and Dale, 2016; Ledger et al., 2021).

Aspects covered could include:

- Roles and responsibilities of the multidisciplinary team
- Personalised maternity care in the homebirth scenario (including choices made by women and birthing people to opt for birth choices outside of universal care pathways)
- Effective communication in all scenarios between the woman or birthing person, the family, midwives, and multidisciplinary team
- Risk management and safety awareness
- Clinical decision making
- Escalation processes (include in drills with paramedic and ambulance staff)
- Development and provision of appropriate equipment and resources
- Reflection on care episodes and incidents
- Human factors and safety awareness
- Implementation of new guidance

Practice Point:
When planning educational activities which involve the use of simulation, attempts should be made to involve all professional groups who might be called upon to attend. This should mean that paramedics, midwives, and sometimes medical staff train together to achieve a better understanding of each other's professional responsibilities, skills, knowledge, and equipment.

Practice Point:
When creating simulation scenarios, consider how this might reflect a family home. Wherever possible, hold educational activities in an area which reflects a non-hospital setting and have access to equipment which replicates that available to the multidisciplinary teams working in the community.

Practice Point:
As part of simulation for pre-hospital and homebirth care, consider live simulation of handover and decision making over the phone. This might reflect a call to the emergency services or update and escalation to the maternity unit.

USING THE EXPERIENCE OF WOMEN TO INFORM EDUCATION

Pregnancy and birth are unique events where beliefs, values, and wishes of women must be respected and considered (NHS England, 2016). As the primary mechanism by which providers of maternity services can monitor service user experience, feedback has a key role to play in helping organisations to track the quality of their services, identify problem areas, and shape service improvements through education and practice development. Feedback from service users has for many years been a significant factor in improving maternity service quality (Wenzel and Jabbal, 2016), and undoubtedly, feedback, both positive and negative, is an essential factor when planning and facilitating educational activities. Using the experiences of homebirth service users provides the opportunity to use their stories to encompass the views, expectations, and needs of women and their babies and to learn directly from women themselves. These in turn can facilitate education which supports flourishing and high-quality homebirth care. Research highlights that those maternity units which demonstrate evident interest in the experiences of the women who use their services and use feedback to improve and address concerns are more likely to provide a high-quality service (Amess and Tyndale-Biscoe, 2014).

In practice, capturing views of service users can be challenging and may not be truly representative of experience of all service users. It is therefore likely that different approaches will be required to collect views from different groups of users whose involvement with maternity care by its very nature usually involves a transient engagement with the service (Wenzel and Jabbal, 2016). The use of a mixed-method approach to the collection of feedback and proactive approaches to seeking the views and opinions of all service users have been found to provide a robust level of information about individual experiences (Wenzel and Jabbal, 2016). It is suggested that these approaches consider local circumstances and are more likely to be representative of the diverse social and ethnic groups within local geographical areas. Sources which can be used to gain direct feedback about experiences of homebirth include:

- Using nominated patient experience representatives responsible for collecting verbal feedback. For example, through the Maternity Voice Partnership forum
- Comment cards given to women where feedback can be given
- Local surveys/patient experience trackers, for example, the Friends and Family Test
- Focus groups or in 'Whose Shoes?' events

- Debriefing services
- Electronic data collection tools. For example, the 'iWantGreatCare' tool where service users can provide feedback anonymously via a tablet (see https://www.iwantgreatcare.org/)

> **Practice Point:**
> Engagement with service users is vital for gaining both positive and negative feedback. Consider how this can be integrated into the development of education with the aim of achieving a safer and more respectful service.

> **Practice Point:**
> Service users should form part of stakeholder groups involved in the design of curricula, guidelines, and educational activities, as well as those directed at service developments. Innovative ways to achieve this, taking into account the specifics of local demographics, should be explored.

> **Practice Point:**
> Consider inviting service users or actors to become involved in simulation activities.

FACILITATING HOMEBIRTH EDUCATION FOR WOMEN/BIRTHING PEOPLE AND THEIR BIRTH PARTNERS

Research has shown that planned homebirth is at least as safe as hospital birth for healthy women with normal pregnancies and is associated with good outcomes for both mothers and babies (Brocklehurst, 2011; Hodnett et al., 2012; Hutton et al., 2019). However, not all women who decide on homebirth will have a straightforward medical or obstetric history and there will be many reasons why women opt to labour and birth their babies at home. Whatever the reason, women will want to prepare for their forthcoming childbirth and the midwife has an important educational role to play in ensuring that women can be provided with unbiased, evidence-based information in an accessible format.

Antenatal education aims to give information, advice, and support on the physiological and emotional aspects of childbirth. Empowerment of knowledge and confidence in the ability to labour and give birth is important. Information on the processes of labour and birth will inevitably be covered but areas such as informed decision making, physical skills for labour such as breathing techniques, pain relief, newborn and postnatal care, infant feeding, and parenting skills may also be included. Conventional group parentcraft classes have the advantage of providing the opportunity to meet other expectant parents but there is inconclusive evidence about efficacy or the most appropriate form of delivery (Brixval et al., 2015). Additionally, there is a wide variation in provision, with many Trusts now providing information via their websites rather than on a face-to-face basis. Group sessions may also not meet the specific individual needs of the woman or birthing person who opts for homebirth and the midwife will need to apply a personalised approach to antenatal education. It may be useful to consider the application of Maslow's (1954) hierarchy of needs (Fig. 2.3)

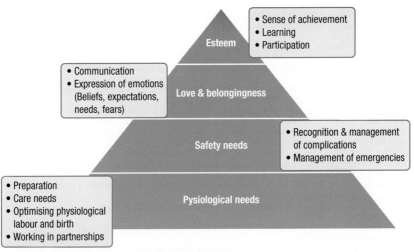

Fig. 2.3 Maslow's hierarchy.

to a woman or birthing person's individual (or a couple's) educational needs as this encompasses the factors which need to be taken into consideration to facilitate an individual's ability to achieve their full potential.

Homebirth education for individual women and their birth partners will often take place in the family home and utilise the opportunities provided by the need to conduct antenatal appointments as well as educational input from a midwife, and women may use a combination of internet resources and privately accessed sources of information or skills for birth such as hypnobirthing or active birth. Areas that could be covered by the midwife could include:

- Making research about homebirth accessible
- Physiological processes of birth – What do labour and birth involve?
- Making a birth plan
- Labour positions and active birth skills
- Emotional preparation – working through expectations and anxieties. How to feel more confident and in control?
- Being able to change their mind at any time
- Safety as an important consideration (including process for transfer should it be necessary)
- Postnatal and newborn care
- Infant feeding
- The role of the birth partner – How can a birth partner(s) help provide support?

Practice Point:
When considering the educational needs of women, this should take a personalised care approach where possible (Gagnon and Sandall, 2007; NHS England, 2016).

CONCLUSION

Development and sustaining education related to homebirth is important if homebirth services are to flourish. Education must be evidence based and aimed at improving service user experience and providing safe, quality care. All healthcare professionals who may be called upon to attend labour and birth in a woman or birthing person's home should ensure that their practice is evidence based and up to date and a collaborative multiprofessional approach is essential. The views and experiences of service users are essential in informing and influencing educational strategies at both local and national levels and facilitators of education should proactively engage with women and their families. In doing so, the provision of the best possible homebirth service can be facilitated, one which empowers not only healthcare professionals but also women, birthing people, and their families for the years to come.

REFERENCES

Amess M, Tyndale-Biscoe J. (2014). What makes a top hospital? Maternity care. Birmingham: CHKS. Available at: www.chks.co.uk/Knowledge-Base

Baby Lifeline (2020). Closing the gap. Prioritising prevention: Urgent investment needed to support multi-professional training in maternity services. Baby Lifeline. February 2020. Available at: https://www.babylifeline.org.uk/wp-content/uploads/2020/11/Closing-the-Gap-FINAL.pdf

BAPM (2022) 'Neonatal Support for Freestanding Midwifery Led Units and Homebirths A Framework for Practice'. British Association of Perinatal Medicine. Available at: https://hubble-live-assets.s3.amazonaws.com/bapm/file_asset/file/1162/MLU_Home_Birth_BAPM_Framework_July_2022.pdf.

Black S. (2018). Obstetric emergencies: Enhancing the multidisciplinary team through simulation. British Journal of Midwifery. 26(2). ISSN (print): 0969-4900. ISSN (online): 2052-4307

British Association of Perinatal Medicine (2022). Neonatal support for freestanding midwifery led units and homebirths: A framework for practice. July 2022. London.

Brixval CS, Axelsen SF, Lauemøller SG, et al. (2015). The Effect of antenatal education in small classes on obstetric and psycho-social outcomes – A systematic review. Syst Rev. 4:20. https://doi.org/10.1186/s13643-015-0010-x

Brocklehurst P, Hardy P, Hollowell J, Linsell L, Macfarlane A, McCourt C, Marlow N, Miller A, Newburn M, Petrou S, Puddicombe D, Redshaw M, Rowe R, Sandall J, Silverton L, Stewart M. (Birthplace in England Collaborative Group) (2011). Perinatal and maternal outcomes by planned place of birth for healthy women with low-risk pregnancies: The Birthplace in England national prospective cohort study. BMJ. 2011 Nov;23(343): d7400. doi: 10.1136/bmj.d7400. PMID: 22117057; PMCID: PMC3223531.

Brown A, Booth C, Hall H. (2012). Emergencies during homebirths. Pract Midwife. 2012 Mar;15(3):11–13. PMID: 22479848.

Gagnon AJ, Sandall J. (2007). Individual or group antenatal education for childbirth or parenthood, or both. Cochrane Database of Systematic Reviews. 2007(3):CD002869. doi: 10.1002/14651858.CD002869.pub2

General Medical Council (2018). Outcomes for graduates. Available at: https://www.gmc-uk.org/education/standards-guidance-and-curricula/standards-and-outcomes/outcomes-for-graduates

Health & Care Professions Council (2014). Standards of proficiency: Paramedics. Available at: standards-of-proficiency—-paramedics.pdf (hcpc-uk.org)

Hermansson E, Mårtensson L. (2010). Empowerment in midwifery context – A concept analysis. Midwifery. 27:811–816. doi: 10.1016/j.midw.2010.08.005

Hodnett ED, Downe S, Walsh D. (2012). Alternative versus conventional institutional settings for birth. Cochrane Database of Systematic Reviews 2012;(8). Art. No.: CD000012. doi: 10.1002/14651858.CD000012.pub4

Hutton EK, Reitsma A, Simioni J, Brunton G, Kaufman K. (2019). Perinatal or neonatal mortality among women who intend at the onset of labour to give birth at home compared to women of low obstetrical risk who intend to give birth in hospital: A systematic review and meta-analyses. EClinicalMedicine. 2019 Jul 25;14:59–70. doi: 10.1016/j.eclinm.2019.07.005. PMID: 31709403; PMCID: PMC6833447.

International Confederation of Midwives (2018). Essential competencies for midwifery practice. Available at: https://www.internationalmidwives.org/assets/files/general-files/2019/02/icm-competencies_english_final_jan-2019-update_final-web_v1.0.pdf

Kings Fund (2008). Safe births: Everybody's business. An independent enquiry into the safety of maternity services in England. Kings Fund: London.

Knowles MS. (1984). Andragogy in action. Applying modern principles of adult education. San Francisco, CA: Jossey Bass.

Komorowski J, Andrighetti T, Benton M. (2017). Modification of obstetric emergency simulation scenarios for realism in a homebirth setting. J Midwifery Womens Health. 2017 Jan;62(1):93–100. doi: 10.1111/jmwh.12527. Epub 2016 Dec 21. PMID: 28002642.

Kumar A, Wallace EM, Smith C, Nestel D. (2019). Effect of an in-situ simulation workshop on homebirth practice in Australia. Women Birth. 2019 Aug;32(4):346–355. doi: 10.1016/j.wombi.2018.08.172. Epub 2018 Sep 13. PMID: 30220576.

Ledger S, Hindle G, McKee A, Smith T. (2021). Mind the gap: An investigation into maternity training for frontline professionals across the UK (2020/21). Baby Lifeline: UK. 2021. Available at: https://www.babylifeline.org.uk/wp-content/uploads/2021/11/Mind-the-Gap-2021-Baby-Lifeline-Full-Report-v1.3.pdf

Ledger S, Hindle G, Smith T. (2018). Mind the gap: An investigation into maternity training for frontline professionals across the UK (2017/18). Baby Lifeline: UK. 2018. Available at: https://www.babylifeline.org.uk/wp-content/uploads/2020/11/Mind-the-Gap-2018.pdf

Maslow AH. (1954). Motivation and personality. New York: Harper and Row.

Miller JL, Avery MD, Larson K, Woll A, VonAchen A, Mortenson A. (2015). Emergency birth hybrid simulation with standardized patients in midwifery education: Implementation and evaluation. J Midwifery Womens Health. 2015 May–Jun;60(3):298–303. Doi: 10.1111/jmwh.12276. Epub 2015 May 11. PMID: 25963413.

Moncrieff G, MacVicar S, Norris G, Hollins Martin CJ. (2020 in press). Optimising the continuity experiences of student midwives: An integrative review. Women and Birth. 34(2021):77–86. https://dx.doi.org/10.1016/j.wombi.2020.01.0071871-5192/

NICE (2017). Intrapartum care for healthy women and babies. National Institute for Health and Care Excellence. Available at: https://www.nice.org.uk/guidance/cg190/chapter/recommendations#pain-relief-in-labour-nonregional (Accessed 29 January 2021).

NHS England (2106). Better births: Improving outcomes of maternity services in England. A five year forward view for maternity care. The National Maternity Review. NHS England. Available at: www.england.nhs.uk/ourwork/futurenhs/mat-review

Norris G. (2008). The midwifery curriculum: Introducing obstetric emergency simulation. British Journal of Midwifery. 16:232–235. doi: 10.12968/bjom.2008.16.4.29047.

Nursing and Midwifery Council (2018). Realising professionalism: Standards for education and training. Part 2: Standards for student supervision and assessment. Available at: https://www.nmc.org.uk/globalassets/sitedocuments/standards-of-proficiency/standards-for-student-supervision-and-assessment/student-supervision-assessment.pdf

Nursing and Midwifery Council (2019). Realising professionalism: Standards for education and training. Part 3: Standards for pre-registration midwifery programmes. Available at: standards-for-pre-registration-midwifery-programmes.pdf (nmc.org.uk)

Nursing and Midwifery Council (2021). What is revalidation. Nursing & Midwifery Council. 26 May 2021 Update. Available at: https://www.nmc.org.uk/revalidation/overview/what-is-revalidation/ (Accessed 16 May 2022).

Pauley T, Dale A. (2016). Train Together to work together: Reviewing feedback of community-based skills drills training for midwives and paramedics. British Journal of Midwifery. 24(6):428–443.

Pritchard A. (2009). Ways of learning: Learning theories and learning styles in the classroom (2nd Edition). New York, NY: Routledge.

Prithishkumar IJ, Michael SA. (2014). Understanding Your Student: Using the VARK Model. Journal of Postgraduate Medicine. 2014 Apr–Jun;60(2):183–186. doi: 10.4103/0022-3859.132337. PMID: 24823519.

Renfrew MJ, McFadden A, Bastos MH, et al. (2014). Midwifery and quality care: Findings from a new evidence-informed framework for maternal and newborn care. Lancet. 2014;384(9948):1129–1145.

Renwick S, Hookes S, Draycott T, et al. (2021). PROMPT Wales Project: National Scaling of an evidence-based intervention to improve safety and training in maternity. BMJ Open Quality. 2021;10:e001280. doi: 10.1136/bmjoq-2020-001280

Resuscitation Council UK (2021). Newborn resuscitation and support of transition of infants at birth guidelines. Available at: https://www.resus.org.uk/library/2021-resuscitation-guidelines/newborn-resuscitation-and-support-transition-infants-birth

Senge, P., et al. (1994) The Fifth Discipline Field Book Strategies and Tools for Building a Learning Organization. Currency Doubleday, New York

Walton C. (2012). The Birthplace in England study: Methods, findings, and evaluation. British Journal of Midwifery. 20(1):22–27.

Wenzel L, Jabbal, J. (2016). User feedback in maternity services. Kings Fund: London. Available at: https://www.kingsfund.org.uk/sites/default/files/field/field_publication_file/User_feedback_maternity_Kings_Fund_Oct_2016.pdf

Winter S. (Editor) (2018). PROMPT course manual. Cambridge University Press: Cambridge.

World Health Organization (2019). Framework for action: Strengthening quality midwifery education for universal health coverage 2030. World Health Organization: Geneva.

CHAPTER 3

PLANNING FOR HOMEBIRTH: ORGANISATIONAL CONSIDERATIONS

Anna Madeley and Carolyn Rooth

Maternity care is a fundamental healthcare service provided in both community and hospital settings. However, although community midwifery is an integral component of maternity services, there is a heavy emphasis on services which are provided within the acute hospital environment, particularly in relation to labour care. Senior managers of maternity services therefore need to consider and evaluate the resources needed to safely provide quality midwifery care in the family home to meet the holistic needs of services users and their families. This includes ways to provide seamless antenatal, intrapartum, and postnatal care in the community and involves facilitation of clear, coordinated communication and pathways for those women and birthing people who opt to have their babies at home. The following chapter is not intended to be an exhaustive list of considerations but aims to provide insight into planning arrangements for safe and effective services when planning and facilitating care for a birth at home.

COMMITMENT TO PROVIDING THE SERVICE CULTURE TRUST PHILOSOPHY

Across the UK, the focus of maternity services has turned to providing personalised care, facilitated practically by midwives, obstetricians, and the wider multidisciplinary team in the form of personalised care and support plans (PCSPs), whilst acknowledging their importance in the provision of safe and empowered perinatal care (NHS England, 2016 Scottish Government, 2017; Welsh Government, 2019) as well as their ability to adapt to both varied clinical settings and different contexts (Burt et al., 2013). For these to apply effectively in relation to true personalised care in relation to homebirth provision, it is imperative that organisational culture is such that there is a commitment to not just the provision of homebirth services but also to respect for all decisions and preferences made by women, inextricably linked to safety (Brintworth and Sandall, 2013; Birthrights, 2017; Ockenden, 2020, 2021). This includes a commitment to continuous improvement in protecting homebirth services and appropriate, humanised, and evidence-based local pathways that enable and respect women's views, needs, and preferences, taking into consideration physiological, psychological, social, cultural, and emotional needs. This might also include arrangements for women who, for whatever reason, choose options outside of guidelines or decline recommended care (see chapter *Homebirth for Women With Complex Needs*). NICE explicitly require that those providing maternity services provide information about available birth settings, including homebirth, that is made available for women either in the immediate locality or neighbouring locations, to enable women and their families to make an informed choice about where they wish to birth their babies (NICE, 2017). Additionally, with the publication of *Better Births* (NHS England, 2016), a robust emphasis has been placed on ensuring that choice, continuity, and control is central to woman-centred care and decision making.

Models of care for providing homebirth will vary from location to location but fall into three main models:

- Continuity of care, a group practice model who provide case loading care for a defined group of women, defined by geographical location, General Practitioner (GP) practice, demographic, or other predefined variables. Each team has potential to provide homebirth service.
- Continuity of care dedicated homebirth teams who caseload women who specifically request a homebirth. (The definition of continuity of care team according to *Better Births* [NHS England, 2016] is a consistent midwifery team, usually between four and eight midwives [although some organisations such as NICE have interpreted this to include anyone providing care as part of the healthcare team; NICE, 2021a, 2021b], who facilitate and provide care for the woman or birthing person throughout pregnancy and labour and postnatally).
- Traditional community service where on-call midwives are allocated to women labouring as they arise.

How such teams are established and operate can have a fundamental effect on the service they provide and outcomes (Brintworth and Sandall, 2013; Noble, 2015; Homer et al., 2017; Cross-Sudworth et al., 2018; Callaghan, Foley, and Olusile, 2019).

> **Practice Point:**
> As a team, is there a shared philosophy for approaching and offering homebirth? Is this reflected across the service in obstetric and neonatal colleagues? Is there a space for reflection and structure debriefing to take place that develops an ongoing philosophy of safe and respectful care?

> **Practice Point:**
> Consider how teams and individual midwives might seek support and reflection on their own practice. Systems should be in place as a part of formal governance and management structures to provide support; however, informal support networks might also be established including buddy systems, discussion groups, and staff debriefing.

However the provision is arranged, practical issues including off-duty planning and rota development to facilitate a 24-hour service are a key consideration, particularly at anticipated periods of high activity. Brintworth and Sandall (2013) suggest that self-managed groups operating within a caseload model, supported by senior management, can foster a positive culture towards homebirth. Staffing of a homebirth service can, however, remain challenging when on-call midwives are used to temporarily supplement gaps in inpatient services, acutely illustrated during the COVID-19 pandemic when many homebirth services were suspended despite evidence suggesting an increase in demand, severely restricting the rights of women to choose their place of birth (Greenfield, Payne-Gifford, and McKenzie, 2021; Nelson and Romanis, 2021), and acute staffing issues in the UK were starkly exposed (Cordey et al., 2022).

Practice Point:

Team and individual midwifery philosophies for care can affect how midwives offer and approach homebirth. It is therefore imperative that these are examined and reflected upon to identify any knowledge gaps. As a midwife, what is your experience of homebirth and how did it make you feel? If you have no experience, does this cause anxiety, and why?

GOVERNANCE AND GUIDELINES

Clinical governance can be defined as:

> ...a framework through which NHS organisations are accountable for continuously improving the quality of their services and safeguarding high standards of care by creating an environment in which excellence in clinical care will flourish.
>
> —Scally and Donaldson, 1998, p. 61

Robust governance requires suitable systems, processes, and leadership to ensure that appropriate mechanisms are in place to monitor, audit, and ensure that patient safety and quality of care are in place. The means by which these are achieved are often framed by the 'seven pillars':

1. Clinical effectiveness and research
2. Risk management
3. Patient and public involvement (PPI)
4. Communication, information, and technology
5. Staffing and staff management
6. Governance structure and audit
7. Education and training

Throughout this book and chapter, these pillars have been discussed directly and indirectly in relation to birth at home; indeed the broad principles now discussed can be applied across any planned service; however, in this context it relates to the planning and implementation of homebirth services.

The development of robust policy, standard operating procedures (SOPs), and guidelines supports effective clinical governance which aim to support the improvement of quality and safe care (Table 3.1).

Table 3.1 Definitions (Frolich and Schram, 2015; NHS England, 2021; RCM, 2022)

STANDARD OPERATING PROCEDURE	GUIDELINE
• Written instruction specifying how to carry out a defined procedure or process. • Appropriate where a safe system of work can only be achieved by undertaking the task in a sequence. • Developed to ensure a standardised, uniform approach and reduce variation in relation to processes and encompass a degree of consistency and standardisation. • Establishes parameters and boundaries of responsibility. • Allows for improvement in auditing and monitoring.	• Systematically developed tool intended for use to assist informed choice and supported decision making. • Describes the woman's condition, care pathway, recommendations for treatment and interventions. • Should be based on best available evidence. • Can be international, national, or local. • May introduce variation in approach to care. • Do not supersede human rights to bodily autonomy. • Can be a gold standard for audit and benchmarking purposes.
Examples for Homebirth Provision: • Continuity of care/community on call • Escalation of obstetric concerns in the community • Safe staffing for homebirth provision • Emergency maternity transfers from community to the hospital • Standard equipment for homebirth	**Examples for Homebirth Provision:** • Monitoring progress in labour • Supporting physiological birth • Facilitating third stage of labour • Pre-labour rupture of membranes • Water birth and use of water in labour

SOPs and guidelines therefore should encapsulate processes and pathways designed to be reliable so far as is practicable, acknowledging that continuous improvement requires periodic review and audit to learn from both episodes of care which demonstrated excellence as well those which require improvement, from the perspective of women, their families, and the staff who support them. Additionally, they should clearly identify roles and responsibilities of stakeholders and methods of both communication and escalation. Where they are well written and developed in a collaborative manner, they can ensure that the best available evidence supports both clinical decision making and also supported decision making for women and their families (Frohlich and Schram, 2015; NICE, 2021c; NHS England, 2021e).

They remain therefore an important element of developing safe governance arrangements and should be viewed in conjunction with other documentation and dynamic procedures. They are fundamental in establishing the scope and local parameters within which a framework of support for midwives, obstetricians, and the wider multidisciplinary team operates. Importantly, they should be designed to support local homebirthing population and guide-supported decision making. When developing local SOPS and guidelines, either to implement wider national or international guidelines or in developing a new service/auditing an existing one, it is fundamental that at all stages, consultation with external and internal stakeholders is undertaken to safeguard governance structures (NICE, 2017). These may include (but not be restricted to):

- **Internal**
  - Providers and commissioners
  - Local Maternity and Neonatal Systems (LMNS) representatives (i.e. Integrated Care Boards)
  - Clinical leadership (Head of Midwifery, Consultant Midwife, Obstetric Clinical Leads)
  - Clinical staff (midwives, obstetricians, neonatologists, maternity support workers)
  - Clinical Risk Management and Governance Representatives including maternity safety champions (NHS Improvement, 2018)
  - Local education and training (Education Dept, Practice Development [Midwives/Nurses])
  - Higher education representatives (Lead Midwife for Education/Link Lecturer for university providing student midwives)
  - GPs
  - Local ambulance Trust representative
- **External**
  - Maternity services liaison committees (MSLC)
  - Maternity voice partnership (MVP)
  - Local National Childbirth Trust (NCT)
  - Non-affiliated lay individuals/parents
  - Community/vulnerable/disadvantaged group representatives
  - Local maternity charities
  - Independent midwives (local to Trusts)
  - Doulas/doula organisations

These factors are fundamental in ensuring not only that the development of SOPs and guidelines remain collaborative, fit for purpose and reflects the population which they serve. Moreover, where establishing or supporting an ongoing homebirth service, supportive management and multi- disciplinary teamwork enhances the safety of the service (Callaghan, Foley and Olusile, 2019). It is worth noting that these documents should stand alongside and complement policies (prescriptive arrangements for an agreed approach to undertaking something, usually by the organisation and expected to be adhered to equally without deviation) and protocols (task-specific approach to a determined scenario or activity, i.e. removal of sutures) (Frohlich and Schram, 2015).

AUDIT, MONITORING, AND CONTINUOUS IMPROVEMENT

Alongside standard national requirements for reporting and audit (Maternity Services dashboard, 2022; MBRRACE-UK, 2022; NPEU, 2022; UKOSS, 2022), it is vital that local systems have mechanisms to monitor and audit any homebirth service and associated guidelines. The aim of audit in this context is to identify where improvements might be made, trends that require targeted interventions, if the service is being provided in line with established governance standards, and resource planning or to identify where the service excels. At a regional level, such data might demonstrate fluctuations in demographics and birth rate that can support future planning activities. Such audits should encompass safety and quality and feed directly back into clinical audit committees, patients' safety forums, and national reporting systems. It is useful for auditing activities to be planned from service inception and feature input from stakeholders to inform which data will be useful for future improvement activities. When planning audits also consider the following:

- What data needs to be collected (demographic of woman, details and outcome of intrapartum care, transfer, use of analgesia, perineal repair, infant feeding etc)
- How often it should take place
- Planning and coordination of the audit
- Responsibilities for planning and undertaking the audit
- How findings are coordinated and fed back into the system and wider stakeholders
- Implementation of recommendations

> **Practice Point:**
> When identifying data that might be collected and audited, how might confidentiality be protected and compliance with the Data Protection Act (2018) assured?

> **Practice Point:**
> Consider at a local level what audit and monitoring data might be useful to feed into your governance structure. How might you feed this back into the service and importantly back to service users?

STAFFING AND RESOURCE MANAGEMENT

The number and skill mix of staff required to provide a safe homebirth service will vary according to the number of homebirths expected, model of care (continuity, traditional), geographical location, acuity, sociodemographic factors, and other organisational requirements. Guidance exists to support planning of safe staffing levels (Ball, Walshbrook, and Royal College of Midwives, 2013; NICE, 2015; RCM, 2016; Birthrate Plus, 2021). It is imperative that this forms a key consideration in planning homebirth services, as staffing shortages have been implicated in reports on poor care and safety of maternity services (Mid Staffordshire NHS Foundation Trust Public Inquiry. (2013.) Kirkup, 2015; Kirkup, 2022; BAPM, 2022; HSCC, 2021; Ockenden, 2021).

Specific guidance from other agencies have begun to make recommendations in relation to safe staffing of a homebirth; for example, the Resuscitation Council UK (RCUK) recommend that two trained professional be present at all homebirths (RCUK, 2021). When planning skills mix for on-call provision, there is an expectation that all midwives be able at the minimum to provide safe universal care for the woman, the fetus, and then neonate (NMC, 2018, 2019) and identify and escalate appropriately using agreed pathways. Any deviation from normal physiological processes or the requirement for emergency care should fall within the midwives' scope of practice.

> **Practice Point:**
> All midwives should be able to initiate any newborn life support in line with recommendations from RCUK (2021). Recommendations from RCUK suggest that at least one person attending a homebirth should have received quality assured training in airway support using mask ventilation as well as chest compressions in a compromised neonate. This would suggest that formal certificated training is a necessity for those who may attend a homebirth (BAPM, 2022).

APPROPRIATE REFERRALS AND ESCALATION

Many women requesting a homebirth will sit within the low-risk model and will not need a referral to obstetric colleagues unless underlying medical or obstetric conditions or history exists or a situation arises that necessitates this such as the identification of gestation diabetes or fetal concerns. The timing of referral to dedicated continuity of care or homebirth teams will be locally decided; however, such pathways should be robust and ensure that they are able to facilitate personalised care planning in the event of any deviation.

> **Practice Point:**
> Once a deviation from the low-risk pathway is identified, then a suitable and timely escalation to the relevant healthcare professional should be made. This might include an obstetrician, senior midwife, consultant midwife, or neonatologist. The role of the multidisciplinary team has been identified as a fundamental part of safe and coordinated care planning including appropriate recognition of when to refer and appropriate escalation featuring heavily in high-profile reports within the UK (Kirkup, 2015; Rowe et al., 2020; Knight et al., 2021; Ockenden, 2021). The timing of these referrals will depend on local arrangements and pre-established pathways as well as personal circumstances. Women are within their rights to decline such referrals (see chapter *Homebirth for Women With Complex Needs*); therefore a respectful approach is required (NMC, 2018).

Conflict between professional groups and women might occur when choices are made that might place the woman or the fetus at risk (Hollander et al., 2016; Jenkinson, Kruske, and Kildea, 2017), or indeed it may simply occur when a homebirth request is made (Sjöblom et al., 2012). Conflict should be avoided and a recognition made that midwives have a responsibility to '*respect, support, and document a person right to accept or refuse care and treatment*' (NMC, 2018, p. 7) and that women have a right to make autonomous decisions about their care. Clear, kind, and respectful conversations should be facilitated with recommendations that remain evidence based, reflecting a culture of respect with NICE (2017) suggesting that all healthcare professionals including senior staff recognise that:

> *... each woman as an individual (is) undergoing a significant and emotionally intense life experience, ... is in control, is listened to and is cared for with compassion, and that appropriate informed consent is sought.*

And that

> *senior staff should demonstrate, through their own words and behaviour, appropriate ways of relating to and talking about women and their birth companion(s), and of talking about birth and the choices to be made when giving birth.*
>
> —NICE, 2017, p. 16

This subject is dealt with in more depth in the chapter *Homebirth for Women With Complex Needs.*

MAKING THE DECISION TO HAVE A HOMEBIRTH

The choice to labour and birth at home may be one that has been made long before conception, but equally many women may not have considered homebirth as an option at all prior to pregnancy. The motivations and reasons for choosing homebirth has been explored globally (Ogden, 1997; Cleeton, 2006; Jouhki, 2012; Murray-Davis et al., 2014; Sassine et al., 2021). These will be highly subjective and personal in nature however common themes are noted to be related to the birth environment and the need to be with trusted supporters (Fordham, 1997; Morison et al., 1998), the retaining and reclaiming of control (Viisainen, 2001; Olafsdottir, Thies-Lagergren, and Sjoblom, 2021), a wish to avoid interventions, restrictions, previous trauma associated with sexual trauma or birth experience, or to actively support their own physiology to birth (Keedle et al., 2015; Garthus-Niegel et al., 2019; Reitsma et al., 2020). It is therefore important that all women are appraised of their options at the very first contact and in a way that is evidence based and unbiased and considers the woman's needs, values, and preferences (UKSC, 2015; NMC, 2018; National Institute for Health and Care Excellence, 2021).

Birth preferences including all options for place of birth should ideally be discussed prior to 28 weeks gestation and the details of such should reflect the information provided in the NICE guidelines for intrapartum care (NICE, 2017) for place of birth. It is imperative that this discussion occurs therefore as early as possible to allow women to digest the information and research supporting birth at home to make an informed choice, but not too early that women are overloaded with information and/or are not yet ready to make a decision (Henshall, Taylor, and Kenyon, 2016).

Research has shown that when considering place of birth, women draw upon sources of information alongside that provided by clinicians, which might include friends, family, social media, and other birth workers including doulas as well as their own experiences of labour and birth (Redshaw and Henderson, 2015; Sayakhot and Carolan-Olah, 2016; Hinton et al., 2018). Hinton's work suggested that midwives were not their main source of information, often due to time constraints and the inability to ask questions despite wishing to have this opportunity. Women in the study lamented that they would have liked to have received information to go away with and evaluate and then return for a discussion to support their decision making. Nevertheless, midwives have an important role in providing information and facilitating conversations in relation to place of birth (Houghton et al., 2008; Pitchforth et al., 2009; Hinton et al., 2018).

Consensus of when to have discussions around homebirth has not been reached; however, an ongoing dialogue can be incorporated into routine antenatal appointments and each maternity contact, remaining mindful of not becoming coercive in discussions. Written information might be provided to take away and review early in pregnancy, with a targeted discussion at a later date (16–24 weeks) to start to explore homebirth as an option when the woman is ready to do so (Henshall, Taylor, and Kenyon, 2016; Cross-Sudworth et al., 2018). This avoids the one-time-only discussions and sustains future lines of communication. Keeping these lines of communication open also means that women can revisit their choices along the pregnancy continuum, maintaining a flexible approach to their choices (Brintworth and Sandall, 2013).

Explicit information regarding the local practicalities of accessing homebirth (as with all birth settings) should be readily available available, offered and recorded clearly, include details of the likelihood of intrapartum care being provided by a known midwife, likelihood of receiving intrapartum one-to-one care (not necessarily by the same midwife for the whole intrapartum period), likelihood of transfer, anticipated transfer times including anticipated issues with ambulance availability and the possibility of delays in reaching obstetric or neonatal support that this might present. This should also include limitations on the care that can be provided by attending midwives in a domestic setting (BAPM, 2022) an obstetric setting (local statistics and details preferably however NICE [2017] provide generic data if no local data available). Information pertaining to the availability of and access to analgesia, access to water, obstetric and neonatal staffing, and theatres (NICE, 2017). How this is achieved will vary from organisation to organisation and should form part of the basis of discussions to support informed choice.

Means by which information and discussion can be provided include:

Leaflets and Written Information: Henshall, Taylor, and Kenyon (2016) found in their review that whilst NICE guidance (NICE, 2017) provides guidance for discussion around place of birth, this is likely impractical in terms of length and time constraints to be able to facilitate discussion. Introductory written information in the form of leaflets to introduce ideas around homebirth can therefore act as a springboard to form the basis of future discussions around the evidence for all places of birth including homebirth but should not be seen as the panacea of information provision to facilitate choice, rather an adjunct to appropriate and facilitative discussion. Leaflets and written information might include evidence for all places of birth and for homebirth, details of local provision, who might attend the birth, how it might affect care, transfer, equipment etc. This could signpost to other organisations and support networks.

Social Media, Mainstream Media, and Internet Resources: Many Trusts now develop resources for access online to support decision making. From a homebirth perspective, this might include explanations of how homebirth works, the practicalities, service users' narratives, what happens if transferred, equipment to provide, analgesia options etc. This might also be expanded to local radio. Mobile apps aimed at providing pregnant women with information on a regular basis have also been developed and introduced as an adjunct to other sources of information (Tripp, 2014).

'Meet the Midwife' Events: Not solely used for those planning homebirth but certainly used to good effect in supporting those considering homebirth are regular 'meet the midwife' events (Cross-Sudworth et al., 2018; Callaghan, Foley, and Olusile, 2019). Those booked for or planning homebirths can attend in person (and increasingly by video call) to meet those clinicians who are likely to provide care at home. These can be used alongside antenatal education to provide a forum for questions and answers, receiving peer support, guidance, and reassurance, particularly when parents invited to return postnatally can discuss with others when things did not necessarily go according to plan (Fage-Butler, 2017; Cross-Sudworth et al., 2018). This also gives a forum for partners and family members who might have anxieties to meet clinicians, view equipment, and importantly access their counterparts in other families.

It is imperative that all options remain accessible and culturally sensitive for all communities likely to access services in the local area. Consideration should be made of social complexities and vulnerabilities that might inhibit and prohibit access to information or events including travel costs and access to the internet and technology.

REFERRAL AND RISK ASSESSMENT

A clear referral pathway should be built into local SOPs and guidelines in order that once a request or decision is made for homebirth, a PCSP can be developed (NHS England, 2021a, 2021b, 2021d). This will be dependent on:

- Local arrangements for homebirth provision (i.e.. dedicated home-birth team, continuity of carer/care team, traditional community team)
- Pregnancy gestation
- Obstetric, medical, psychological, or fetal risk assessment (usually referred to 'low-risk' or 'high-risk' pathway)
- Maternal requests, needs, choices, and preferences

As discussed in Chapter 1, *The Evidence for Homebirth*, for primiparous and multiparous women who are deemed at low risk of complications, birth at home is a safe option and that choice should be supported (NICE, 2017). A clear and ongoing risk assessment should be undertaken and reviewed at periodic intervals, beginning at the booking-in appointment (or when homebirth is requested). This will focus initially and then revisited throughout the pregnancy on biopsychosocial risk criteria-based assessment of suitability to recommend birth at home with ongoing assessment of risk usually undertaken at every contact. Any deviation should be identified and escalated appropriately in discussion with the woman or birthing person. Additionally, risk assessment should include local data including reasons for transfer from home to hospital, time taken from 999 call to attendance, and overall transfer time. This will support informed decision making alongside the biopsychosocial risk criteria.

Specific homebirth risk assessment at or around 36 weeks of pregnancy should be undertaken with the woman and her family to consider the following (list not exhaustive) (Table 3.2):

Women who present with obstetric, medical, or other risk factors that might present concerns in pregnancy and labour and postnatally should be recommended to birth in an environment with access to obstetric and neonatal care including theatres (NICE, 2017, 2021a; BAPM, 2022). Some women, however, will make an informed decision to decline this recommendation (see chapter *Homebirth for Women With Complex Needs*). Ongoing assessment considerations should include risks to health and wellbeing of the woman, clear risk pathways which include process of escalation, and a clear process for escalation when issues arise that might move the woman from a low-risk pregnancy to one that might be considered high risk.

Practice Point:
How will any risk assessment be communicated to the wider homebirth team or maternity team? Consider any access or safety issues that might present and need to be communicated to the on-call midwife prior to attending. This might be a folder on labour ward with a copy of the 36-week assessment, a digital spreadsheet with specific issues identified that can be accessed by the labour ward coordinator triggering the on-call midwife. Should include full name, address (including postcode), contact telephone numbers, estimated date or birth, gravida and parity, and any risk factors or outside of guidance plans.

Practice Point:
Is there a standardised approach to continuous and ongoing risk assessment and appropriate escalation pathways should this occur at a homebirth? How is this communicated to women?

Practice Point:
It might be useful to invite any planned doulas to attend discussions and birth planning at 36 weeks in order to foster good working relationships.

Table 3.2 Specific Homebirth Risk Assessment

BIRTH PLANNING AND PREFERENCES	LOGISTICAL ISSUES
• Pregnancy so far and individualised considerations/ specific birth plan • Use of birth planning tools/decision making aids • When homebirth is no longer recommended • Option to change their mind at any time • Equipment they need to provide • Food and hydration and its importance in labour • Birth positions • Analgesia including TENS and aromatherapy • What to expect • Monitoring of fetal and maternal wellbeing • Third stage management – active or physiological • Vitamin K discussion including routes of administration • Perineal trauma – indications for transfer and repair at home • Perineal protection during birth • Indications for transfer and how this will be communicated • Routinely offered interventions and monitoring during labour and birth • Who will observe the sex of the baby (if not already known) • Any cultural considerations for midwives to respect • Skin-to-skin contact preferences • Who will cut the cord? Methods of tying the cord • Anticipated method of feeding	• Preference for student midwives to attend or not • Anticipated location of birth within the home environment • Location for water and soap for handwashing • Location for equipment and newborn resuscitation station • Prepacked birth bag being ready to go for both the woman and the neonate (in case of transfer) • When to call a midwife and how – telephone numbers of agreed contacts, i.e. labour ward • What a midwife at a homebirth can and cannot do logistically (managing expectations) • Emergencies and how transfer works • Estimated time from home to hospital and anticipated transfer times • Provide where possible local data of transfer reasons and times from call to attendance and transfer times from home to hospital • Who is going to be in attendance? • Other children/pets/mothers/friends/doulas • Who will look after children if they are at home? • Logistics of a pool (including location and who fills it!) • Midwife safety and wellbeing (including basic needs, food, water etc) • What happens if the homebirth cannot be facilitated? • Travel directions and parking arrangements for midwives and paramedics • Means of indicating house if call is in dark or middle of the night

> **Practice Point:**
> Many women will express preferences for birth at home early in pregnancy, whilst others may not wish to make definitive plans until later in pregnancy. It is advisable therefore to guide a two way discussion regarding flexible birth preferences regarding place of birth, informed by the woman s needs, wants and preferences and what matters most to them. Moreover recognising and assuring women that whilst they might decide for homebirth or specific request, they can, at any point in pregnancy or in labour, change their minds and come into hospital.

Risk assessment during the intrapartum period at predefined intervals as well as dynamically is essential and any deviation from normal should be escalated without delay by predefined pathways and guidelines (NICE, 2017; NHS England, 2019; NICE, 2021c) (see chapters *Labour at Home, 1st Stage* and *Labour and Birth at Home, 2nd and 3rd Stage*).

RECORD KEEPING

The NMC Code (2018) requires, that record keeping is clear and accurate, ensuring records they are contemporaneous (as far as is possible, or if not possible, documented as soon after an event as possible), reflect any issues that arise and how they have been escalated and to whom, avoiding any false information, correcting any errors in an appropriate manner whilst ensuring that entries in documentation are clearly attributed to the individual making the entry, without jargon or abbreviations. Additionally, methods of keeping records confidential. Arrangements outside those normally employed within the organisation for birth notifications, NHS number, notification of the GP, and subsequent provision of documents to allow birth registration should be included in homebirth SOP and information provided to the woman postnatally.

> **Practice Point:**
> Consider how the move to digital record keeping might be affected by birth at home. How are records kept? Do you need Wi-Fi access and a power supply? What safety issues might this raise in the event of a pool labour and birth?

> **Practice Point:**
> Consider how you might record the withholding consent to or declining a treatment or intervention. See also chapter *Homebirth for Women With Complex Needs.*

SETTING, ENVIRONMENT, AND EQUIPMENT

PERSONAL SAFETY CONSIDERATIONS FOR THE MIDWIFE

Individual midwives must take responsibility for their own safety alongside institutional arrangements for supporting safe lone working. Consider the following issues when discussing care plans for the safety of midwives:

- Is the local community and destination unknown to you or will you need to spend time finding the location? Perhaps a strategically placed coloured light or a unique way to identify the house in the small hours of the morning if difficult to find.
- Are there areas of the geographical area covered that might not be considered safe?
- Might wearing a uniform in areas that might make you feel unsafe cause problems?
- Not leaving equipment visible in cars. Consider signs that state nothing is left in vehicles (including drugs or valuables) and park where possible where you can see the vehicle.
- Access to a physical map rather than satellite navigation might be useful.
- Distance from car parking to the house for manual handling of equipment.
- Method of ensuring colleagues know your whereabouts dependent on local procedures and lone working policies. Some services have engaged lone working call centres to achieve this or panic alarms. However the information of knowing the midwife's whereabouts is achieved, it is essential that this forms part of personal risk assessment and safety auditing.
- Ensure that mobile phones are charged, that you carry a charger, and that your car is fuelled or charged.
- The ability to decide if you should take your second midwife with you if you have concerns about your personal safety in any location will be dependent on local arrangements and your own judgement.

> **Practice Point:**
> Some women may live in locations that require some specific planning considerations planning. For example, house and canal boats, high-rise flats and apartments, city centre locations, mobile communities etc. This might present some individualised challenges which need to be taken into account when planning care. The key is early and personalised discussions.

> **Practice Point:**
> Personal safety also involves recognition of any situation where decision making might be impaired for any reason including tiredness, traumatic events, or difficult situations. Consider what arrangements might be needed to arrange handover to other clinicians in the event of these occurring.

> **Practice Point:**
> Consider how colleagues who may not be used to community or homebirth working might feel when lone working, either when encountering logistical and environmental issues but also when making clinical decisions outside the confines of a hospital. Whilst individual registrants have a responsibility to identify skills and professional development needs (NMC, 2018), an established support mechanism such as buddy systems may help, access to Professional Midwifery Advocates, mentoring of colleagues, and robust documented arrangements for personal safety might also be established. Periodic review of its usefulness should be undertaken.

HOMEBIRTH BAGS AND EQUIPMENT

Until relatively recently, standardised equipment lists or configurations of equipment for those facilitating homebirth did not exist, and it remains the responsibility of the NHS Trust to identify the necessary equipment to be carried and brought. The equipment therefore required for the standard intrapartum care or transfer of the compromised newborn baby and/or woman will be dependent on local geography and demographics and will vary between areas. An online survey undertaken by the Baby Lifeline charity alongside the Royal College of Midwives identified that a third of midwife respondents reported problems with non-standardisation of equipment including unsafe containers and bags (30%), containers and bags not meeting the needs of the midwife (40%), and equipment lacking in everything needed to facilitate birth in the community, including emergency scenarios (27%), with a shocking 35% of respondents reporting having to source and pay for their own containers (35%) (Ledger, 2019). The subsequent development of bespoke homebirth bags followed the recommendations of an expert working group convened by Baby Lifeline, which included a multidisciplinary team of midwifery, obstetric, paramedic, and neonatologists alongside advice provided by RCUK (RCUK, 2011; BAPM, 2022).

RECOMMENDED CONTENTS FOR HOMEBIRTH BAGS

Regardless of whether NHS Trusts purchase a standardised commercially available bag or develop their own equipment bags, it is imperative that the following be considered:

- Equipment and bags should contain all equipment necessary to facilitate safe birth in the community including any emergencies and taking into consideration the local population.
- The bags and containers should be so designed to ensure that manual handling is taken into consideration and that they can be safely transported and lifted and that a manual handling assessment is undertaken with reference to individual capabilities (Health and Safety Executive, 1992).
- The contents and practicalities of the equipment should be reviewed on a regular basis with those who use them to ensure that they remain appropriate and that any changes are communicated effectively.
- Arrangements should be made for restocking, cleaning, and routine checking, and auditing of this built into governance procedures and guidelines for birth at home. This can include a checklist which should be dated, signed, and retained for audit purposes.
- Consider how those new to the team be orientated to the equipment and bags.
- When undertaking training, skills, and drills, use the bags and the equipment to develop a familiarity with them.
- Where possible, carry laminated copies of algorithms and checklists for emergencies to support good communication.

A separate section should be included for relevant paperwork which should include:

- Blood request forms including rhesus-negative forms
- Prescription chart (acknowledging that electronic prescribing or charts may be in place)
- Intrapartum, postnatal, and neonatal notes
- Laminated script for calling an ambulance
- Obstetric and neonatal emergency checklists
- List of useful numbers

If developing a Trust-specific homebirth bag, consider how the bag is to be laid out. Grouping elements of equipment together by use is a common method, that is, birth/delivery pack, suturing, or universal maternal care (Tables 3.3–3.8), universal neonatal care, etc., as well as by obstetric emergency: maternal resuscitation, postpartum haemorrhage etc. Consideration could be given to colour-coding the elements or clearly labelling the containers or pouches for ease of identification. The following are recommended equipment lists:

Table 3.3 Universal Maternal Care and Labour

- Birth/delivery pack
- Sterile instruments including cord scissors (if autoclavable, container for transportation)
- Sterile gloves
- Sharps box/bin
- Placenta disposal container
- Clinical waste disposal bag/container
- Personal Protective Equipment (eyewear/visor/masks/aprons/nonsterile gloves)
- Torch/headlamp
- Incontinence pads
- Sphygmomanometer with appropriate sized cuffs
- Stethoscope
- Pulse oximeter*
- Thermometer* (human and pool)
- Pinards stethoscope
- Fetal doppler/Sonicaid
- Spare batteries for electrical equipment
- Sanitary towels
- Amnihook
- Water-based lubricant
- Mid-stream urine bottles/urinalysis sticks

*Calibrated in line with Trust requirements.

Table 3.4 Emergency Neonatal Care and Labour

- Self-inflating bag and valve mask – 500 mL with 40 cm blow off valve
- Round soft silicone masks ×2 of each, preterm and term baby sizes
- Laryngoscope handle with long and short blade (0,00)
- Laryngeal mask for neonates >34/40 >2000 g
- Oropharyngeal airway for neonates <34/40 (sizes 0,00,000)
- Portable suction (manual or electronic)
- Paediatric suction catheters (×2)
- Soft suction catheters 12/14FG
- Syringes 5 mL (×2)
- Fixing tapes
- Spare bulbs/batteries for laryngoscope
- Gauze squares
- Pulse oximeter neonatal probe

*Calibrated in line with Trust requirements.
(RCUK, 2011, 2021)

Table 3.5 Universal Neonatal Care and Labour

- Scales*
- Oral and IM vitamin K syringes
- Spare cord clamps ×2
- Disposable tape measure
- Identification labels
- Clock/stopwatch
- Hats

*Calibrated in line with Trust requirements.

Table 3.6 Maternal Collapse and Adult Resuscitation

- Adult bag and valve mask/pocket mask
- Adult identification and allergy wrist bands
- Non-rebreather high-flow oxygen mask with associated tubing with connectors for portable oxygen
- Adult oropharyngeal airways

Table 3.7 IV Access, Bloods, Urinary Catheterisation, and Fluids

- IV wide bore cannula
- Blood bottles/vacutainer equipment
- Giving sets/Octopus/3-way tap
- Crystalloid fluids for fluid resuscitation and bladder filling
- Flushes
- Indwelling urinary catheter with urometer/bag
- Intermittent urinary catheters/bungs/clamp
- 20 mL, 10 mL, and 5 mL syringes
- 21 g needles/drawing needles
- Swabs
- Fixings, dressings, and gauze

Table 3.8 Suturing

- Instruments
- Sterile perineal repair pack
- Drapes
- X-ray detectable swabs
- Sterile water
- Suture material (Vicryl Rapide 2.0)

> **Practice Point:**
> Arrangements should be in place to maintain an inventory of equipment which includes calibration (scales, thermometers, sphygmomanometers). This should identify weekly, monthly, and annual checks and be audited as part of governance policies.

> **Practice Point:**
> Midwives who carry homebirth equipment must take responsibility for ensuring that daily checks of bags and equipment are undertaken and records of these checks are kept and maintained. After a homebirth the midwife must ensure that all equipment is rechecked and any used equipment replaced as needed.

MEDICINES, DRUGS, AND MIDWIVES EXEMPTIONS

The drugs and medicines carried for use at a homebirth will vary dependent on NHS Trust, scope of midwifery practice, and local arrangements for analgesia (see table 3.9). Ambulance trusts also vary across the UK in relation to the drugs carried for maternity attendance; therefore it is imperative that communication between ambulance trusts and local maternity trusts be coordinated and mutual understanding of each other's capabilities and equipment documented (see chapters *Transfer and Multidisciplinary Working* and *Emergencies*). the range of pharmacological pain relief options available to the woman should be a key feature in antenatal discussions t guide infromed decision making and should, include local arrangements for requesting and using opoids such as pethidine. Whilst pethidine remains a midwife's exemption, many Trusts are reluctant to provide opioids at home due to their side effects. Notwithstanding, consideration should be given to how to facilitate the provision of pethidine as analgesia in labour. This might be achieved using:

- A guideline/SOP that facilitates the midwife being responsible for obtaining the
  pethidine at the point of onset of labour, transporting to the home at the point of early labour, and then subsequent administration or responsibility for returning/disposal
- The woman obtaining independently from the GP, storing at home for administration by the midwife, and then disposing via community or hospital pharmacy.

In any of the above cases clear and unambiguous information should be provided to the woman for the supply, administration, and disposal of the drug including any anticipated side effects and emergency care. In all cases the midwife is responsible for ensuring that all drugs they are carrying are stored and carried safely, supplied, checked, and administered in line with local arrangements and that arrangements for documentation are robust.

Storage and transportation of medical gases such as Entonox and oxygen should be undertaken in line with local and national arrangements and guidelines followed regarding obtaining from pharmacy and returning empty cylinders. For many midwives working within the NHS they will transport their own cylinders for use when called to a homebirth; however, some Trusts provide a cylinder directly to women planning a homebirth or a community pharmacy will provide this. However, this is undertaken locally; these arrangements should be made explicit in information provided to women at the antenatal planning stage. BAPM (2022) guidance suggests that separate gas sources be available for both the woman and the neonate (pressure limited) should they both require resuscitation. Consideration therefore should be given to midwives carrying oxygen as part of their homebirth equipment.

Table 3.9 Medical Gases and Drugs for Homebirth

Intrapartum Analgesia
- Entonox
- Pethidine
- Paracetamol (woman can provide this)

Third Stage Management
- Syntocinon/synthetic oxytocin

Postpartum Haemorrhage
- Syntometrine
- Ergometrine
- Misoprostol
- Carboprost (Hemabate)
- Tranexamic acid (TXA)

Other Emergency Drugs
- Oxygen

Suturing
- Lidocaine 1%

Neonatal
- Vitamin K

EQUIPMENT AND RESOURCES FOR PROVISION BY THE WOMAN/FAMILY

This will vary from provider to provider; however, in general, these will likely be (Table 3.10).

STAFF SAFETY (PHYSICAL AND PSYCHOLOGICAL)

Staff safety and wellbeing is fundamental to being able to plan and provide effective care at home. Considerable emphasis is placed on issues around supporting homebirth outside of guidelines or for women with complex needs (see chapter *Homebirth for Women With Complex Needs*); however, there are some essential issues that must be addressed and planned for outside of these more complex issues. As discussed in chapter *Homebirth in Undergraduate, Postgraduate and Clinical Education* around ensuring competence and ongoing competence in providing community-based intrapartum care, midwives might feel vulnerable in attending and providing care where this is outside their frame of reference or experience, particularly where they have little exposure to homebirth in education or preceptorship. The availability and access to a Professional Midwife Advocate (PMA) can support individual practitioners and are an important resource to assist midwives in working through difficult issues as well as assisting with individual and group developmental needs.

TRAINING AND PREPARATION/PRECEPTORSHIP

Ideally exposure to homebirth and pre-hospital care will have been undertaken as part of pre-registration programmes and then again through continuing professional development and updates post registration. Sadly this is variable across the UK; indeed, reports into the provision of maternity training overall highlight the need to standardise how maternity training is assessed, provided, funded, and accessed (Ledger et al., 2018). Much in-service training relates to the development of skills and the management of emergency situations rather than meeting the needs of local populations and the healthcare professional that are called to attend homebirth. This extends to homebirth being potentially neglected within preceptorship programmes, where clinical practice often appears to focus on care provided in hospital environments. The development and implementation of continuity of carer models (Sandall et al., 2016; NHS England, 2021c) suggests that more of a focus is required to support preceptor midwives (Welsh Government, 2014; NHS Scotland, 2020; NMC, 2020) (see chapter *Homebirth in Undergraduate, Postgraduate and Clinical Education*).

COMMUNICATION

Factors that influence communication need to be continually evaluated; these include communication between professionals within the immediate environment or in hospital and communication with the woman and her family. Women and their families should remain at the centres of decision making which involves clear and effective communication with them. This can be challenging where issues around languages, disabilities, and communication difficulties are present; however, this should form part of the ongoing risk assessment and care plan (BAPM, 2022). The use of a

Table 3.10 Suggested Equipment and Resources List for Woman to Provide

PHYSICAL RESOURCES	PROXIMITY RESOURCES
• Surface coverings (*shower curtains/sheeting/old sheets/dust sheets*) • Birth pool including lining (with associated pumps) • Disposable sieve (for use in pool) • Clothing for woman to labour and birth in/ transfer in • Towels (for use around pool and for wrapping baby) • Torch and batteries • Fan • Food and drinks for labouring woman and birth attendants • Mirror (preferably new/and not glass) • Sanitary/maternity towels • Paracetamol and ibuprofen* • TENS machine • Birthing ball/mobility aids • Music/speaker • Aromatherapy/homeopathy • Birth plan/preferences • Working landline/charged mobile phone with signal • Power point to charge mobile phone • Nappies • Hat and clothes for baby • Packed hospital bag in case of transfer to hospital (maternal and baby) • Camera	• A flat surface for a neonatal resuscitation station, preferably to allow the clinician to stand (*dining table, coffee table, worktop*) • Dedicated radiator to warm towels and baby clothes, or hot water bottle in absence of radiator. • Pre-determined/identified location for birth, i.e. front room, bedroom, pool (notwithstanding this may change) • Identified location for midwife parking and ambulance access • Cot with dressing • Location to store clinical equipment when not in use • Location to facilitate suturing if necessary

Table 3.11 Example SBAR (NHS Institute for Innovation and Improvement, 2010)

Situation	• Who you are? • Where you are calling from? • What the concern is – specifics of the situation including woman's/patient's name, immediate concerns including abnormal signs?
Background	• Significant medical and obstetric history • Date of attendance • Allergies, lab results of note, relevant observations • Relevant biopsychosocial issues
Assessment	• Clinical impressions or concerns • Observations
Recommendation	• What you need or want to happen? • Suggestions • Clarify expectations

recognised communication tool between professionals that facilitates good communication in a variety of situations, such as SBAR (see table 3.11) (NHS Institute for Innovation and Improvement, 2010), is recommended, with this also being included in skills and drills. The use of a closed-loop system of communication is also recognised as an effective method of avoiding miscommunication and takes into consideration any human factors in the situation (NHS Institute for Innovation and Improvement, 2010).

> **Practice Point:**
> When evaluating potential communication challenges with the woman and her family, consideration should be given at the care planning phase to manage expectations, the potential for and means of transfer from home to a clinical environment, logistical issues including geographical consideration, children, language barriers, and disabilities. These should not be used as reasons for not recommending homebirth but should be planned for in the event of any issues (Table 3.11).

Any deviations from normal physiological processes should be escalated and referred by agreed pathways and methods. Local arrangements for such escalation should take into consideration out-of-hours advice and referral mechanisms, whom and how to call for advice or assistance, which receiving hospital in the event of transfer and conveyance arrangements, and importantly when to call. This involved careful consideration of how this will be achieved including use of mobile phones, house phones, and telemedicine (BAPM, 2022).

> **Practice Point:**
> A standardised method of communication in relation to transfer to a receiving hospital should form part of an established pathway, developed in conjunction with local ambulance services. This is of consideration with remote and rural locations (see *Remote and Rural, Highlands and Islands Geographical Considerations*). When undertaking skills and drills, testing this should form part of the evaluation and feedback loop (BAPM, 2022).

REMOTE AND RURAL, HIGHLANDS, AND ISLANDS GEOGRAPHICAL CONSIDERATIONS

For many supporting and facilitating birth at home, geographical location of services will have little bearing on the provision of service; however, for some, this might need careful consideration and planning. Of note are those births taking place in remote and rural locations, including island locations.

The extent to which these considerations feature within labour and birth planning will be influenced by a variety of factors, and related to transfer:

- The distance for a midwife to travel from their point of call out to the labouring woman.
- The anticipated distance and time from the location of labour and birth to the nearest midwife-led birthing or obstetric/neonatal unit (dependent on reason for transfer).
- The provision of and arrangements for ambulance transfer for whatever reason, that is, maternal request, analgesia, labour progression, or obstetric/neonatal emergency.
- The type of vehicle needed for transfer, that is, air or road transfer.

As the need for transfer is largely unpredictable, each homebirth service provider will need to develop robust guide-lines for supporting transfer when needed (see also chapter *Transfer and Multidisciplinary Team Working*). Whilst the need for and means of transport to an obstetric unit will need to feature within discussions and risk assessment planning for all women, this is of particular importance when a delay might be anticipated due to the geographical location of the birth (BAPM, 2022). This is not to say that this should preclude labour and birth at home. Midwives are well situated to provide emergency care for women at home and, as discussed within this book, should possess the necessary skills and equipment to confidently administer emergency care, including dynamic risk assessment and escalation to protect both maternal and fetal wellbeing. The woman's needs and values should feature within these discussions and preparations, agreeing on which elements of any situation her immediate partner can assist in.

It may be useful to develop service user leaflets and resources to support decision making and provide critical information. These should be co-created and reflect needs of the demographic of the local population (i.e. leaflets, web resources, translation services and documents).

Newborn Life Support Considerations

The BAPM Framework for Practice in relation to Neonatal Support for MLU and Homebirths (2022) acknowledge that remote and rural locations might create challenges in timely transfer to a medical facility by 999 transfer, and accordingly, they suggest that specialist neonatal retrieval arrangements will need to be in place. Such arrangements will require planning and pathways pre-established within the local communities and services; however, it is critical that women and their families are aware of the following:

- Limitations exist in relation to the immediate care that can be provided by attending clinicians.
- This might create a significant delay in reaching assistance and specialist medical support.
- Expected and anticipated timescales to reach the woman and neonate and the risks are associated with long delays.

(BAPM, 2022)

Organisational Considerations for Remote and Rural Locations

It is vital that the multidisciplinary team providing care for transfers and counselling women regarding place of birth are involved in the development of guidelines and procedures that support the safer transfer of women in remote and rural locations and that they can train and learn alongside with those clinicians called upon to support women at home. Skills and drills should include these scenarios as well as human factors related to their situation.

When devising the on-call off duty, it is important to consider how midwives will be relieved in the event of a long labour, particularly where travel distances are such that forward planning is needed. This also includes consideration of student midwives who are placed within a continuity team or otherwise.

Electronic Equipment and Communication Considerations

With the move towards a digitised health service, documentation methods are increasingly being implemented that require good Wi-Fi/internet access and mobile telephone service. This is also an important consideration when identifying how an ambulance is to be summoned in the event of an emergency. Ask the woman and her family the extent to which phone signal is available and where any dead spots might be encountered. If the planned location does not have good mobile phone signal, then a house phone will be required. Some houses may have a landline but it isn't used for telephone communication; therefore ensuring that a handset is available to plug into the landline jack is vital, alongside checking that this works and outgoing calls can be made.

Where the Trust has electronic notes, does this have to be connected to a consistent Wi-Fi signal or is work done offline on a laptop and then uploaded when arriving at a hospital? If this is the case, will this affect any information necessary to support the birth or delay handover either in an ambulance or at the hospital?

Directions

Regardless of the location of a birth, but particularly important in the case of remote and rural locations, directions to and from the planned location of birth should be carefully mapped and described. This should be undertaken early enough in the planning process to ensure that in the event of an unfamiliar midwife or ambulance is required it can be shared. Consider paper copies circulated to key team members and emergency vehicles. Remember that satellite navigation is only as good as its data and many anecdotal stories exist of Sat Navs sending unwary drivers down dead ends, rivers, mountain roads, and fields! This is the same for web-based maps. These might be useful to print and attach to directions but check that they are accurate.

Other things to consider when planning directions:

- You may be familiar with the area, but colleagues and students may not.
- Try to avoid shortcuts and dangerous local cut-throughs when providing directions
- Be clear about where parking is situated and if there is a walk anticipated after parking – how far, and will you need help with equipment?
- Make a note of any roads or areas where road surfaces are treacherous or challenging and poorly lit, potholes or precipitous drops, or when needing to crossing ford.
- When developing directions, try to avoid using generic terms such as 'turn left at the white church' or 'turn right at the road sign' – these might be plentiful and unhelpful.
- Ask the woman and her family to make the location of the birth as visible as possible, either by lighting or other means.

ANIMALS

If the birth is to take place in a domestic premises within an agricultural setting, that is, a farm or smallholding, consider the likelihood of coming into contact with farm animals. Although it is unlikely that you will meet cows, sheep, and other livestock it is important to be familiar with your settings and, where this is likely, build this into your plan. Consider appropriate footwear and somewhere to wash your hands. Much more likely is the presence of working dogs or other animals or birds such as cats or geese. Ensure that you have conversations about how comfortable you are with animals, and the need to avoid some areas to maintain hygiene. It might be necessary to ask for specific areas to be excluded from the area in which the birth takes place.

PERSONAL SAFETY

Many remote and rural areas can be affected by extreme weather conditions. In addition to the generic personal safety arrangements detailed at the beginning of this chapter, equipment should be carried to support any lone working midwife who may become stranded, or breakdown, should this occur. You may wish to consider carrying the following:

- Torch with spare batteries
- Water to consume
- Snacks/emergency food
- Car charger for mobile phone (with emergency numbers pre-programmed)
- An envelope with details of the midwife and next of kin/emergency contact/whom to contact at their place of work, breakdown services number (perhaps in glove compartment)
- Snow shovel (if working in areas where likely to be affected)
- A warm blanket
- Change of socks/clothing/coat
- Breakdown triangle

A dynamic risk assessment of the needs and safety of the midwife as a lone worker will inform other needs such as additional local arrangements for equipment.

REFERENCES

Ball, J., Walshbrook, M. and Royal College of Midwives (2013) 'Working with Birthrate Plus'. Royal College of Midwives.

BAPM (2022) 'Neonatal support for freestanding midwifery led units and homebirths – A framework for practice'. British Association of Perinatal Medicine. Available at: https://hubble-live-assets.s3.amazonaws.com/bapm/file_asset/file/1162/MLU_Home_Birth_BAPM_Framework_July_2022.pdf.

Birthrate Plus (2021) Birthrate Plus® Methodology. Birthrateplus.co.uk. Available at: https://birthrateplus.co.uk/an-overview-of-methodology-and-its-development-within-the-uk/.

Birthrights (2017) Human Rights in Maternity Care. Birthrights. Available at: http://www.birthrights.org.uk/library/factsheets/Human-Rights-in-Maternity-Care.pdf.

Brintworth, K. and Sandall, J. (2013) 'What makes a successful homebirth service: an examination of the influential elements by review of one service', Midwifery, 29(6), pp. 713–721. Available at: https://doi.org/10.1016/j.midw.2012.06.016.

Burt, J. et al. (2013) 'Care plans and care planning in long-term conditions: a conceptual model', Primary Health Care Research & Development, 15, pp. 342–354.

Callaghan, F., Foley, C. and Olusile, M. (2019) 'Setting up a homebirth service in East London: lessons learned and reflections on the first year', British Journal of Midwifery, 27(9), pp. 507-513.

Cleeton, E.R. (2006) 'Birthing autonomy: women's experiences of planning homebirths', Birth (Berkeley, Calif.), 33(4), pp. 339–339. Available at: https://doi.org/10.1111/j.1523-536X.2006.00135_1.x.

Cordey, S. et al. (2022) '"There's only so much you can be pushed": Magnification of the maternity staffing crisis by the 2020/21 COVID-19 pandemic', BJOG: An International Journal of Obstetrics and Gynaecology, 129(8), pp. 1408–1409. Available at: https://doi.org/10.1111/1471-0528.17203.

Cross-Sudworth, F. et al. (2018) 'Creating a dedicated homebirth service: results of a 3-year pilot', British Journal of Midwifery, 26(3), pp. 164–170. Available at: https://doi.org/10.12968/bjom.2018.26.3.164.

Data Protection Act (2018). Data Protection Act 2018. [online] GOV.UK. Available at: <https://www.gov.uk/government/collections/data-protection-act-2018> [Accessed 24/03/23].

Fage-Butler, A.M. (2017) 'Risk resistance: constructing homebirth as morally responsible on an online discussion group', Health, Risk & Society, 19(3–4), pp. 130–144. Available at: https://doi.org/10.1080/13698575.2017.1327038.

Fordham, S. (1997) 'Women's views of the place of confinement', British Journal of General Practice, 47(415), pp. 77–81.

Frohlich, J. and Schram, R. (2015) 'Clinical guidelines: hindrance or help for respectful compassionate care?', in S. Byrom and S. Downe (eds) The Roar Behind the Silence. London: Pinter and Martin, pp. 119–126.

Garthus-Niegel, S. et al. (2019) 'Posttraumatic stress symptoms following childbirth: associations with prenatal attachment in subsequent pregnancies', Archives of Women's Mental Health, 23(4), pp. 547–555. Available at: https://doi.org/10.1007/s00737-019-01011-0.

Greenfield, M., Payne-Gifford, S. and McKenzie, G. (2021) 'Between a rock and a hard place: considering "freebirth" during Covid-19', Frontiers in Global Women's Health, 2, p. 5. Available at: https://doi.org/10.3389/fgwh.2021.603744.

Health and Safety Executive (1992) Manual Handling Operations Regulations 1992, as amended by the Health and Safety (Miscellaneous Amendments) Regulations 2002. SI 2002/2174 The Stationery Office 2002 ISBN 0 11 042693 2

Henshall, C., Taylor, B. and Kenyon, S. (2016) 'A systematic review to examine the evidence regarding discussions by midwives, with women, around their options for where to give birth', BMC Pregnancy and Childbirth, 16(1), p. 53. Available at: https://doi.org/10.1186/s12884-016-0832-0.

Hinton, L. et al. (2018) 'Birthplace choices: what are the information needs of women when choosing where to give birth in England? A qualitative study using online and face to face focus groups', *BMC Pregnancy and Childbirth*, 18(12), pp. 1–15.

Hollander, M. et al. (2016) 'Women refusing standard obstetric care: maternal fetal conflict or doctorpatient conflict?', *Journal of Pregnancy and Child Health*, 03. Available at: https://doi.org/10.4172/2376-127X.1000251.

Homer, C.S. et al. (2017) 'Midwifery continuity of carer in an area of high socio-economic disadvantage in London: a retrospective analysis of Albany Midwifery Practice outcomes using routine data (1997–2009)', *Midwifery*, 48, pp. 1–10. Available at: https://doi.org/10.1016/j.midw.2017.02.009.

Houghton, G. et al. (2008) 'Factors influencing choice in birth place – An exploration of the views of women, their partners and professionals', *Evidence-Based Midwifery*, 6(2), pp. 59-64.

HSCC (2021) *House of Commons Health and Social Care Committee: The Safety of Maternity Services in England*. London: House of Commons.

Jenkinson, B., Kruske, S. and Kildea, S. (2017) 'The experiences of women, midwives and obstetricians when women decline recommended maternity care: a feminist thematic analysis', *Midwifery*, 52, pp. 1–10.

Jouhki, M.-R. (2012) 'Choosing homebirth – The women's perspective', *Women and Birth: Journal of the Australian College of Midwives*, 25(4), pp. e56–e61. Available at: https://doi.org/10.1016/j.wombi.2011.10.002.

Keedle, H. et al. (2015) 'Women's reasons for, and experiences of, choosing a homebirth following a caesarean section', *BMC Pregnancy Childbirth*, 15(1), pp. 206–206. Available at: https://doi.org/10.1186/s12884-015-0639-4.

Kirkup, B. (2015) *The Report of the Morecambe Bay Investigation*. London: The Stationary Office.

Kirkup, B. (2022) *Reading the signals. Maternity and neonatal services in East Kent – the Report of the Independent Investigation*. London: Department of Health and Social Care. Available at: https://assets.publishing.service.gov.uk/government/uploads/system/uploads/attachment_data/file/1111992/reading-the-signals-maternity-and-neonatal-services-in-east-kent_the-report-of-the-independent-investigation_print-ready.pdf (Accessed: 24/03/23)

Knight, M. et al. (2021) *Saving Lives, Improving Mothers Care – Lessons Learned to Inform Maternity Care From the UK and Ireland Confidential Enquiries Into Maternal Deaths and Morbidity 2017–19*. Oxford: National Perinatal Epidemiology Unit, University of Oxford.

Ledger, S. (2019) 'Safer maternity care: addressing variation in community midwifery', *British Journal of Midwifery*, 27(8), pp. 476-477.

Ledger, S. et al. (2018) 'Mind the gap: an investigation into the training gap between NHS Trusts in England'. BabyLifeLine. Available at: https://www.babylifeline.org.uk/wp-content/uploads/2020/11/Mind-the-Gap-2016.pdf.

Maternity Services dashboard (2022). Available at: https://digital.nhs.uk/data-and-information/data-collections-and-data-sets/data-sets/maternity-services-data-set/maternity-services-dashboard.

MBRRACE-UK (2022) *MBRRACE-UK: Mothers and Babies: Reducing Risk Through Audits and Confidential Enquiries Across the UK*. Available at: https://www.npeu.ox.ac.uk/mbrrace-uk.

Mid Staffordshire NHS Foundation Trust Public Inquiry. (2013). *Report of the Mid Staffordshire NHS Foundation Trust Public Inquiry: Executive summary* (HC 947). The Stationery Office. https://assets.publishing.service.gov.uk/government/uploads/system/uploads/attachment_data/file/279124/0947.pdf

Morison, S. et al. (1998) 'Constructing a homebirth environment through assuming control', *Midwifery*, 14(4), pp. 233–241. Available at: https://doi.org/10.1016/S0266-6138(98)90095-X.

Murray-Davis, B. et al. (2014) 'Deciding on home or hospital birth: results of the Ontario choice of birthplace survey', *Midwifery*, 30(7), pp. 869–876. Available at: https://doi.org/10.1016/j.midw.2014.01.008.

National Institute for Health and Care Excellence (2021) 'Antenatal care for uncomplicated pregnancies'. National Institute for Health and Care Excellence.

Nelson, A. and Romanis, E.C. (2021) 'The medicalisation of childbirth and access to homebirth in the UK: Covid-19 and beyond', *Medical Law Review*, 29(4), pp. 661–687. Available at: https://doi.org/10.1093/medlaw/fwab040.

NHS England (2016) 'National maternity review. Better Births'. NHS England.

NHS England (2019) 'Saving Babies Lives Version Two: a care bundle for reducing perinatal mortality'. NHS England. Available at: https://www.england.nhs.uk/wp-content/uploads/2019/03/Saving-Babies-Lives-Care-Bundle-Version-Two-Updated-Final-Version.pdf.

NHS England (2021a) *Comprehensive Model of Personalised Care*. england.nhs.uk. Available at: https://www.england.nhs.uk/personalisedcare/comprehensive-model-of-personalised-care/.

NHS England (2021b) *Maternity Choice and Personalisation*. england.nhs.uk. Available at: https://www.england.nhs.uk/mat-transformation/choice-and-personalisation/.

NHS England (2021c) *Maternity Transformation Programme*. england.nhs.uk. Available at: https://www.england.nhs.uk/mat-transformation/.

NHS England (2021d) 'Personalised care and support planning guidance. Guidance for local maternity systems'. NHS England. Available at: https://www.england.nhs.uk/wp-content/uploads/2021/03/B0423-personalised-care-and-support-planning-guidance-for-lms.pdf. [Accessed 24/03/23].

NHS England (2021e) *Shared Decision Making*. england.nhs.uk. Available at: https://www.england.nhs.uk/shared-decision-making/.

NHS Improvement (2018) 'A guide to support maternity safety champions'. NHS Improvement. Available at: https://www.england.nhs.uk/wp-content/uploads/2020/08/Maternity_safety_champions_13feb.pdf.

NHS Institute for Innovation and Improvement (2010) 'Safer Care. SBAR Situation • Background • Assessment • Recommendation Implementation and Training Guide'. NHS Institute for Innovation and Improvement. Available at: https://www.england.nhs.uk/improvement-hub/wp-content/uploads/sites/44/2017/11/SBAR-Implementation-and-Training-Guide.pdf.

NHS Scotland (2020) 'Scottish Preceptorship Framework'. NHS Education for Scotland. Available at: https://learn.nes.nhs.scot/42348/preceptorship.

NICE (2015) 'Safe midwifery staffing for maternity settings'. National Institute for Health and Care Excellence. Available at: https://www.nice.org.uk/guidance/ng4.

NICE (2017) 'Intrapartum care for healthy women and babies.' National Institute for Health and Care Excellence. Available at: https://www.nice.org.uk/guidance/cg190/chapter/recommendations#pain-relief-in-labour-nonregional.

NICE (2021a) 'Antenatal care for uncomplicated pregnancies'. National Institute for Health and Care Excellence.

NICE (2021b) 'Postnatal care'. National Institute for Health and Care Excellence. Available at: https://www.nice.org.uk/guidance/ng194/chapter/Recommendations#organisation-and-delivery-of-postnatal-care.

NICE (2021c) 'Shared decision making'. National Institute for Health and Care Excellence. Available at: https://www.nice.org.uk/guidance/ng192/resources/caesarean-birth-pdf-66142078788805.

NMC (2018) 'The Code: professional standards of practice and behaviour for nurses, midwives and nursing associates'. Nursing and Midwifery Council.

NMC (2019) *Standards for Proficiency for Midwives*. London: Nursing and Midwifery Council. Available at: https://www.nmc.org.uk/globalassets/sitedocuments/standards/standards-of-proficiency-for-midwives.pdf.

NMC (2020) 'Principles of preceptorship'. Nursing and Midwifery Council. Available at: https://www.nmc.org.uk/standards/guidance/preceptorship/.

Noble, S. (2015) 'Promoting homebirth: intermediate homebirth report', *British Journal of Midwifery*, 23(4), pp. 276–280. Available at: https://doi.org/10.12968/bjom.2015.23.4.276.

NPEU (2022) *UK Midwifery Study System (UK-MidSS), UK Midwifery Study System*. Available at: www.npeu.ox.ac.uk/ukmidss.

Ockenden, D. (2020) *Emerging Findings and Recommendations From the Independent Review of Maternity Services at the Shrewsbury and Telford Hospital NHS Trust*. London: Her Majestys Stationary Office, pp. 1–38. Available at: https://assets.publishing.service.gov.uk/government/uploads/system/uploads/attachment_data/file/943011/Independent_review_of_maternity_services_at_Shrewsbury_and_Telford_Hospital_NHS_Trust.pdf.

Ockenden, D. (2021) *Findings, Conclusions and Essential Actions From the independant Review of Maternity Services at the Shrewsbury and Telford Hospital NHS Trust*. London: House of Commons.

Ogden, J. et al. (1997) 'Women's memories of homebirth 3–5 years on', *British Journal of Midwifery*, 5(4), pp. 208–211.

Olafsdottir, O.A., Thies-Lagergren, L. and Sjoblom, I. (2021) 'Being in charge in an encounter with extremes. A survey study on how women experience and work with labour pain in a Nordic homebirth setting', *Women and Birth: Journal of the Australian College of Midwives*, 34(2), pp. 122–127. Available at: https://doi.org/10.1016/j.wombi.2020.01.015.

Pitchforth, E. et al. (2009) '"Choice" and place of delivery: a qualitative study of women in remote and rural Scotland', *BMJ Quality & Safety*, 18(1), pp. 42–48.

RCM (2016) 'RCM guidance on implementing the NICE safe staffing guideline on midwifery staffing in maternity settings'. Royal College of Midwives. Available at: https://www.rcm.org.uk/media/2369/rcm-guidance-on-implementing-the-nice-safe-staffing-guideline-on-midwifery-staffing-in-maternity-settings.pdf.

RCM (2022) Care outside guidance. Caring for those women seeking choices that fall outside guidance. Royal College of Midwives. Available at: https://www.rcm.org.uk/media/5941/care_outside_guidance.pdf.

RCUK (2011) 'Equipment used in homebirth'. Resuscitation Council UK. Available at: https://www.resus.org.uk/library/quality-standards-cpr/equipment-used-homebirth.

RCUK (2021) 'Newborn resuscitation and support of the transition of infants at birth Guidlines'. Resuscitation Council UK.

Redshaw, M. and Henderson, J. (2015) 'Safely delivered: a national survey of women's experience of maternity care 2014'. National Perinatal Epidemiology Unit, University of Oxford.

Reitsma, A. et al. (2020) 'Maternal outcomes and birth interventions among women who begin labour intending to give birth at home compared to women of low obstetrical risk who intend to give birth in hospital: a systematic review and meta-analyses', *EClinicalMedicine*, 21, pp. 100319–100319. Available at: https://doi.org/10.1016/j.eclinm.2020.100319.

Rowe, R. et al. (2020) 'Intrapartum-related perinatal deaths in births planned in midwifery-led settings in Great Britain: findings and recommendations from the ESMiE confidential enquiry', *BJOG: An International Journal of Obstetrics & Gynaecology*, 127(13), pp. 1665–1675. Available at: https://doi.org/10.1111/1471-0528.16327.

Sandall, J. et al. (2016) 'Midwife-led continuity models versus other models of care for childbearing women', *Cochrane Database of Systematic Reviews* [Preprint], 4. Available at: https://doi.org/10.1002/14651858.CD004667.pub5.

Sassine, H. et al. (2021) 'Why do women choose homebirth in Australia? A national survey', *Women and Birth: Journal of the Australian College of Midwives*, 34(4), pp. 396–404. Available at: https://doi.org/10.1016/j.wombi.2020.06.005.

Sayakhot, P. and Carolan-Olah, M. (2016) 'Internet use by pregnant women seeking pregnancy-related information: a systematic review', *BMC Pregnancy and Childbirth*, 16(1), p. 65. Available at: https://doi.org/10.1186/s12884-016-0856-5.

Scally, G. and Donaldson, L.J. (1998) 'Clinical governance and the drive for quality improvement in the new NHS in England', *BMJ*, 317(7150), pp. 61–65. Available at: https://doi.org/10.1136/bmj.317.7150.61.

Scottish Government (2017) *The Best Start: A Five-Year Forward Plan for Maternity and Neonatal Care in Scotland*. Edinburgh: Scottish Government.

Sjöblom, I. et al. (2012) 'A provoking choice – Swedish women's experiences of reactions to their plans to give birth at home', *Women and Birth: Journal of the Australian College of Midwives*, 25(3), pp. e11–e18. Available at: https://doi.org/10.1016/j.wombi.2011.07.147.

Tripp, N. et al. (2014) 'An emerging model of maternity care: Smartphone, midwife, doctor?', *Women and Birth*, 27(1), pp. 64–67. Available at: https://doi.org/10.1016/j.wombi.2013.11.001.

UKOSS (2022) *UK Obstetric Surveillance System (UKOSS), UKOSS*. Available at: https://www.npeu.ox.ac.uk/ukoss.

UKSC (2015) *Montgomery v Lanarkshire Health Board*.

Viisainen, K. (2001) 'Negotiating control and meaning: homebirth as a self-constructed choice in Finland', *Social Science & Medicine*, 52, pp. 1109–1121.

Welsh Government (2014) 'Core principles for preceptorship'. Welsh Government. Available at: http://www.nwssp.wales.nhs.uk/sitesplus/documents/1178/Final%20Report%20for%20Preceptorship.pdf.

Welsh Government (2019) *Maternity Care in Wales – A Five Year Vision for the Future (2019–2024)*. Cardiff: Welsh Government. Available at: maternity-care-in-wales-a-five-year-vision-for-the-future-2019-2024.pdf (gov.wales).

CHAPTER 4

HOME ALONE – CHOOSING FREEBIRTH

Dr Mari Greenfield and Dr Claire Feeley

Some women and other birthing people in the UK choose to give birth at home, without healthcare professionals present, a practice which is known as 'freebirthing'. Sometimes those people will choose to have antenatal care, postnatal care, or both, either from the NHS or from an independent provider, and choose just to give birth without a midwife or other healthcare professional present. Other people will decline all medical perinatal care and also freebirth. The choice to freebirth is sometimes confused with other situations in which people may not seek antenatal care or may choose to give birth alone, and we will begin this chapter by defining what a freebirth is and is not.

The rates of freebirth in the UK are unknown, meaning that it is challenging to establish the mortality and morbidity outcomes. Estimates that are produced sometimes include figures for babies who are born before arrival (BBA), but as BBA births are usually unplanned, these figures are unlikely to be an accurate representation of freebirth outcomes. Freebirth has historically been understudied in both the academic and medical literature; however, research does tell us about who chooses to freebirth, and why. In this chapter we will examine this research to draw out the common factors and provide information about the legalities of freebirth.

Lastly, we will examine the practical issues that women and birthing people choosing to freebirth face and look at how perinatal services and individual practitioners can work positively to support them.

WHAT A 'FREEBIRTH' IS AND IS NOT

Freebirth, sometimes known as 'unassisted birth', broadly means an active decision to birth without trained health professionals present but where maternity care is readily available (Feeley and Thomson, 2016a). While definitions may differ amongst those who choose to freebirth, perinatal researchers, and midwifery organisations, the key feature of freebirth is the willing decision by the person giving birth. Therefore those who feel forced to opt out of maternity care are not included in this definition – for example, women who are 'not ordinarily resident' may fear being charged for maternity care and/or the consequences of not being able to pay for their care (Feldman et al., 2019), but their decision not to use perinatal services would not fit the definition of freebirth. In addition, it is important to distinguish freebirthing from other situations such as concealed pregnancy, pervasive pregnancy denial, or coercive reproductive control.

In a concealed pregnancy the birthing woman or other birthing person is aware they are pregnant but chooses to keep this fact hidden, including from those closest to them (Murphy Tighe and Lalor, 2016a). They may take great care to avoid the pregnancy being detected by wearing only a limited wardrobe or restrictive clothes, isolating themselves from family and friends, and even moving away (Murphy Tighe and Lalor, 2016a). Motivations for concealing a pregnancy are varied and include teenage pregnancies, infidelity, domestic violence, rape, and incest (Hatters Friedman, Heneghan, and Rosenthal, 2007; Porter and Gavin 2010; Murphy Tighe and Lalor, 2016b). Concealing a pregnancy is not illegal, but concealing a birth, or a stillbirth, is illegal (Offences against the Person Act, 1861).

Pervasive pregnancy denial is a rare phenomenon wherein a pregnant person is either entirely unaware or cannot accept that they are pregnant (Barnes, 2022). However, denial may only persist for part of the pregnancy, as in situations when someone is genuinely unaware that they are pregnant (Barnes, 2022). There is no consistent demographic profile for those who experience pervasive pregnancy denial, but there are linking symptoms such as the absence or misattribution of pregnancy symptoms (Barnes, 2022). There again are those experiencing reproductive coercion and abuse such as forced pregnancies and births, which are often linked to other forms of intimate partner violence (Tarzia and Hegarty, 2021). Reproductive coercion and abuse could include coercion into place and method of birth, and therefore potentially coerced freebirth.

Concealed or denied pregnancies and reproductive coercion are of concern to healthcare professionals due to negative outcomes for the baby, including attachment difficulties (Barnes, 2022), an increased rate of abandonment (which may cause death), and direct neonaticide (Murphy Tighe and Lalor, 2016c). Freebirth is not associated with these outcomes, but if the differences between these situations are not understood by healthcare professionals, unnecessary safeguarding referrals or actions may occur (Feeley and Thomson, 2016b; Plested and Kirkham, 2016; Medway NHS Trust, 2021). Those choosing freebirth are aware of their pregnancy, not in denial or being coerced. The reasonable concerns that healthcare professionals have relating to concealed pregnancies, pervasive pregnancy denial, or reproductive control do not apply to birthing women and people who are making the active choice to freebirth.

Babies who are 'born before arrival' (BBA) are also not freebirthed. BBAs occur either when the parent(s) were intending to birth in the hospital or birth centre, but the baby arrived before they could get there; or during a planned homebirth where the midwife did not arrive before the baby. In the former case this might be caused by insufficient support and triage, for example, if the parent was deemed to be 'not in established labour' and sent home (Shallow,

2016). In the latter case a midwife might not arrive at a planned homebirth before the baby was born either because of a precipitous labour, where the baby was born very quickly, or because insufficient staffing levels meant a midwife was not dispatched in time to arrive and support the birth. A defining feature in these situations is that the parent(s) did not intend for the birth to happen without a healthcare professional present. Parents may often experience BBAs as distressing (Shallow, 2016). However, because of the societal stigma associated with freebirth, some parents who planned to freebirth may call the midwife shortly after the birth, stating that the labour was precipitous – a 'planned BBA' – to avoid suspicion and undue interference by health professionals (Feeley and Thomson, 2016b).

Furthermore, issues arise when homebirth services or birth centres are suspended, often due to staffing or resource issues (O'Boyle, 2016). These issues were compounded by the pandemic with a high number of homebirth service suspension and birth centre closures (Romanis and Nelson, 2020; Brigante et al., 2022), which, alongside significant partner restrictions in hospital, led to a rise in freebirthing (Romanis and Nelson, 2020; Greenfield, Payne-Gifford and McKenzie, 2021; Schröder et al., 2021). While we believe these unassisted births appear on the surface to fit the definition of freebirth proposed above, we suggest that these parent(s) were not making an active, willing choice to freebirth, as the only other options available to the parent(s) were unacceptable to them.

> **Practice Point:**
> In a situation where a midwife is told by someone that they are choosing to freebirth due to NHS policies, practices, or service restrictions, the midwife has a professional duty to support and advocate for care within maternity services, to ensure that they receive care that they want. This may include seeking input from a consultant midwife or leader to cocreate a complex care plan (as described in Chapter Homebirth in the presence of complex needs). In cases where Trusts are unable to provide a specific service (e.g. a homebirth due to staffing), or where there is a lack of expertise within the Trust (e.g. vaginal breech or twin birth), they should consider employing an independent midwife to facilitate the birthing woman or person's wishes. The use of honorary contracts for independent midwives has had some success at Chelsea and Westminster NHS Foundation Trust.

The common feature in all of the situations above is that a freebirth has not been chosen by the birthing parent. Rather, in each situation the situation of birthing without a healthcare professional present has been imposed by an external force, whether that is a financial situation, a controlling partner or family member, or NHS maternity services.

WHO CHOOSES TO FREEBIRTH, AND WHY?

Research into freebirth is a relatively recent development, and there are significant gaps in our knowledge about the rates, demographics, and outcomes for freebirth. Existing studies focus on the motivations of women in Western nations such as the UK (Feeley and Thomson, 2016a; Greenfield, Payne-Gifford, and McKenzie, 2021), Ireland (O'Boyle, 2016), Canada (Cameron, 2012), Australia (Jackson, Dahlen, and Schmeid, 2012; Jackson, Schmeid, and Dahlen, 2020), Norway (Henriksen et al., 2020), and the Netherlands (Holten and de Miranda, 2016), and non-binary people and trans men in the UK (LGBT Foundation, 2022; Oakes-Monger and Pearce, 2021) and the USA (Spencer-Freeze, 2008). Collectively, these studies highlight a range of reasons why people decide to freebirth, including a previous traumatic birth (Jackson, Dahlen, and Schmeid, 2012), dissatisfaction with the care offered by perinatal services (Henriksen, Nordström, Nordheim, Lundgren, and Blix, 2020), and an inherent belief in the undisturbed physiological processes of birth (Feeley and Thomson, 2016a). Being unable to access care based on 'logistics' and the geographical distance to a maternity unit (Kornelsen and Stefan, 2006) and limitations on homebirths have also been shown to play a role in women's decision-making (O'Boyle, 2016), and new research highlights that freebirth may be more common amongst lesbian, bisexual, pansexual and Queer women, non-binary people, and trans men (Greenfield, Payne-Gifford, and McKenzie, 2021; Oakes-Monger and Pearce, 2021; LGBT Foundation, 2022). We will look at these reasons individually.

LACK OF CHOICE

Autonomy and the right to make choices about your own body are important motivating factors amongst those choosing freebirth (Feeley and Thomson, 2016b). When homebirth services are not provided or are only available for some people, freebirth may be chosen because it is the only way to retain such bodily autonomy (O'Boyle, 2016). My own research (Mari) shows that during the UK pandemic, when many birth centres were closed and many homebirth services were suspended, the lack of choice contributed to people considering freebirth (Greenfield, Payne-Gifford, and McKenzie, 2021). Although all pregnant people in the UK should have a choice of where to give birth (National Maternity Review, 2016), not all maternity services have resumed after the pandemic, meaning that choices continue to be limited for many.

PREVIOUS EXPERIENCES

Previous traumatic experiences with NHS maternity care are common reasons for opting to freebirth (McKenzie, Robert, and Montgomery, 2020). Around 30% of women in the UK experience childbirth as a traumatic event (Ayers, 2014) (no figures are available for trans men or non-binary people), and the care received during birth contributes significantly to this high rate (Watson et al., 2021). A number of research studies have found that previous poor intrapartum care, whether or not it resulted in birth trauma, has motivated some women to plan a freebirth in a subsequent pregnancy (Jackson, Dahlen, and Schmied, 2012; Jackson, Schmied and Dahlen, 2020). Poor care, in this context, includes coercion and bullying into giving 'consent' to unwanted tests, procedures, and interventions, or in other circumstances no consent given at all (Reed, Sharman, and Inglis, 2017; Forsberg, 2019). Poor care also includes disrespectful care such as being spoken to rudely, scolded, shouted at, or 'told off' (van der Pijl et al., 2022). Similarly, receiving care which is perceived as poor or uncaring in the current pregnancy has been shown to motivate some people to consider freebirth (Greenfield, Payne-Gifford, and McKenzie, 2021). More widely, previous negative experiences with healthcare professionals in settings other than perinatal care have been reported as a factor motivating some trans men and non-binary people to choose to freebirth (LGBT Foundation, 2022).

Fear of being unsupported in upcoming birthing decisions or facing obstructive practices to receiving their preferred care may disenfranchise some expectant parents, preventing them from using services, and/or compounding pre-existing trauma (Feeley and Thomson, 2020; Greenfield and Marshall, 2022). Understanding the significant and lifelong impact that birth trauma can have and acknowledging the role of maternity care as a factor which can both cause and protect against birth trauma is important for all healthcare practitioners and is something that must be considered in relation to this pregnancy when caring for those planning a freebirth, as there is the potential to cause (further) trauma.

Undisturbed Physiological Birth

Many people who choose to freebirth share a belief that an undisturbed physiological birth provides the best physical and emotional experience for both the mother or other birthing parent and for the new baby (Miller 2009; Lundgren 2010; Feeley and Thomson 2016a). This is often accompanied by a belief that most healthy pregnant people are capable of giving birth without medical intervention (Miller, 2009; Lundgren, 2010; Feeley and Thomson 2016a; Rigg, Schmied, Peters and Dahlen, 2017) – an ideal which is also embedded in UK midwifery philosophy (Feeley and Thomson, 2016a). Yet as McKenzie and Montgomery (2021) report, achieving a truly undisturbed physiological birth within the context of the increasing medicalisation of birth within the UK can be difficult; however, it is the usual birth experience amongst those who choose to freebirth. Norton's systematic review tells us that amongst those who choose to freebirth:

'Women frequently recognised that, within standard maternity care, risk assessments were carried out using a framework not corresponding to their perception of risk'. (Norton, 2020)

Indeed, disturbing a physiological birth is rarely discussed as a risk within NHS literature. While freebirth is not without risk, the research from those opting for freebirth shows that they typically weigh up these risks against the risks of seeking care from providers who may not be supportive or skilled to support physiological birth (Feeley and Thomson, 2016a; Plested and Kirkham, 2016), and/or the risks of hospital birth, where evidence demonstrates medical interventions are routine and commonplace (Seijmonsbergen-Schermers et al., 2020; NHS Digital, 2022), thus reducing the chance of an undisturbed birth. These differences in assessments of risks are one motivation for choosing freebirth, with the belief that it offers the best opportunity for an undisturbed physiological birth.

Demographics of Freebirth

Statistics regarding freebirth are not routinely collected in the UK; therefore it is not clear whether this decision pertains to particular groups. Previous research has mostly reported findings from white middle-class heterosexual women (Feeley and Thomson, 2016a, 2016b; Holten and de Miranda, 2016; Jackson, Dahlen and Schmeid, 2020; O'Boyle, 2016; Plested and Kirkham, 2016; Henriksen et al, 2020); however, two recent pieces of work have reported freebirths amongst different demographic populations (Greenfield, Payne-Gifford and McKenzie, 2021; LGBT Foundation, 2022). In research I (Mari) conducted during the pandemic I collected demographic data and qualitative responses to questions about how birth plans had changed from over 1750 new or expectant parents in the UK. Bisexual, lesbian, and pansexual respondents made up 4.2% of all respondents but made up 13.9% of the respondents who said they were considering freebirth (Greenfield, Payne-Gifford, and McKenzie, 2021). This was the first piece of research showing a link between sexual orientation and freebirth, and further research is needed to investigate whether this finding continues outside of the pandemic. In separate research conducted with 121 trans men and non-binary people who had given birth in the UK, it was found that 30% of their respondents had not accessed midwifery support at any point during their pregnancy(s) or births (LGBT Foundation, 2022) and that this rose to 46% amongst Black and Brown non-binary people and trans men.

This research also pointed out that some non-binary people and trans men may conceal their pregnancies from the public, engaging in some behaviours common to cis women who conceal their pregnancies such as wearing a limited wardrobe and may also experience fear of the consequences of their pregnancy being revealed in a public location. However, their motivation may be entirely different to the motivation of cis women who conceal their pregnancies, in that they may fear for their own or their unborn baby's safety if their pregnancy is publicly recognised. In this situation those close to the pregnant person are likely to be aware of the pregnancy – it is a concealment which is limited to the public sphere. Therefore the concerns about concealed or denied pregnancies cited above are not relevant in these situations, but this important difference is not referenced in any NHS policies we are aware of.

What's the Common Factor?

The motivations for choosing to freebirth may seem disparate, but they do share a common feature. Whether the pregnant person has wished to give birth at home with midwives or in a birth centre, has wanted an undisturbed physiological birth, or has just wanted a non-traumatic birth or a birth in which their gender or sexual orientation is respected, perinatal services available in the UK have been unable to provide the support that women and birthing people desire.

LEGALITIES (IN THE UK)

ANTENATAL

In the UK a fetus does not have legal rights. Pregnant women and other pregnant people retain their full legal rights to bodily autonomy throughout pregnancy, including the right to consent to or decline offered healthcare (Human Rights Act, 1998). It is illegal to administer healthcare to any adult with mental capacity without their consent, and this includes whilst they are pregnant (Human Rights Act, 1998). As soon as a baby is born, the baby has full legal rights too, but treatment cannot be administered to a pregnant woman or other pregnant person without their consent solely on the grounds that it would benefit the unborn baby.

Choosing to freebirth, and choosing to accept or decline any antenatal care, is therefore a legal right for every pregnant person with mental capacity in the UK (AIMS, 2013; Birthrights, 2017; Royal College of Midwives, 2020). All perinatal care, all midwifery care, all scans, all tests, and all appointments with an obstetrician are optional in the UK. Pregnant women and other pregnant people are not obliged to accept any perinatal care; however, choosing not to, in the current climate, risks undue cause for concern by health professionals (Feeley and Thomson, 2016b; Plested and Kirkham, 2016), and there are even NHS policies which contradict this legal right (Feeley and Thompson, 2016b; Schiller, 2016). In part, this is based on hypervigilance amongst perinatal healthcare professionals about safeguarding concerns, based on a belief that not attending appointments for offered perinatal care is associated with issues such as (but not exclusive to) domestic violence, significant substance misuse, human trafficking, and child neglect/abuse (University Hospital Wishaw, 2020; Payne and Matthews, 2022).

While guidance in the UK clearly states midwives should not consider a freebirth alone as a safeguarding concern (Royal College of Midwives, 2020), some midwives may also receive contradictory advice from their employer, or from a local organisation with a safeguarding role (Thomas, 2013; North Yorkshire Safeguarding Children Partnership, 2021). Some maternity professionals and Trusts have wrongly claimed freebirthing as illegal (Feeley and Thomson, 2016b; Plested and Kirkham, 2016; Medway NHS Trust, 2021) causing much distress and inappropriate safeguarding referrals and policy interventions.

Practice Point:
In a situation where local policies require a midwife to make a safeguarding referral due to a choice to freebirth only, the midwife has a professional duty to challenge this policy. This may include seeking support from a consultant midwife or leader to ensure that local policies are in accordance with relevant legislation such as the Human Rights Act (1998), allowing all midwives to adhere to the professional guidance issued by RCM.

Against this backdrop of local policies which sometimes contradict legal rights, it is unsurprising that participants in freebirth research report mixed experiences of choosing to freebirth. Many of their negative experiences occur when healthcare professionals are unaware of the fact that freebirth is a legal choice, or where healthcare professionals decide to follow incorrect guidance from their employer rather than their professional bodies' guidance. Referral to Children's Services on the grounds of 'safeguarding' is a common experience.

> *I was offered another appointment with the consultant but declined, saying I'd go back to my midwife if I wanted anything else. In spite of this, another appointment was made for me, and when I didn't go to it, it was used as an excuse to refer me to social services. I don't see how I can default on an appointment I didn't make, but that was the reason given (Claire, interview).*
>
> —Feeley and Thomson, 2016b

Further tension between women and other pregnant people's legal rights and NHS policies may arise from 'late booker' policies. If someone has initially decided that they do not wish to receive any antenatal care but during pregnancy has then decided that they would like to receive some care or would like specific tests or scans, they are likely to be considered as 'late bookers', rather than as freebirthers who wish to exercise their right to consent to some maternity care. All NHS Trusts have policies which flag late booking as a concern, because it may indicate a pregnancy which was until recently concealed or denied. A similar situation may arise for those who do not want antenatal care or a midwife present at the birth but would like to access postnatal services.

The positive or negative experiences of freebirthers who choose some antenatal care are shared, often via social media, with others who are considering or planning a freebirth, and these experiences – along with NHS policies – may affect whether those planning a freebirth choose to opt into any antenatal or postnatal care. This means that one negative experience potentially leads to a number of parents declining care that they might otherwise have wanted.

INTRAPARTUM

Confusion around legalities about who may be present at a freebirth has sometimes arisen due to misunderstandings of the law. Article 45 (Nursing and Midwifery Order, 2001) serves to protect families from unregulated, unlicensed medical professionals. Confusion arises because the word 'attend' is used within the Nursing and Midwifery Order (2001), and 'attend' has two meanings in English. The legislation does not preclude birth partners, doulas, or family members from being present at freebirths, but it would be a criminal offence for them to assume a health professional role (Nursing and Midwifery Order, 2001):

> It is illegal for anyone present during the labour or birth, to be undertaking the roles of a midwife or doctor. According to Article 45 of the Nursing and Midwifery Order (2001), it is a criminal offence for anyone other than a midwife or registered doctor to "attend" a woman during childbirth, except in an emergency. Birth partners, including doulas and family members, may be present during childbirth, but must not assume responsibility, assist or assume the role of a midwife or registered medical practitioner or give midwifery or medical care in childbirth.
>
> —Royal College of Midwives, 2020

POSTNATAL

It is a legal requirement all births are 'notified' to the relevant authorities, by someone present at the birth, and within legal timeframes (Notification of Births Act, 1907). If a midwife completes the notification, they must do so within 6 hours of a birth; if anyone else completes the notification it must be within 36 hours of a baby being born. For those who choose to freebirth, complying with this law can be difficult. Notification must be sent to the Child Health Information Service, via the local Child Health Unit. However, there is no centralised list of Child Health Units, and as they are a service usually dealing with healthcare professionals rather than parents, their contact details are not often published. Finding the correct details can be difficult, and parents may have to contact their local maternity services to obtain the details. If maternity services refuse to give these details to parents, they could unintentionally fall foul of the law. Even where maternity services are willing to provide the details, someone contacting maternity services in later pregnancy or just after birth may run the gauntlet of late booking or concealed pregnancy policies, depending on the interpretation of the individual who answers their query. Birth notification is the first legal requirement, the second being registering a birth, when a baby is named and receives their birth certificate (Gloucestershire Hospitals NHS Trust, 2021).

SUPPORTING FREEBIRTH

Most people who choose to freebirth will have some contact with maternity services, and so with midwives. Their experiences of midwifery care and/or interactions with midwives have potential long-term implications; positive, supportive interactions promoting respectful, dignified care is likely to have a positive impact (Watson et al., 2021). Conversely, negative, hostile interactions can generate mistrust in both individual maternity professionals and the wider services, fostering disengagement with any or all services (Byrne et al., 2017). Therefore it is vital that all maternity professionals (midwives or obstetricians, health visitors, paramedics etc.) understand how to constructively support those opting to freebirth, should they share this intention. Guidance from the Royal College of Midwives (RCM) acknowledges the midwife's role is to provide information regarding the benefits of antenatal and intrapartum care while ensuring the conversations are centred on the needs and decisions of those choosing freebirth (Royal College of Midwives, 2020).

The collaborative and flexible approach RCM recommends has been taken up in a new NHS patient information leaflet for those considering freebirth (Cambridge University Hospitals NHS Trust, 2022; Gloucestershire Hospitals NHS Trust, 2021), which acknowledges freebirthing as a right and maternity care as an opt-in. Both the leaflet and the RCM approach signal a shift away from paternalistic assumptions and the negative connotations associated with this birthing choice, instead focussing on 'good' midwifery (and wider maternity) care – supportive, respectful, relational care. Relational care involves establishing a relationship in which a midwife is truly listening to the woman or other pregnant person and understanding why a freebirth is preferred. This kind of care does include being aware of the potential for a situation being presented as a freebirth being something else, in which case this care pathway will become irrelevant. Good midwifery care does include considering safeguarding responsibilities, but these are not the focus of the care. Where a midwife is clear that a freebirth is planned, good care involves offering options which facilitate choices, for both the birth itself and discussing preferences for antenatal and postnatal care. Typically (but not always) such care would include a complex care plan detailing the information the midwife has provided based on the woman's decision-making (for more information on complex care planning, see Chapter Homebirth in the presence of complex needs). All documentation should include the risk, benefits, alternatives, and contingencies should unexpected issues arise during the labour or birth (e.g. thick meconium). Midwives may require support for themselves and organisations should provide meaningful non-punitive support:

> If a midwife is caring for a woman planning to have an unassisted birth or wishing to have a homebirth with risk factors that would suggest she would be safer to give birth in a hospital, the midwife should be offered the opportunity to discuss their concerns and plan of care with their manager. Midwives will also benefit from seeking support through midwifery supervision or professional midwifery advisors (PMA) or other peer support.
>
> —Royal College of Midwives, 2020

We welcome this recognition that midwives who are providing care in specialist situations may need additional support from managers and peers. Currently, following the guidance provided above would mean providing care which is 'outside of (local) guidelines' in all NHS Trusts that we are aware of. One way to resolve this situation is to create Trust-specific guidance for the provision of care when a midwife becomes aware that a freebirth is planned.

Providing relational, meaningful care whereby hospital Trusts proactively support their staff to support these choices has the potential to create a psychologically safe environment for all concerned. It is possible, through good relationships, that a planned freebirth may become a planned attended birth, but that is not the only outcome which

Table 4.1 Benefits of Creating a Local Care Pathway for Those Planning a Freebirth

Within the Trust:

Opportunity to ensure all staff are aware of the legalities of freebirth.

Opportunity to ensure all staff are aware of the differences between freebirth, concealed pregnancies, denied pregnancies, and reproductive coercion.

Midwives who become aware of a planned freebirth will have a clear pathway to refer to, and new policies will not have to be invented ad hoc.

Midwives following the pathway have reassurance that this care is not 'outside of guidelines', and that they will be supported.

The importance of thoroughly documenting all discussions can be conveyed.

More people planning a freebirth may choose to access some antenatal/postnatal care, which may improve outcomes.

Opportunity to build in appropriate supervision and support for midwives caring for those planning a freebirth.

For Expectant Parents:

Reassurance that choosing to opt into some care is both possible and safe.

Understanding that an individualised care plan which could facilitate their birth choices may be possible.

Greater understanding of why safeguarding is a consideration when determining whether a pregnancy or freebirth is concealed, denied, or coerced, alongside reassurance that freebirth will not be subject to inappropriate safeguarding referrals.

Reassurance that choosing to contact Maternity Services in an emergency is possible, even if they have chosen not to opt into any antenatal care prior to that point.

Builds trust in midwives and the Maternity Service even before contact is initiated.

would be deemed successful in this model. If the midwife has been able to establish a relationship of trust with the parent(s), and they have been supported to accept the antenatal and/or postnatal care of their choice, choose to freebirth, and are confident that they can contact the maternity services if they choose or need to, then the episode of care is also successful. We suggest that hospital Trusts co-produce local care pathways and guidelines to ensure maternity professionals are supported to authentically support those who choose to freebirth. A collaborative document may have several benefits, outlined in Table 4.1.

CONCLUSIONS

Freebirth is a legal choice available to all pregnant people who have mental capacity in the UK, and they can have partners, family and friends, and doulas present to support them during birth. Reasons for choosing to freebirth are varied, complex, and multifaceted. Current confusion about the legalities of freebirth, as well as policies which equate freebirth with pregnancy concealment and pervasive pregnancy denial, and practices which encourage midwives to report those planning a freebirth as safeguarding risk, are likely to traumatise parents and discourage future engagement with maternity services. We encourage instead the development of Trust-specific policies for midwives encountering those planning a freebirth. Such policies should prioritise relationship building between midwives and expectant parents and facilitate parents' choices (Table 4.2).

Table 4.2 Freebirth Myths

MYTH	REALITY
Freebirth is illegal	Freebirth is legal in the UK. This has been affirmed by all relevant authorities, many times. However, misinformation is still frequently given, including by some official bodies.
People who choose to freebirth are careless, irresponsible, and care only about their experience not their baby	Freebirths may be chosen for a variety of reasons, including a lack of choice within NHS services, previous traumatic birth or other health experiences, a physiological belief in undisturbed birth combined with a belief that the NHS cannot provide this, fear of homophobia or transphobia, or a misunderstanding of or fear connected to charges that having a midwife-attended birth may bring.
	'Wanting the best and safest' for both the birthing person and their baby was the core motivation for choosing freebirth in one piece of research (Jackson, Schmied, and Dahlen, 2020).

Table 4.2 Freebirth Myths—cont'd

MYTH	REALITY
Doulas can't attend freebirths	Doulas (and anyone else the birthing person chooses) can be present at a freebirth. They may not perform actions that would only be performed by a midwife or other medical professional. The performing of medical actions is the legal meaning of 'attend' in this context.
Partners can be prosecuted for being at a freebirth	Partners can be present at a freebirth, and as this is entirely legal, they cannot be prosecuted for it. If they were to perform actions that would only be performed by a midwife or other medical professional, they could potentially be prosecuted.
Wider family and friends can be prosecuted for attending a freebirth	The birthing person can have anyone they like present at a freebirth. Friends, family, neighbours, pets – anyone. No one would be breaking the law unless they performed actions that would only be performed by a midwife or other medical professional.
Unassisted or 'wild' pregnancies are the same as concealed pregnancies	A concealed pregnancy is concealed from everyone (or almost everyone) close to the woman or other pregnant person. Choosing not to tell healthcare professionals you are pregnant is not concealing a pregnancy, as healthcare professionals have no legal right to know the contents of a uterus. Some people who do conceal a pregnancy from those close to them may also not conceal the pregnancy from healthcare professionals for the full duration of the pregnancy.
People choosing freebirth won't want any care from perinatal services	Some people who choose to freebirth will not want any antenatal or postnatal care. Others may want standard NHS antenatal and/or postnatal care, and some people may choose to accept some offered care and decline parts of it. Blanket policies which treat freebirthers and those who might be concealing a pregnancy or experiencing pervasive pregnancy denial in the same way are dangerous. They may discourage those planning a freebirth from accessing wanted antenatal or postnatal care, and this may reinforce this myth.
Midwives supporting people who choose freebirth are breaking the Nursing and Midwifery Council's Code of Conduct	Midwives have a legal responsibility to uphold and respect any legal decisions that a pregnant person makes about their antenatal or intra-partum care, including freebirth. Documents from the NHS Maternity Transformation Hub, the Royal College of Midwives, and the Nursing and Midwifery Council all affirm that midwives should offer care and support to people who are choosing to freebirth. Refusing to support someone because they are choosing to freebirth, or making a referral to Children's Services solely because someone is planning/has had a freebirth is a potential breach of the Nursing and Midwifery Code of Conduct.
Parents can decline all care for a baby	Babies have no legal rights until they are born. From the moment that they are born, they have full legal rights to appropriate healthcare. Parents can decline routine care for healthy babies that they do not wish their child to have, including being weighed at birth, receiving immunisations and vitamin K injections, and newborn tests such as the heel prick test and the Newborn and Infant Physical Examination (NIPE). If a baby is unwell, they have a legal right to healthcare. Whether parents can decline treatment generally depends on the severity of the illness. If agreement between the parent(s) and the healthcare professional about a particular treatment or what is in the child's best interests cannot be reached, the courts can always be asked to make a decision, but they are unlikely to be involved in decisions about treatments for minor illnesses. In an emergency, when an illness or injury is severe or life-threatening, where treatment is vital and waiting for parental consent would place the child at risk, healthcare professionals can legally administer treatment to a baby without parental consent (General Medical Council, 2018).

REFERENCES

AIMS (2013). Freebirth and the law. *AIMS Journal*. 25(4). 0256-5004 [Date accessed: 9 September 2022]. Available at: https://www.aims.org.uk/journal/item/freebirth-and-the-law

Ayers, S. (2014). Fear of childbirth, postnatal post-traumatic stress disorder and midwifery care. *Midwifery*, 30(2), pp. 145-8. doi:10.1016/j.midw.2013.12.001

Barnes, D.L. (2022). Towards a new understanding of pregnancy denial: the misunderstood dissociative disorder. *Arch Womens Ment Health*, 25, pp. 51–9. doi:10.1007/s00737-021-01176-7.

Birthrights (2017). *Unassisted Birth Factsheet.* Birthrights. [Date accessed: 9 September 2022]. Available at: https://www.birthrights.org.uk/factsheets/unassistedbirth/

Brigante, L., et al. (2022). Impact of the COVID-19 pandemic on midwifery-led service provision in the United Kingdom in 2020–21: findings of three national surveys. *Midwifery*, 112. doi:10.1016/j.midw.2022.103390.

Byrne, V., Egan, J., Mac Neela, P., and Sarma, K. (2017). What about me? The loss of self through the experience of traumatic childbirth. *Midwifery*, 51, pp. 1–11. doi: 10.1016/j.midw.2017.04.017.

Cambridge University Hospitals NHS Trust (2022). *Maternity Information for Those Considering Giving Birth Unassisted by a Midwife.* [Date accessed: 9 September 2022]. Available at: https://www.cuh.nhs.uk/patient-information/maternity-information-for-those-considering-giving-birth-unassisted-by-a-midwife/

Cameron, H.J. (2012). *Expert on Her Own Body: Contested Framings of Risk and Expertise in Discourses on Unassisted Childbirth: Master's Thesis Lakehead University.* [Date accessed: 31 August 2022]. Available at: https://knowledgecommons.lakeheadu.ca/handle/2453/526.

Feeley, C. and Thomson, G. (2016a). Why do some women choose to freebirth in the UK? An interpretative phenomenological study. *BMC Pregnancy Childbirth*, 16, pp. 1–12. doi:10.1186/s12884-016-0847-6

Feeley, C. and Thomson, G. (2016b). Tensions and conflicts in 'choice': womens' experiences of freebirthing in the UK. *Midwifery*, 41, pp. 16–21. doi:10.1016/j.midw.2016.07.014

Feeley, C. and Thomson, G. (2020). 'Understanding women's motivations to, and experiences of, freebirthing in the UK', in Dahlen, H., Kumar-Hazard, B. and Schmied, V. (eds.). *Birthing outside the system: The canary in the coalmine.* Routledge, London. doi:10.4324/9780429489853.

Feldman, R., Hardwick, J., Cleaver Malzoni, R., Bragg, R., and Harris, S. (2019) Duty of Care? The impact on midwives of NHS charging for maternity care, *Maternity Action.* [Date accessed: 3 April 2023]. Available at: https://www.maternityaction.org.uk/wp-content/uploads/DUTY-OF-CARE-with-cover-for-upload.pdf

Forsberg, L. (2019). 'Childbirth, consent, and information about options and risks' in Pickles, C. and Herring, J. *Childbirth, Vulnerability and Law: Exploring Issues of Violence and Control.* Routledge, London.

General Medical Council (2018). 0–18 years: *guidance for all doctors.* [Date accessed: 3 April 2023]. Available at: https://www.gmc-uk.org/ethical-guidance/ethical-guidance-for-doctors/0-18-years

Gloucestershire Hospitals NHS Trust (2021). *Maternity Information for Those Considering Giving Birth Unassisted by a Midwife.* [Date accessed: 9 September 2022]. Available at: https://www.gloshospitals.nhs.uk/media/documents/Unassisted_birth_leaflet_FINAL_110521_1.pdf

Greenfield, M. and Marshall, A. (2022). Big Birthas – The effect of being labelled 'high-BMI' on women's pregnancy and birth autonomy. *MIDIRS Midwifery Digest*, 32(1), pp. 25–30.

Greenfield, M., Payne-Gifford, S., and McKenzie, G. (2021). Between a rock and a hard place: considering 'freebirth' during Covid-19. *Front Women's Health*, 2. doi:10.3389/fgwh.2021.603744.

Hatters Friedman, S., Heneghan, A., and Rosenthal, M. (2007). Characteristics of women who deny or conceal pregnancy. *Psychosomatics*, 48(2), pp. 117–122. doi:10.1176/appi.psy.48.2.117.

Henriksen, L., et al. (2020). Norwegian women's motivations and preparations for freebirth – A qualitative study. *Sex Reprod Healthc*, 25, 100511. doi:10.1016/j.srhc.2020.100511.

Holten, L. and de Miranda, E. (2016). Women's motivations for having unassisted childbirth or high-risk homebirth: an exploration of the literature on 'birthing outside the system'. *Midwifery*, 38, pp. 55–62. doi:10.1016/j.midw.2016.03.010.

Human Rights Act (1998). c.42. London: HMSO. [Date accessed: 9 September 2022]. Available at: https://www.legislation.gov.uk/ukpga/1998/42/contents

Jackson, M., Dahlen, H., and Schmeid, V. (2012) Birthing outside the system: perspectives of risk amongst Australian women who have high risk homebirths. *Midwifery*, 28, pp. 561–567. doi:10.1016/j.midw.2011.11.002.

Jackson, M.K., Schmied, V., and Dahlen, H.G. (2020). Birthing outside the system: the motivation behind the choice to freebirth or have a homebirth with risk factors in Australia. *BMC Pregnancy Childbirth* 20, p. 254. doi:10.1186/s12884-020-02944-6.

Kornelsen, J. and Stefan, G. (2006). The reality of resistance: the experiences of rural parturient women. *J Midwifery Women's Health*, 51, pp. 260–265. doi:10.1016/j.jmwh.2006.02.010

LGBT Foundation (2022). *Trans and non-binary experience of maternity services.* LGBT Foundation, Manchester. [Date accessed: 31 August 2022]. Available at: https://dxfy8lrzbpywr.cloudfront.net/Files/97ecdaea-833d-4ea5-a891-c59f0ea429fb/ITEMS%2520report%2520final.pdf

Lundgren, I. (2010). Women's experiences of giving birth and making decisions whether to give birth at home when professional care at home is not an option in public health care. *Sex Reproduct Healthc*, 1(2), pp. 61–66.

McKenzie, G., and Montgomery, E. (2021). Undisturbed physiological birth: insights from women who freebirth in the United Kingdom. *Midwifery*, 101. doi:10.1016/j.midw.2021.103042.

McKenzie, G., Robert, G., and Montgomery, E. (2020). Exploring the conceptualisation and study of freebirthing as a historical and social phenomenon: a meta-narrative review of diverse research traditions *Med Humanit*, 46, pp. 512–524. doi:10.1136/medhum-2019-011786.

Medway NHS Trust (2021). [Date accessed: 31 August 2022]. Comment originally at: https://www.facebook.com/medwaymaternity/photos/a.851590238522471/1365182103829946/; Screenshot available at: https://twitter.com/ResearchDoula/status/1353790221012369408

Miller, A.C. (2009). 'Midwife to myself': birth narratives among women choosing unassisted homebirth. *Sociol Inq*, 79(1), pp. 51–74.

Murphy Tighe, S. and Lalor, J.G. (2016a). Concealed pregnancy and newborn abandonment: a contemporary 21st century issue – Part 1. *Pract Midwife*, 19(6). pp. 12-5. PMID: 27451485.

Murphy Tighe, S. and Lalor, J.G. (2016b). Concealed pregnancy: a concept analysis. *J Adv Nurs*. doi:10.1111/jan.12769.

Murphy Tighe, S. and Lalor, J.G. (2016c). Concealed pregnancy and newborn abandonment: a contemporary 21st century issue – Part 2. *Pract Midiwfe*, 19(7). pp. 14-6. PMID: 27652438.

National Maternity Review (2016). *Better Births, Improving Outcomes of Maternity Services in England*. [Date accessed: 2 August 2022]. Available at: https://www.england.nhs.uk/wp-content/uploads/2016/02/national-maternity-review-report.pdf

NHS Digital (2022). *Maternity Services Monthly Statistics, May 2022*. [Date accessed: 3 September 2022]. Available at: https://digital.nhs.uk/data-and-information/publications/statistical/maternity-services-monthly-statistics/may-2022-experimental-statistics

North Yorkshire Safeguarding Children Partnership (2021). *Concealed, denied or late presentation of pregnancy*. North Yorkshire Safeguarding Children Partnership. [Date accessed: 9 September 2022]. Available at: https://www.safeguardingchildren.co.uk/professionals/procedures-practice-guidance-and-one-minute-guides/concealed-denied-or-late-presentation-of-pregnancy-2/

Notification of Births Act, 1907. (7 Regnal & 7 Edw. c. 40) London:HMSO [Date accessed: 3 March 2023]. Available at: https://www.legislation.gov.uk/ukpga/Edw7/7/40

Norton, J. (2020). Why women freebirth: a modified systematic review. *MIDIRS Midwifery Digest*, 30(4), pp. 509–514.

Nursing and Midwifery Order (2001). (SI 2002: 253) Article 45. London: HMSO. [Date accessed: 9 September 2022]. Available at: https://www.legislation.gov.uk/uksi/2002/253/contents

O'Boyle, C. (2016). Deliberately unassisted birth in Ireland: understanding choice in Irish maternity services. *Br J Midwife*, 24(3). doi:10.12968/bjom.2016.24.3.181

Oakes-Monger, T. and Pearce, R. (2021). 'Inequalities in perinatal healthcare for trans people in England', in *Converging Crises in Transgender Activism, Health, and Rights in 2021*. Transgender Professional Association for Transgender Health.

Offences Against the Person Act (1861). (24 & 25 Vict. c.100). London: HMSO. [Date accessed: 31 August 2022]. Available at: https://www.legislation.gov.uk/ukpga/Vict/24-25/100/section/60

Payne, L. and Matthews, L. (2022). *Missed antenatal appointments and women declining antenatal care management guideline*. University Hospitals of Leicester. [Date accessed: 9 September 2022] Available at: https://secure.library.leicestershospitals.nhs.uk/PAGL/Shared%20Documents/Missed%20Antenatal%20Appointments%20UHL%20Obstetric%20Guideline.pdf

Plested, M. and Kirkham, M. (2016). Risk and fear in the lived experience of birth without a midwife. *Midwifery*, 38, pp. 29–34. doi:10.1016/j.midw.2016.02.009.

Porter, T. and Gavin, H. (2010). Infanticide and neonaticide: a review of 40 years of research literature on incidence and causes. *Trauma, Violence and Abuse*, 11(3), pp. 99–112. doi:10.1177/1524838010371950.

Reed, R., Sharman, R., and Inglis, C. (2017). Women's descriptions of childbirth trauma relating to care provider actions and interactions. *BMC Pregnancy Childbirth*, 17(21). doi:10.1186/s12884-016-1197-0.

Rigg, E.C., Schmied, V., Peters, K., and Dahlen, H.G. (2017). Why do women choose an unregulated birth worker to birth at home in Australia: a qualitative study. (2017). *BMC Pregnancy Childbirth*, 17(99). doi:10.1186/s12884-017-1281-0.

Romanis, E.C. and Nelson, A. (2020). Homebirthing in the United Kingdom during COVID-19. *Med Law Int*, 20(3), pp. 183–200. doi:10.1177/0968533220955224.

Royal College of Midwives (2020). *RCM Clinical Briefing Sheet: 'freebirth' or 'unassisted childbirth' during the COVID-19 pandemic*. Royal College of Midwives. [Date accessed: 9 September 2022]. Available at: https://www.rcm.org.uk/media/3923/freebirth_draft_30-april-v2.pdf

Schiller, R. (2016). The women hounded for giving birth outside the system. *The Guardian*, 26 October 2016. [Date accessed: 9 September 2022]. Available at: https://www.theguardian.com/lifeandstyle/2016/oct/22/hounded-for-giving-birth-outside-the-system

Schröder, K., et al. (2021). Concerns about transmission, changed services and place of birth in the early COVID-19 pandemic: a national survey among Danish pregnant women. The COVIDPregDK study. *BMC Pregnancy Childbirth*, 21(664). doi:10.1186/s12884-021-04108-6.

Seijmonsbergen-Schermers, A.E., et al. (2020) Variations in use of childbirth interventions in 13 high-income countries: a multinational cross-sectional study. *PLoS Med*, 17(5), e1003103. doi:10.1371/journal.pmed.1003103. PMID: 32442207.

Shallow, H. (2016). 'Are you listening to me?: An exploration of the interactions between mothers and midwives when labour begins: a feminist participatory action research study', PhD thesis, University of the West of Scotland, Glasgow.

Spencer-Freeze, R. (2008). 'Born free: unassisted childbirth in North America', PhD Thesis University of Iowa. doi:10.17077/etd.gqjehps0.

Tarzia, L., Hegarty, K. (2021). A conceptual re-evaluation of reproductive coercion: centring intent, fear and control. *Reprod Health*, 18(87). doi:10.1186/s12978-021-01143-6

Thomas, M. (2013). Freebirth and Social Services. *AIMS Journal*, 25(4)

University Hospital Wishaw. (2020). *Guidance for non-attendance at antenatal clinics*. NHS Lanarkshire. [Date accessed: 9 September 2022]. Available at: https://nhslguidelines.scot.nhs.uk/media/1937/non-attendance-at-antenatal-clinics-and-letter-september-2020-2.pdf

van der Pijl, M.S.G.R., et al. (2022). Disrespect and abuse during labour and birth amongst 12,239 women in the Netherlands: A national survey. *Reprod Health*, 19(160). doi:10.1186/s12978-022-01460-4.

Watson, K., White, C., Hall, H., and Hewitt, A. (2021). Women's experiences of birth trauma: a scoping review. *Women Birth*, 34(5), pp. 417–424. doi:10.1016/j.wombi.2020.09.016.

CHAPTER 5

FIRST STAGE OF LABOUR AT HOME

John Pendleton

INTRODUCTION

Although labour and birth represent only one moment in the continuum from conception and pregnancy to parenthood, it is perhaps considered the gateway between the two states and is the subject of much anticipation. The homebirth midwife therefore has an important role to play in helping the woman or birthing person, their partners, and support network to navigate this transformational process. Intrapartum care in hospitals places emphasis on the mechanistic process of labour, whereas choosing to labour and birth at home is often in recognition of the equal importance of psychological safety (Olza et al., 2020). It is by foregrounding this understanding that the homebirth midwife is able to practice most effectively and in synergy with the needs and wants of those who have made an informed decision to have a homebirth. Whilst acknowledging the phenomenon of the '*ever narrowing window of normality*' (Scamell & Alaszewski, 2012), this chapter focuses on intrapartum care for term singleton pregnancies without additional complexities that may require input from obstetricians. Nevertheless, many of the core principles of intrapartum care at home are readily transferable to support the needs of a diversity of midwifery caseloads.

LABOUR AS A NEUROHORMONAL EVENT

The uterus is a large muscular organ which has been held back throughout pregnancy from contracting – known as 'myometrial quiescence' – under the influence of a cocktail of hormones, chiefly progesterone (McNabb, 2017, p. 563). Labour can be considered the onset of uterine activity to begin the process of expelling the fetus. What causes the onset of labour – or myometrial activation – is still under-researched and poorly understood (Coad & Dunstall, 2012, p. 318; Jackson et al., 2020, p. 449). What is generally accepted is that labour is the gradual activation of myometrial activity which is influenced by complex interactions between the stretching of the uterus at term and signals from the maturing fetus which in turn activate maternal receptors and pathways for dynamic hormonal activity (Coad & Dunstall, 2012, p. 320; Howie & Watson, 2017, p. 374). This activity will control the strength and length of uterine contractions as well as the maternal and fetal responses.

There does appear to be clear evidence of a strong correlation between 'chronic anxiety, heightened levels of fear, pain perception' and dystocia (McNabb, 2017, p. 571). On the one hand, the release of oxytocin in conjunction with the formation of oxytocin receptors in the myometrium is essential for efficient rhythmic uterine activity. This activity works in symbiosis with the release of melatonin which enhances relaxation and minimises cognitive stimulation. Both processes are central to optimising birth physiology and are stimulated by the woman or birthing person feeling safe and secure. On the other hand, the sustained and excessive release of catecholamines, principally adrenaline (McNabb, 2017, p. 573), can be triggered when the woman or birthing person feels that they are in danger or excessively anxious. This is not only the antagonist to oxytocin release but also reduces blood flow to the uterus with consequent prolongation of labour (Howie & Rankin, 2017, p. 399), causing a positive feedback mechanism between increased perception of pain and labour complications. For the homebirth midwife creating optimal conditions for this hormonal cascade to flourish should guide all activity – or inactivity – and decision making and will inform the discussion on how to effectively support women and birthing people throughout this chapter.

THE 'STAGES' OF LABOUR

It has been acknowledged that the concept of 'stages' of labour is arbitrary. Myles' textbook describes the division of birth into discrete phases as 'a rather pedantic, medically ascribed view, as labour is obviously a continuous process' (Jackson et al., 2020, p. 449). It seems likely that the division of birth into discrete phases originated in the 17th century when scientific enquiry sought to understand the birthing body in mechanistic terms (Pendleton, 2019; Reed, 2021, p. 154), whereas in reality, the transition from pregnancy to labour is a highly individual process and for many, particularly those who have not birthed before, there is no abrupt transition into labour (Coad & Dunstall, 2012, p. 318). Nevertheless, the 'stages' of labour are easily understandable concepts and helpful in explaining to women and birthing people complex physiological processes as well as making them intelligible to students and midwives. In fact, midwives *must* understand these concepts when devising plans of care and organising resources in line with local and national guidelines. The initial stages of labour are divided into the 'latent' and 'established' first stage of labour by National Institute for Health and Care Excellence (NICE) (2014), and as they form the basis for all Local NHS Trust guidelines, these terms will be used here. What is important is that midwives and birth workers keep in mind that the embodied experience of labour and birth is likely to feel very different from the textbook definitions and to allow for individualised care in response to this. Continuity of care and carer models and homebirth midwifery in general hold this at the very core of their philosophical underpinnings and are embedded in current standards of education for student midwives in the UK (Nursing & Midwifery Council, 2019) (see chapter *homebirth in undergraduate, postgraduate and clinical education*). This is what will help prevent trying to replicate in the domestic arena the conditions of a hospital birth (Charles, 2018a, p. 128) by rigidly following guidelines which are primarily designed to meet the needs of organisational efficiency in obstetric-led units.

CARE IN THE LATENT FIRST STAGE OF LABOUR

The latent phase is arguably more easily conceptualised as the liminal space between pregnancy and labour. McNabb (2017, p. 571) describes a period of 4 weeks at the end of pregnancy which is crucial to optimising and preparing the woman or birthing person for physiological birth. Relaxation and increased periods of sleep enhance myometrial activity and changes in the cervix in preparation for labour under the influences of oxytocin and melatonin and have also been associated with shorter labour and reduced perceptions of pain.

Practice Point:
Knowledge of this represents an important opportunity to inform women and birthing people about the need to rest more in the final weeks of pregnancy. For example, many people in paid employment choose to continue working as long as possible into their pregnancy in order to maximise paid maternity leave to spend more time with their baby. They may spend what little time is left available to them before the baby is born making final practical preparations and 'nesting activity' at a time when they could be sleeping and relaxing, neglecting their important roles in birth physiology.

Many organisational guidelines place emphasis on healthcare professionals determining the onset of labour. The onset of labour – latent or established – can only really be determined in retrospect. NICE (2014) defines the latent phase as a period of time, which may not be continuous, where there are painful contractions leading to cervical change up to 4 cm of dilatation. Perceptions of pain, however, are subjective, can provoke anxiety, and are arguably unhelpful when trying to affirm birth as an empowering and transformative event rather than a pathological state to be endured. The use of vaginal examinations as a diagnostic tool is equally problematic. Like all interventions, vaginal examinations to establish cervical dilatation carry risks (Christopher et al., 2019; Gluck et al., 2020), can be experienced as painful and/or uncomfortable (Lewin et al., 2005), and are often inaccurate (Nizard et al., 2009) and subjective (Buchmann & Libhaber, 2007). Furthermore, there is no international consensus on the correlation between cervical dilatation and the onset of active labour – the World Health Organization (2018, p. 35) adopt a definition of 5 cm dilatation and there is increasing evidence that cervical dilation rapidly increases from 5 to 6 cm (Oladapo et al., 2017). Vaginal examinations can also undermine birth physiology if the woman or birthing person perceives their own embodied experience as inadequate to diagnose labour. They should therefore be offered sparingly and only if the findings are necessary to inform ongoing plans of care. Furthermore, uterine activity that causes the cervix to shorten and flatten out (efface) can take up to a week to occur (Coad & Dunstall, 2012, p. 337) and this process is more noticeable in nulliparous women and birthing people than those who have laboured before.

Practice Point:
Defining the onset of labour at home represents both a challenge and an opportunity for the homebirth midwife. Good antenatal education is key to preparing women and birthing people in advance to recognise and understand these changes and thus minimise potential anxiety when they start to occur. This will avoid release of excessive catecholamines which will interrupt oxytocin and decrease or cease uterine activity, causing 'prolonged' labour and the cascade of interventions that are likely to ensue (increased need for early analgesia, admission to hospital for augmentation and/or epidural analgesia and their sequelae [Iobst et al., 2019]). This education should ideally take place prior to 34 weeks of pregnancy to minimise activation of the neocortex in absorbing new information at a time when this needs to be reducing in activity (McNabb, 2017, p. 571). Birth supporters and partners should be integral to this conversation.

Other common symptoms indicating that labour is imminent are low backache, loose bowel movements, increased vaginal discharge, a blood-stained show, and spontaneous rupture of membranes (SROM) (Walsh, 2017, p. 597; Charles, 2018b, p. 5). SROM can precede labour in up to 19% of term pregnancies (Walsh, 2017, p. 597). Contiguous with this is the 'effacement' of the cervix as it prepares to open up to admit the fetus.

Practice point:
If SROM is suspected and reported, then the midwife should visit to confirm it and assess maternal wellbeing and a baseline set of observations to exclude maternal infection as well assessing fetal wellbeing. Confirmation by speculum is only necessary if there is any doubt as to whether SROM has occurred; current NICE (2014) guidance advises induction of labour 24 hours after SROM if labour does not occur spontaneously.

THE INITIAL PHONE CALL

Once the woman or birthing person suspects that labour has started, they will need to make contact with their midwife. This represents a crucial moment to influence and sets the tone for ongoing interaction and trust with their caregivers.

Most studies on the initial phone contact between women and birthing people and maternity services are predicated on the premise of delaying admission to hospital to avoid the cascade of interventions that may follow (Walsh, 2012, p. 46) rather than as part of an integrated homebirth service. Many NHS Trusts triage people booked for homebirths when calling 'out of hours' via Labour Ward co-ordinators based on obstetric-led units. Triaging on a labour ward often requires the person triaging to be observed and overheard, which may pressurise them to conform to standardised advice whilst juggling competing demands. This may mean limiting conversation to meet acceptable time limits, and limited training in the skill can cause anxiety (Spiby et al., 2014; Bailey et al., 2019). Very often, the tone of the conversation is 'not ready yet' and a lack of recognition of the important physiological changes that are already occurring.

> **Practice Point:**
> If you are a homebirth practitioner, what support can you offer to colleagues to more effectively handle phone calls from women and birthing people planning to birth at home who may be in early labour? How can you enhance the learning for student midwives in this area to better prepare them for autonomous practice?

Very often, there is a discrepancy between the labouring person's perception of onset of labour and that of the healthcare professional. What matters are the needs of the person at the moment that they make contact with midwifery services. It has been argued that encouraging women and birthing people to 'carry on' without the assistance of a midwife can be empowering and reassuring (Janssen et al., 2009); others, however, may find it distressing. Evidence suggests that it is the act of being heard and listened to sympathetically which is more important to the labouring person than the content of the advice (Myhre et al., 2021). In their meta-synthesis of 11 papers Eri et al. (2015) identified that women were sensitive to the way they were spoken to on the phone, valuing being heard as an individual whilst fearing being exposed as silly or 'making a mistake' about being in labour. This can be overcome by reassurance from a trusted midwife.

> **Practice Point:**
> Whilst it is possible for the midwife to make an initial assessment, create a plan of care including whether to attend imminently or not, and provide support via the phone and increasingly via video calls (Spiby et al., 2019; Faucher & Kennedy, 2020), it is also known that home visits are likely to provide a more positive labour experience overall (Janssen & Desmarais, 2013). When a homebirth midwife is 'on call', they might like to consider liaising with the labour ward co-ordinator, explaining that they are happy to be contacted by any labouring person and have the initial conversation themselves. Midwives can then directly affirm with the women or birthing person that what they are experiencing is important and offer them a direct line for further support or offer a home visit if requested and/ or likely to be beneficial. In this way it is possible to avoid the disempowering experience of being told by a midwife that what they are experiencing is not labour and thus starting the relinquishing of agency on the part of the labouring person in favour of the midwife rather than nurturing a relationship based on partnership (Janssen et al., 2009).

Most midwives will be familiar with a system which has attempted to do good by keeping labouring people away from maternity services until clearly in active labour because this is the system that they are likely to have trained within. It may be hard to switch to a different way of thinking when working in a continuity of care or caseload system, particularly when there is a persistent threat of homebirth services being suspended in order to centralise services on an obstetric unit due to low staffing levels. What is clear is that there is a tension between the needs of the organisation and what women and birthing people who plan on birthing at home need.

SHOULD I STAY OR SHOULD I GO?

Having made the decision to conduct a home visit, it may not always be necessary or beneficial to remain at home. Deciding on when to stay and when to go is really only a debate when the woman or birthing person is considered to be in the latent phase of labour and needs to be made holistically, assessing the needs of the individual and the wider context. The initial phone call will have given the midwife some clue as to the progress of labour. If they were calm on the phone and able to converse through most of the contraction, and if the contractions are irregular or infrequent, then first principle on arrival is to minimise disruption to environment. It would be wise to only take essential equipment into the home whilst making an initial assessment – for example, baby scales and Entonox can be left in the car until needed or confident that labour is established but neonatal resuscitation equipment, a birth pack, and equipment for managing a postpartum haemorrhage should be with the midwife to avoid being 'caught out'. Midwives may choose to leave this equipment outside the room while making their initial assessment and have a separate bag with sphygmomanometer, stethoscope, and Pinard (and Doppler) along with what is required for record keeping (paper notes or laptop) for immediate use. If the environment is calm and birth does not appear to be imminent, then the priority is to establish a rapport with the woman or birthing person and their partner and others present (see chapter *Antenatal Planning*).

There may be operational practicalities to consider. For example, the midwife may decide it is safe and in the best interests of the woman or birthing person to leave until there is a change in the intensity and frequency of uterine activity. However, if there is only capacity within the team to support one birth, there is a risk that the midwife may get called to another birth in the interim and be unable to return to the original labourer. There may also be pressure to support episodes of high activity on an obstetric unit or birth centre if co-ordinators are aware that the midwife is not actively engaged in supporting a homebirth. In short, the midwife must consider if they can offer reassurance that they will be able to return when wanted or when labour is considered more established. This should at least be part of the informed discussion the midwife has with the woman or birthing person before it is agreed that they should leave the home. Midwives working in the UK have a professional obligation to make the needs of those accessing midwifery care their primary concern (Nursing and Midwifery Council, 2018), and therefore assessment on whether continuous support is required needs to be made holistically by the midwife. For some women who are distressed and anxious or need additional support, it may be appropriate to stay even if they do not yet meet the criteria for being in established labour. If the midwife does confirm that the woman or birthing person is in established labour, then they must remain at the home and ensure that continuous one-to-one midwifery care is provided.

CARE IN ESTABLISHED FIRST STAGE OF LABOUR

THE 'BASICS' – ENVIRONMENT, MOBILISATION, NUTRITION, AND HYDRATION

Environment

The importance of 'creating' an optimal environment for physiological birth to occur is recognised by the foundational midwifery textbooks (Walsh, 2017, p. 594; Charles, 2018b, p. 2; Jackson et al., 2020, p. 457). Whilst this may present a challenge for midwives working in hospitals, this is only because they are having to recreate what already exists in a home environment: an environment which provides a sense of safety and security and which the woman, birthing person, and her partner have control over in terms of heat, lighting, music, or quiet and in which they move around in response to their instinctive needs which are governed by the flow of birth hormones. Midwives need to ensure that they minimise disruption or medicalising this environment by unnecessary overt and prominent display of equipment such as resuscitation equipment, instruments, and weighing scales. Certainly, during the first stage of labour it is safe to 'follow' the lead of the woman or birthing person as they move around their space. Undisturbed labours with spontaneous onset usually occur at night-time, with the peak time of birth occurring on average at Change to 4 am (Howie & Watson, 2017), suggesting that darkness and peace are important components of optimal hormonal flow.

> **Practice Point:**
> Midwives may want to wear soft-soled shoes and turn off any alarms or ring tones on their phones to minimise noise which can 'pull' a woman or birthing person out of their 'birth zone'. A small torch or possibly a head torch and a fob watch with luminescent face can be useful for record keeping in dim lighting.

One fixed element of the environment will be if women and birthing people choose to labour in a birthing pool. This is discussed in detail in chapter *Labour and Birth in Water* but will certainly require the pool to be located somewhere where the floor can support the weight of it when full, that has access to water for filling it up, and that has room for the midwife and partner to manoeuvre around it as required, likely to be downstairs in a living or dining room.

Mobilisation and Positioning

It is now widely accepted that movement in labour can be useful to support birth physiology, shorten labour times, and reduce the need for obstetric interventions (Lawrence et al., 2013a; NICE, 2014). It is also clear that this is more easily facilitated in the home environment as opposed to on an obstetric unit where the bed takes centre stage. The general principle is that midwives should not undermine the woman or birthing person's instinctive movements for fear of pulling them out of the 'zone' by engaging their cognitive brain to listen to excessive instructions and undermining their faith in their body's ability to birth their baby. The woman or birthing person is likely to move freely around the home, using furniture to support themselves during contractions and resting in between contractions if the transition to active birth is lengthy. This is supported by birth physiology as gravity enables descent of the presenting part and application to the cervix. A well-applied presenting part will trigger an efficient positive feedback mechanism as it presses down on the cervix, causing a neuroendocrine reaction to produce the oxytocin needed for further contractions in a continuous rhythmic cycle (Lawrence et al., 2013b). Adopting upright positions including seating, kneeling, and standing has been shown to reduce the duration of labour by up to 90 minutes (Lawrence et al., 2013b). As contractions become more co-ordinated and intense, the woman or birthing person is likely to stay in one place where they feel safe and secure, adjusting position in response to urges within her body. Most of the time, this will not require any intervention from the midwife unless the woman or birthing person becomes distressed or actively seeks support. Simkin and Ancheta (2017) offer a comprehensive guide to the pros and cons of particular positions in labour. The most common reason for a woman or birthing person seeking guidance is when a fetus is in the occipito-posterior (OP) position. It is estimated to impact 25% of labours, with 10% not rotating to occipito-anterior (OA) for delivery (Guittier et al., 2016). It is more common in first-time labours, although once again, most research is based on care in obstetric units which in themselves may aggravate the incidence of this malpresentation by limiting mobility and the use of epidurals. Nevertheless, the rotation to an OA position can be prolonged with significant lower back pain causing maternal anxiety and distress. Simkin and Ancheta (2017) advocate encouraging the woman or birthing person to adopt kneeling, forward leaning, or hands-and-knees (all fours) positions.

Research has been unable to prove a causal link between these positions and rotation of fetus but does suggest that they are acceptable and comfortable for women and birthing people (Guittier et al., 2016) and allow for access to the lower back for massage. It is also important to recognise that with experience, midwives themselves will develop intuitive understanding of the ability of different positions to alleviate discomfort, which, although not yet researched and part of evidence-based practice, less experienced midwives can learn from.

> **Practice Point:**
> It is important when suggesting alternative positions to do so in a manner which does not signal to the woman or birthing person that they are trying to control labour and thereby undermine the labourer's faith in the body's ability to birth their baby. Midwives should also not over-emphasise their potential to influence the duration or intensity of labour in order not to create false expectations.

Food and Drink

The concept of restricting food and drink from labouring women and birthing people originates from obstetric-led practice, which feared the possibility of pulmonary aspiration with a general anaesthetic should an emergency caesarean be required (Fraser & Francis, 2016, p. 84). A 2013 Cochrane review rejected the idea that women and birthing people at low risk of complications should be prevented from eating and drinking according to their appetite and needs. This should now be standard practice in all settings (Singata et al., 2013) and is supported by current NICE guidance (2014), although there is some empirical and anecdotal evidence that the fear of aspiration continues to influence midwifery practice (Tadaumi et al., 2020).

There is limited evidence regarding what women and birthing people actually want to eat and drink in labour, although gastric motility in labour is reduced, meaning women and birthing people are likely to be less hungry and there is evidence that they often choose not to eat in labour, with appetite diminishing further as labour progresses (Fraser & Francis, 2016, p. 91). Food with high levels of fibre and fat aggravates delayed gastric emptying (Howie & Watson, 2017, p. 379), so it may be beneficial to avoid them in favour of fruit, nutritious snacks, and soups.

> **Practice Point:**
> It is helpful to remind women and birthing people of the option to eat and drink and make sure that suitable snacks are bought in advance and readily available to them. This is likely to be more beneficial in the latent phase, particularly if prolonged. Encouraging food and drink beyond their natural appetite and thirst in established labour is likely to increase the risk of vomiting due to the reduced gastric motility and should be discouraged.

Care in Labour and Ongoing Assessment: the Other Basics

Despite the advance in knowledge facilitated by an ever-expanding evidence-based approach to midwifery care, knowledge of birth physiology remains the primary evidence base for the midwife in caring for those at low risk of complications and in that sense, little has changed from the advice given in Myles textbook of 1961:

> Refrain from unnecessary interference... Complications should be prevented where possible, recognized early and dealt with promptly.
>
> —Myles, 1961, p. 260

Whilst the emphasis on early recognition of pathophysiology and deviations from the norm is rightly enshrined in NICE and Trust guidelines, there should be equal focus from the attending midwife on *prevention* of avoidable complications arising in the first place.

Midwifery Presence

The way support is offered can be highly individual based on the personality of the midwife and the needs of the labouring person. One ethnographic study of one-to-one care in labour showed this dynamic interplay in action. Women observed labouring at home in this study took themselves off to another room or the bathroom when they needed privacy (Sosa et al., 2018). Equally, midwives benefitted from 'time out' to eat, drink, and reflect on how best to continue their support by removing themselves briefly to another room. Although the study looked at support from midwives in both birthing centres and at homebirths, there was a consensus that the midwives in all labours were generally successful in knowing when to be physically close and present to offer support and when to withdraw but be close at hand, what the authors term a 'subdued presence'. Borrelli et al. (2016) describe this as the difference between physical presence and 'immediately available presence' or 'peaceful presence' (Sjöblom et al., 2014), whereby, once the initial relationship is established, women and birthing people may alternate between needing to spend time alone or with their partner safe in the knowledge that the midwife is available and will appear intermittently to provide assurance that labour was progressing well. Key to the establishment of this relationship was a mutual trust – from the birthing person in the midwife's skills, knowledge, and experience and from the midwife to the woman and birthing person in trusting them to follow their instincts and their body's ability to labour. As labour progresses from early to established to advanced labour, there is a concomitant move away from the labouring woman or birthing person being sociable and interactive to turning inward and even feeling separate from external stimuli, sometimes described as withdrawing to an 'inner space' (Olza et al., 2018) or 'inner focus' (Olza Id et al., 2020). The need for the midwife to be physically present is likely to increase as the intensity of the labour increases. There is also evidence that quiet but repeated reassurance and confirmation that all was well, what Leap (2010, p. 24) has termed 'midwifery mutterings', is beneficial at this stage and does not require in-depth explanation or reasoning or verbal exchanges, which would disrupt this altered state.

Practice Point:
For the less experienced homebirth midwife whose intrapartum education and/or experience has come from obstetric units, it may take some time to develop this instinct and they would benefit from working in partnership with another homebirth midwife where possible to observe and learn this dynamic.

Summary of Routine Observations in Active First Stage of Labour:
Offer intermittent auscultation of fetal heart using a Pinard or Doppler after a contraction for at least 1 minute, at least every 15 minutes, and record it as a single rate
Record the following observations during the first stage of labour:
Half-hourly documentation of frequency of contractions
Hourly pulse
4-Hourly temperature and blood pressure
Frequency of passing urine
Offer a vaginal examination 4-hourly or if there is concern about progress or in response to the woman's wishes

---

(NICE: National Institute for Health and Care Excellence, 2014)

Working With 'Endogenous Opiates'

Once uterine activity becomes co-ordinated and rhythmic in nature, the cervix dilates. The period of involuntary myometrial activity, lasting up to a minute, has become known as a 'contraction' and is described as painful, resulting from ischaemia in the uterine muscle (Coad & Dunstall, 2012, p. 337). Women and birthing people experience a rise in pain threshold from 30 weeks onwards which increases dramatically in labour originating from placental steroids (McNabb, 2017, p. 565) and the sedative effect of increased melatonin levels. During labour, there is also a concomitant release of 'endogenous opiates', peptides which act to inhibit pain transmission (Coad & Dunstall, 2012, p. 355). Conversely, anticipation of pain can cause fear and anxiety and can lead to a cascade of physiological and neuroendocrinal responses already discussed, contributing to a decrease in uterine contractions, increase in risk of hypoxia to fetus, and feelings of panic and nausea (Howie & Rankin, 2017, p. 402). This is important information to share with women and birthing people in advance so that they can feel reassured of their body's increased ability to tolerate pain.

All analgesia brings risks and benefits and therefore the general principle should be to start with the least invasive approach and gradually increase in line with women and birthing people's wishes and needs. Clearly, methods that support the uninterrupted hormonal cascade are aligned with a homebirth philosophy and complementary therapies and water immersion (see chapter *Labour and Birth in Water*) may be sufficient to ensure adequate comfort and pain relief. Transcutaneous electrical nerve stimulation (TENS) machines are portable, battery-operated devices attached by wires to a series of electrode pads which are placed at key points on the lower back. Like massage, they use the 'gate control theory' to modify pain signals between touch receptors at base of spine and the transfer of signals along myelinated fibres inside the spinal cord to and from the brain (Coad & Dunstall, 2012, p. 354). TENS has been evaluated as safe, effective in relieving pain, and acceptable to users (Thuvarakan et al., 2020) but needs to be started in early labour with a low frequency in order to stimulate endogenous opiates with higher frequencies used as labour progresses to block the pain signals (Howie & Rankin, 2017, p. 404).

Practice Point:
If a woman or birthing person chooses to use a TENS machine, then they will need to have one available prior to the start of labour, have a supply of batteries, and be familiar with how to apply pads and operate it in advance of labour. When midwives are making initial assessments either via telephone, video conference, or a home visit they can encourage the labouring person to apply the TENS machine early on; they will need the assistance of a birth companion to help apply the pads; as this is incompatible with immersion in water, they also need to be reminded to remove them if taking a bath.

Entonox and Exogenous Opioids

Entonox (50% oxygen and 50% nitrous oxide) is usually the first pharmacological analgesic recommended to labouring women and birthing people who request it and can be offered in the home environment. It is self-administered by the labourer via a handheld mouthpiece attached to a portable cannister. The labourer should begin to inhale the gas at the first sign of a contraction; in this way the maximum benefit of the analgesic properties of the gas will coincide with the peak of the contraction (Howie & Rankin, 2017, p. 405). They should breathe slowly and deeply through the mouthpiece until the contraction has faded, as overventilation can cause them to feel dizzy and provoke fetal hypoxia (Jordan, 2010, p. 81). In general, there are no known serious side effects for the physiologically stable or fetus and it can be discontinued immediately with no prolonged unpleasant sensations. It can be used in combination with other drugs or when labouring in water, but the midwife must be present at all times when Entonox is being used.

> **Practice Point:**
> Midwives should ensure cannisters of Entonox are transported, so the length of the cannisters runs parallel with the width of the car to avoid the risk of them being shunted forward at speed and causing maximum damage in case of a traffic accident. It is recommended that cannisters are stored horizontally and above 10°C for at least 24 hours before use, and they should not be left in cars during colder weather to avoid the risk of separation (Jordan, 2010, p. 85).

Pethidine is the strongest analgesic that can be offered at a homebirth. It can be administered intramuscularly, takes up to 20 minutes to act, and lasts up to 4 hours but can cause nausea and drowsiness (Howie & Rankin, 2017, p. 405) and so should not be used when labouring in water. NICE (2014) state that opioids should be available in all settings and an antiemetic should also be administered. The woman or birthing person will need to obtain these themselves via their general practitioner in readiness (Charles, 2018a, p. 129). Pethidine crosses the placenta causing decreased fetal heart rate variability with maximum exposure to the fetus 2–3 hours after administration. A baby born at this time is likely to experience respiratory depression with increased risk of the need for neonatal resuscitation. Birth within 1 hour or after 6 hours of administration greatly reduces this risk (Jordan, 2010, p. 88), but the unpredictability of birth means many midwives are reluctant to offer it for fear of having to manage neonatal resuscitation at home – the expectations of the woman or birthing person need to be considered carefully and sensitively well in advance of labour if there is a possibility that they will be attended in labour by a midwife who feels unable to administer pethidine.

> **Practice Point:**
> If administering pethidine, the midwife should consider calling for a second midwife to join them in case birth progresses more rapidly than anticipated and any resuscitation can be managed appropriately.

Intermittent Auscultation

Intermittent auscultation of the fetal heart is part of the package of 'routine' observations advocated by NICE (2014) once labour is considered established and any complications which might necessitate more continuous monitoring have been excluded. Safe and effective intermittent auscultation is part of a holistic assessment of fetal wellbeing and is comprised of the following:
- Fetal movements should be discussed and documented. If there is a reported decrease in fetal movements as assessed subjectively by the mother or pregnant person, advice by the RCOG is for auscultation via handheld doppler to establish fetal viability followed by admission to hospital for CTG monitoring for a minimum period of 20 minutes (Royal College of Obstetricians and Gynaecologists, 2011) to confirm fetal wellbeing.
- Prior to auscultation, a full abdominal examination should be undertaken to establish fundal height, position, presentation, and engagement of the fetus. This will also help determine the position for auscultation (Johnson & Taylor, 2016, p. 10).
- Either a Doppler or a Pinard can be used – a Pinard allows the midwife to hear the fetal heart directly (Baston, 2020, p. 264) but can be uncomfortable for the midwife and the labourer. A Doppler can allow others to also hear the fetal heart, does not require the labouring person to adopt a semi-recumbent position, and, if waterproof, can be used for labour in water (Read, 2018, p. 62).
- Palpation of the maternal radial pulse enables the midwife to differentiate it from the fetal heart; auscultation should last for 1 minute immediately after a contraction for 1 minute and the average heart rate recorded, not the range (NICE, 2014).
- If a deceleration is heard or the fetal heart rate is either below 110 bpm or above 160 bpm, then these are indications for transfer for continuous monitoring (NICE, 2014).
- Auscultation should be conducted every 15 minutes in the first stage of established labour.

BIRTH COMPANIONS

Perhaps one of the unique benefits for many women and birthing people is that freed from the visiting restrictions of hospitals, they can choose to surround themselves – or not – with trusted companions, doulas, in-laws, pets, and/or their children. For the confident homebirth midwife, being part of this community can be one of the joys of the job. They can take some of their cues for how to be around the woman or birthing person from them as most people choose a birthing partner that has 'knowledge and an emotional connection with a woman that a midwife would not be able to develop within their short relationship' (Sosa et al., 2018). For many – but not all – this will be their partner. A meta-ethnography of male partners indicates that men would like to be acknowledged as a valuable presence and a wish to be actively involved in providing support as well as advocating for the needs of their partner (Johansson et al., 2015). Keeping partners updated may be valued as well as providing more directive suggestions if appropriate as to how partners can provide physical support such as back massage, adopting positions which allow them to be physically close and supportive to partners. Whereas birthing women and people have made conscious decisions to birth at home and therefore have invited midwives to attend to support and facilitate their needs, studies have shown that men look to healthcare professionals for permission' to not only be present in the birth space, but own it (Johansson et al., 2015). This needs to be achieved by empowering birth supporters without adopting paternalistic/maternalistic tones which can be infantilising and impose the midwife as 'in charge' – collaboration and partnership is key.

There are a few practical considerations which should be negotiated in advance. Some people choose to birth at home to avoid being separated from their other children so that these children can learn about birth and bond with their sibling (Sjöblom et al., 2006; Jouhki et al., 2017). Nevertheless, there will need to be another adult in the home who can care for these siblings if the mother or person does not want them around at points in labour, if the children become bored or distressed, and most obviously, if there is a need to move from home to hospital at any point.

> **Practice Point:**
> There is little research on pets at homebirths and a lot will depend on the individual circumstances. It is sensible for parents to be advised that they need to set up a safe space for their dog(s) to retreat to – behind a stair gate or in a separate room – if they become overstimulated or feel anxious. Certainly, this will be beneficial in general, as babies should never be left unattended in the presence of a dog. Midwives who are allergic to pets should have antihistamines at hand and it is reasonable to ask a birth companion to put pets in a separate room if they are going to aggravate allergic reactions.

One final point, midwives should be mindful of who is present and what their relationship is to the woman or birthing person with an understanding of whether their presence is wanted or needed by them. This is particularly important when attending a homebirth for someone who is not previously known to the homebirth or caseloading team or who has recently moved from out of area. Developing a 'professional curiosity' (Burton & Revell, 2018) for such situations is an important skill to develop to help identify women and birthing people who are vulnerable or may be at risk. Midwives should record the names and relationships of those present within the birth records and if there are concerns follow up as soon as possible with enquiries to a multi-agency safeguarding hub or specialised safeguarding midwives to discuss any concerns.

SELF-CARE

Midwifery is arguably the only health or professional service which expects its members, almost exclusively female, to enter an unfamiliar environment at any hour of the night or day on their own to potentially meet strangers for the first time. Therefore, it is important for midwives to familiarise themselves with and follow lone worker policies where they exist. Where someone is in labour and not previously known to maternity services – and therefore no prior assessment has been able to take place – it would be reasonable to consider attending in pairs rather than alone. Either way, it is important for the midwife attending to ensure that a colleague knows of their whereabouts and to phone to check in with them at pre-agreed intervals. Employers have a duty to provide a safe workplace which, for community workers, can include training in de-escalation techniques or provision of lone-worker devices, so it's important for midwives to keep up to date with technology and training provided (Royal College of Midwives, 2018). Regardless of the instinct to provide care to vulnerable women and birthing people, midwives must safeguard themselves first.

> **Practice Point:**
> If the environment is unfamiliar and a midwife feels threatened by individuals, they should ensure they have a clear exit route, don't go upstairs, and make an excuse to go to the car to get further equipment where they can safely summon further help.

Food and drink is not just an important consideration for the person in labour – the midwife and any other birth supporters will need to stay alert and able to function over a prolonged period of time and will often be working antisocial hours and unable to take meals at normal times. This can lead to increased weight gain and caffeine consumption, which in turn can lead to ongoing sleep disturbance (Peplonska et al., 2015; Centofanti et al., 2018). Caffeinated drinks should be drunk moderately and avoided towards the end of a shift. Midwives should also have a selection of healthy food and snacks available for when on call. There is evidence that half of the midwives feel dehydrated most of the time when working and delay emptying their bladder, which can impair decision making and cause low mood along with increasing risks to physical wellbeing (Royal College of Midwives, 2021). The general rule should be to drink to thirst, up to around 2 L of fluid per day, to avoid symptoms of dehydration.

In an era where social media is an important way of sharing news and experiences, midwives are increasingly having to recognise that they may be filmed as part of their work for sharing on the internet by parents. The NMC (2018) have published social media guidance but this primarily relates to registrants managing their own social media profiles rather than being included in other people's content. There is little practical guidance on this matter, but midwives do have a right to privacy and any recording of midwives or birth workers must be with consent (Caddell & Game, 2022). If this is of concern to any member of the midwifery team, this should be discussed in advance with the woman or birthing person. It should be documented within antenatal and birth records what has been agreed to avoid any ill feeling at the time of labour and birth when emotions are heightened.

Finally, if midwives do find themselves tiring, it can certainly be beneficial and reasonable to call the second midwife sooner rather than later. A fresh perspective can provide reassurance and confidence to carry on (Bedwell et al., 2015), something which midwives are likely to do repeatedly in a birth centre or labour ward but are not readily available to the homebirth midwife. What must be negotiated is who is the lead carer in this situation so that the labouring woman or birthing person knows whom to listen to and respond to.

CONCLUSION

The first point of contact with the woman or birthing person in labour is crucial in determining the quality of the birth experience and how the labour will progress. Awareness of how women and birthing people feel and behave is key to the midwife being able to identify how best to support birth physiology and work with neuroendocrine activity (Olza et al., 2020) rather than solely relying on seemingly objective markers such as cervical dilatation and frequency of contractions to identify progress in labour and meet the needs of the birthing woman or person. Similarly, whilst carrying out the schedule of routine observations, it is important, equal emphasis should be placed on the psychosocial elements of caring for someone in labour as well as being mindful of facilitating involvement of the wider network of birth supporters and family who may be present at a homebirth. All of this can present unique rewards but also challenges for the homebirth midwife. Self-care, often neglected in midwifery, needs to be equally prioritised so that 'partnership' working (International Confederation of Midwives, 2014) with those in the care can be fostered for safe and effective practice and birth outcomes.

REFERENCES

Bailey, C. M., Newton, J. M., & Hall, H. G. (2019). Telephone triage in midwifery practice: A cross-sectional survey. *International Journal of Nursing Studies, 91*, 110–118. https://doi.org/10.1016/J.IJNURSTU.2018.11.009

Baston, H. (2020). Antenatal care. In J. Marshall & M. Raynor (Eds.), *Myles textbook for midwives* (17th ed., pp. 246–274). Elsevier.

Bedwell, C., McGowan, L., & Lavender, T. (2015). Factors affecting midwives' confidence in intrapartum care: A phenomenological study. *Midwifery, 31*, 170–176. https://reader.elsevier.com/reader/sd/pii/S0266613814002046?token=D48454E4AA7B01FC2ED84DE7D-323B8659775CE05B0077AE81DAD4A7B71BB78931B1DE08E5A74C6F6E98FDBDD00298AF3&originRegion=eu-west-1&originCreation=20220215103551

Borrelli, S. E., Spiby, H., & Walsh, D. (2016). The kaleidoscopic midwife: A conceptual metaphor illustrating first-time mothers' perspectives of a good midwife during childbirth. A grounded theory study. *Midwifery, 39*, 103–111. https://doi.org/10.1016/j.midw.2016.05.008

Buchmann, E. J., & Libhaber, E. (2007). Accuracy of cervical assessment in the active phase of labour. *BJOG: An International Journal of Obstetrics & Gynaecology, 114*(7), 833–837. https://doi.org/10.1111/J.1471-0528.2007.01386.X

Burton, V., & Revell, L. (2018). Professional curiosity in child protection: Thinking the unthinkable in a neo-liberal world. *The British Journal of Social Work, 48*(6), 1508–1523. https://doi.org/10.1093/BJSW/BCX123

Caddell, M., & Game, E. (2022). Socially acceptable. *Midwives*, Vol. 25, 36–37.

Centofanti, S., Banks, S., Colella, A., Dingle, C., Devine, L., Galindo, H., Pantelios, S., Brkic, G., & Dorrian, J. (2018). Coping with shift work-related circadian disruption: A mixed-methods case study on napping and caffeine use in Australian nurses and midwives. *Chronobiology International, 35*(6), 853–864. https://doi.org/10.1080/07420528.2018.1466798

Charles, C. (2018a). Homebirth. In V. Chapman & C. Charles (Eds.), *The midwife's labour and birth handbook* (4th ed., pp. 123–154). Wiley Blackwell.

Charles, C. (2018b). Labour and normal birth. In V. Chapman & C. Charles (Eds.), *The midwife's labour and birth handbook* (Vol. 4, pp. 1–48). Wiley-Blackwell.

Christopher, U., Goldy, S. J., Oral, B. J., & Rose, A. C. (2019). Multiple vaginal examinations and early neonatal sepsis. *International Journal of Reproduction, Contraception, Obstetrics and Gynecology, 8*(3), 876–882. https://doi.org/10.18203/2320-1770.IJRCOG20190848

Coad, J., & Dunstall, M. (2012). *Anatomy and physiology for midwives* (3rd ed.). Churchill Livingstone Elsevier.

Eri, T. S., Bondas, T., Gross, M. M., Janssen, P., & Green, J. M. (2015). A balancing act in an unknown territory: A metasynthesis of first-time mothers' experiences in early labour. *Midwifery, 31*(3), e58–e67. https://doi.org/10.1016/J.MIDW.2014.11.007

Faucher, M. A., & Kennedy, H. P. (2020). Women's perceptions on the use of video technology in early labor: Being able to see. *Journal of Midwifery & Women's Health, 65*(3), 342–348. https://doi.org/10.1111/JMWH.13091

Fraser, D., & Francis, J. (2016). Nutrition and hydration in labour. In S. Arulkumaran (Ed.), *Best practice in labour and delivery* (pp. 84–92). Cambridge University Press. https://doi.org/10.1017/9781316144961.009

Gluck, O., Ganer Herman, H., Tal, O., Grinstein, E., Bar, J., Kovo, M., Ginath, S., & Weiner, E. (2020). The association between the number of vaginal examinations during labor and perineal trauma: A retrospective cohort study. *Archives of Gynecology and Obstetrics, 301*(6), 1405–1410. https://doi.org/10.1007/S00404-020-05552-Z/TABLES/4

Guittier, M. J., Girard, V. O., de Gasquet, B., Irion, O., & Boulvain, M. (2016). Maternal positioning to correct occiput posterior fetal position during the first stage of labour: A randomised controlled trial. *BJOG: An International Journal of Obstetrics and Gynaecology, 123*(13), 2199–2207. https://doi.org/10.1111/1471-0528.13855

Howie, L., & Rankin, J. (2017). Pain relief in labour. In J. Rankin (Ed.), *Physiology in childbearing with anatomy and related biosciences* (pp. 399–410). Elsevier.

Howie, L., & Watson, J. (2017). The onset of labour. In J. Rankin (Ed.), *Physiology in childbearing with anatomy and related biosciences* (4th ed., pp. 373–380). Elsevier.

International Confederation of Midwives. (2014). *Core document philosophy and model of midwifery care.* www.internationalmidwives.org

Iobst, S. E., Breman, R. B., Bingham, D., Storr, C. L., Zhu, S., & Johantgen, M. (2019). Associations among cervical dilatation at admission, intrapartum care, and birth mode in low-risk, nulliparous women. *Birth, 46*(2), 253–261. https://doi.org/10.1111/BIRT.12417

Jackson, K., Anderson, M., & Marshall, J. E. (2020). Physiology and care during the first stage of labour. In J. Marshall & M. Raynor (Eds.), *Myles textbook for midwives* (17th ed., pp. 447–499). Elsevier.

Janssen, P. A., & Desmarais, S. L. (2013). Women's experience with early labour management at home vs. in hospital: A randomised controlled trial. *Midwifery, 29*(3), 190–194. https://doi.org/10.1016/J.MIDW.2012.05.011

Janssen, P., Nolan, M. L., Spiby, H., Green, J., Gross, M. M., Cheyne, H., Hundley, V., Rijnders, M., de Jonge, A., & Buitendijk, S. (2009). Roundtable discussion: Early labor: What's the problem? *Birth, 36*(4), 332–339. https://doi.org/10.1111/J.1523-536X.2009.00361.X

Johansson, M., Fenwick, J., & Premberg, Å. (2015). A meta-synthesis of fathers' experiences of their partner's labour and the birth of their baby. *Midwifery, 31*(1), 9–18. https://doi.org/10.1016/j.midw.2014.05.005

Johnson, R., & Taylor, W. (2016). *Skills for midwifery practice* (4th ed.). Elsevier.

Jordan, S. (2010). *Pharmacology for midwives: The evidence base for safe practice* (2nd ed.). Palgrave Macmillan.

Jouhki, M. R., Suominen, T., & Åstedt-Kurki, P. (2017). Giving birth on our own terms – Women's experience of childbirth at home. *Midwifery, 53*, 35–41. https://doi.org/10.1016/J.MIDW.2017.07.008

Lawrence, A., Lewis, L., Hofmeyr, G. J., & Styles, C. (2013a). Maternal positions and mobility during first stage labour. *Cochrane Database of Systematic Reviews, 2013*(10). https://doi.org/10.1002/14651858.CD003934.PUB4/INFORMATION/EN

Lawrence, A., Lewis, L., Hofmeyr, G. J., & Styles, C. (2013b). Maternal positions and mobility during first stage labour. *Cochrane Database of Systematic Reviews, 2013*(10). https://doi.org/10.1002/14651858.CD003934.PUB4/MEDIA/CDSR/CD003934/IMAGE_N/NCD003934-CMP-001-17.PNG

Leap, N. (2010). The less we do, the more we give. In M. Kirkham (Ed.), *The midwife-mother relationship* (2nd ed., pp. 17–37). Palgrave Macmillan.

Lewin, D., Fearon, B., Hemmings, V., & Johnson, G. (2005). Women's experiences of vaginal examinations in labour. *Midwifery, 21*(3), 267–277. https://doi.org/10.1016/J.MIDW.2004.10.003

McNabb, M. (2017). Physiological changes from late pregnancy until the onset of labour. In S. Macdonald & G. Johnson (Eds.), *Mayes' midwifery* (15th ed., pp. 562–585). Elsevier.

Myhre, E. L., Lukasse, M., Reigstad, M. M., Holmstedt, V., & Dahl, B. (2021). A qualitative study of Norwegian first-time mothers' information needs in pre-admission early labour. *Midwifery, 100*, 103016. https://doi.org/10.1016/J.MIDW.2021.103016

Myles, M. (1961). *A textbook for midwives* (4th ed.). E & S Livingstone Ltd.

NICE: National Institute for Health and Care Excellence. (2014). *Intrapartum care for healthy women and babies: Clinical guideline 190.* www.nice.org.uk/guidance/cg190

Nizard, J., Haberman, S., Paltieli, Y., Gonen, R., Ohel, G., Nicholson, D., & Ville, Y. (2009). How reliable is the determination of cervical dilation? Comparison of vaginal examination with spatial position-tracking ruler. *American Journal of Obstetrics and Gynecology, 200*(4), 402.e1-402.e4. https://doi.org/10.1016/J.AJOG.2009.01.002

Nursing & Midwifery Council. (2018). *Guidance on using social media responsibly.*

Nursing & Midwifery Council. (2019). *Standards of proficiency for midwives.* www.nmc.org.ukStandardsofproficiencyformidwives1

Nursing and Midwifery Council. (2018). *The Code: Professional standards of practice and behaviour for nurses, midwives and nursing associates.* https://doi.org/10.1111/1471-0528.14930

Oladapo, O. T., Diaz, V., Bonet, M., Abalos, E., Thwin, S. S., Souza, H., Perdon, G., Souza, J. P., & Ulmezoglu, A. M. (2017). Cervical dilatation patterns of 'low-risk' women with spontaneous labour and normal perinatal outcomes: A systematic review. *BJOG.* https://doi.org/10.1111/1471-0528.14929

Olza, I., Leahy-Warren, P., Benyamini, Y., Kazmierczak, M., Karlsdottir, S. I., Spyridou, A., Crespo-Mirasol, E., Takács, L., Hall, P. J., Murphy, M., Jonsdottir, S. S., Downe, S., & Nieuwenhuijze, M. J. (2018). Women's psychological experiences of physiological childbirth: A meta-synthesis. *BMJ Open, 8*, 20347. https://doi.org/10.1136/bmjopen-2017-020347

Olza, I., Uvnas-Moberg, K., Ekström-Bergström, A., Leahy-Warren, P., Karlsdottir, S. I., Nieuwenhuijze, M., Villarmea, S., Hadjigeorgiou, E., Kazmierczak, M., Spyridou, A., & Buckley, S. (2020). Birth as a neuro-psycho-social event: An integrative model of maternal experiences and their relation to neurohormonal events during childbirth. *PLoS ONE, 15*(7 July). https://doi.org/10.1371/JOURNAL.PONE.0230992

Olza Id, I., Uvnas-Moberg, K., Ekströ M-Bergströ, A., Leahy-Warren, P., Karlsdottir, I., Nieuwenhuijze, M., Villarmea Id, S., Hadjigeorgiou, E., Kazmierczak, M., Spyridou, A., & Buckley Id, S. (2020). *Birth as a neuro-psycho-social event: An integrative model of maternal experiences and their relation to neurohormonal events during childbirth.* https://doi.org/10.1371/journal.pone.0230992

Pendleton, J. (2019). What role does gender have in shaping knowledge that underpins the practice of midwifery? *Journal of Gender Studies, 28*(6). https://doi.org/10.1080/09589236.2019.1590185

Peplonska, B., Bukowska, A., & Sobala, W. (2015). Association of rotating night shift work with BMI and abdominal obesity among nurses and midwives. *PLoS One, 10*(7). https://doi.org/10.1371/JOURNAL.PONE.0133761

Read, B. (2018). Fetal heart rate monitoring in labour. In V. Chapman & C. Charles (Eds.), *The midwife's labour and birth handbook* (4th ed., pp. 61–74). Wiley Blackwell.

Reed, R. (2021). *Reclaiming childbirth as a rite of passage.* Word Witch Press.

Royal College of Midwives. (2018). *RCM employment relations publication: Lone worker guidance.* www.rcm.org.uk

Royal College of Midwives. (2021). *Hydration – Know your rights and responsibilities in the workplace.*

Royal College of Obstetricians and Gynaecologists. (2011). *Reduced Fetal Movements Green-top Guideline No. 57.*

Scamell, M., & Alaszewski, A. (2012). Fateful moments and the categorisation of risk: Midwifery practice and the ever-narrowing window of normality during childbirth. *Health, Risk & Society, 14*(2), 207–221. https://doi.org/10.1080/13698575.2012.661041

Simkin, P., & Ancheta, R. (2017). The labor progress toolkit part 1: Positions and movements. In *The labor progress handbook: Early interventions to prevent and treat dystocia* (4th ed., pp. 277–326). Wiley Blackwell.

Singata, M., Tranmer, J., & Gyte, G. M. L. (2013). Restricting oral fluid and food intake during labour. *The Cochrane Database of Systematic Reviews, 2013*(8). https://doi.org/10.1002/14651858.CD003930.PUB3

Sjöblom, I., Idvall, E., Lindgren, H., Blix, E., Kjaergaard, H., Olofsdottir, O. A., Hildingsson, I., Thies-Lagergren, L., Radestad, I., & Lundgren, I. (2014). Creating a safe haven – Women's experiences of the midwife's professional skills during planned homebirth in four Nordic countries. *Birth, 41*(1), 100–107. https://doi.org/10.1111/BIRT.12092

Sjöblom, I., Nordström, B., & Edberg, A. K. (2006). A qualitative study of women's experiences of homebirth in Sweden. *Midwifery, 22*(4), 348–355. https://doi.org/10.1016/J.MIDW.2005.11.004

Sosa, G. A., Crozier, K. E., & Stockl, A. (2018). Midwifery one-to-one support in labour: More than a ratio. *Midwifery, 62*, 230–239. https://doi.org/10.1016/J.MIDW.2018.04.016

Spiby, H., Faucher, M. A., Sands, G., Roberts, J., & Kennedy, H. P. (2019). A qualitative study of midwives' perceptions on using video-calling in early labor. *Birth, 46*(1), 105–112. https://doi.org/10.1111/BIRT.12364

Spiby, H., Walsh, D., Green, J., Crompton, A., & Bugg, G. (2014). Midwives' beliefs and concerns about telephone conversations with women in early labour. *Midwifery, 30*(9), 1036–1042. https://doi.org/10.1016/J.MIDW.2013.10.025

Tadaumi, M., Sweet, L., & Graham, K. (2020). A qualitative study of factors that influence midwives' practice in relation to low-risk women's oral intake in labour in Australia. *Women and Birth, 33*(5), e455–e463. https://doi.org/10.1016/J.WOMBI.2019.11.004

Thuvarakan, K., Zimmermann, H., Mikkelsen, M. K., & Gazerani, P. (2020). Transcutaneous electrical nerve stimulation as a pain-relieving approach in labor pain: A systematic review and meta-analysis of randomized controlled trials. *Neuromodulation, 23*(6), 732–746. https://doi.org/10.1111/NER.13221

Walsh, D. (2012). *Evidence and skills for normal labour and birth: A guide for midwives* (2nd ed.). Routledge.

Walsh, D. (2017). Care in the first stage of labour. In S. Macdonald & G. Johnson (Eds.), *Mayes' midwifery* (17th ed., pp. 586–613). Elsevier.

World Health Organization. (2018). *Intrapartum care for a positive childbirth experience WHO recommendations.* http://apps.who.int/bookorders.

SECOND AND THIRD STAGES OF LABOUR AT HOME

Becky Louise Westbury

CHAPTER 6

INTRODUCTION

The aim of this chapter is to provide discussion points and guidance in relation to the second and third stage of labour at home. Defined as the period between signs of full dilatation, the baby being visible, or expulsive surges and the birth of the baby (NICE, 2022b), the second stage of labour is physiologically the same during home birth, however subtle care differences may be noticed. Similar can be said for the third stage of labour (the time from the baby's birth to the birth of the placenta and membranes (NICE, 2022b). This chapter will explore the considerations, differences, and additional opportunities of providing care during the second and third stages of labour at home, whilst drawing on the authors own experiences and observations as well as those of midwives who regularly support home birth (Images 1 and 2).

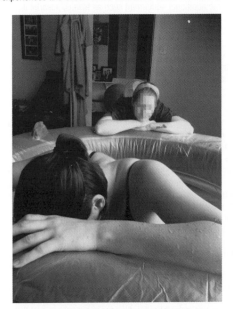

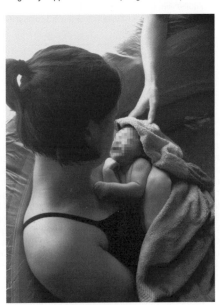

Image 1 Community midwife Lisa supports a woman for whom she is named midwife to have a VBAC in the pool at home

Image 2 Baby Idris is born

PRACTICAL AND EQUIPMENT CONSIDERATIONS

One of the subtle differences between home and hospital birth which must be addressed first and foremost, and which all clinicians must respect, is the power shift between care giver and care receiver. We are guests at a home birth, entering the family's home, their space where they live and love. Always be mindful that we are guests. It is a true privilege to support a birthing woman or person in their own home, as they are often more instinctive and less inhibited than in hospital/midwife-led units.

> **Practice Point:**
> Enter the home quietly and unobtrusively, so as not to disrupt a woman or birthing person's oxytocin, or the nest they have created. Be guided by what you see; if there is a pile of footwear by the front door, then take your shoes off.

The practicalities of home birth equipment differ across health boards and trusts in the UK (see chapter *Planning for Home birth*). In some areas each community midwife carries a full home birth kit including Entonox, some areas have a home birth vehicle that is used by the on-call midwife, and some areas deliver equipment to the homes of women and birthing people when they plan their home birth. Nevertheless, for any home birth there will be a require-ment for the midwives to bring equipment into the home. This equipment will need to be easily accessible and ideally close to where birth is anticipated to take place, although it's not unheard of to have to relocate all of your kit in a hurry because the woman or birthing person is all of sudden pushing somewhere else, such as on the toilet! A widely adopted safety practice amongst midwives attending home births is to set up a neonatal resuscitation area once they have ascertained that established birth is underway; this is recommended by the Resuscitation Council UK to be on a 'designated elevated surface' (2021). This ensures that should an emergency occur it can be responded to swiftly, and by selecting an elevated location, any resuscitation can be undertaken without discomfort. This may be a coffee table, dining room table, kitchen worktop, or dressing table. Such a station can be set up on the floor but be careful not to tread on equipment.

Practice Point:
When selecting a location for the resuscitation, consider ensuring that it remains outside the eye line of the labouring woman so as not to distract from labour. You may wish to cover the station with a towel or a muslin to achieve the same aim whilst allowing it to remain accessible at all times.

Additionally, families may have been asked to provide some additional equipment such as towels, absorbent pads, shower curtains, or tarpaulins to protect sofas and floors, and a placenta/vomit/urine bucket etc.

Practice Point:
Familiarise yourself well with your kit prior to supporting a home birth. Have emergency equipment to hand, a neonatal resuscitation station ready, and baby scales out to weigh blood loss.

One of the things that simultaneously many midwives enjoy and challenge them about home birth is that each birth is in a very different setting and environment. This encourages and requires midwives to think on their feet and remain dynamic and effective problem solvers when supporting and suggesting different birth positions and where to locate equipment; indeed, this also can create challenges when planning for transfer in the event of an emergency or otherwise. Continuity of care and carer is widely recognised as having numerous benefits for women and birthing people (Sandall et al, 2016). For those planning a home birth, it is vital for enabling adequate support with decision making and planning for home birth. In a hospital or birth centre setting equipment and kit are in a uniform environment, and all midwives will know exactly where to find things. In the home setting, how-ever, this will vary. Remaining mobile can be supported by easy access to stairs to climb, kitchen worktops to sway against, dining chairs to straddle, banisters to support squats, sofas to kneel on, and so much more that probably would not be possible in many hospital settings. Additionally, there can be access to outdoor spaces such as gardens and balconies, which is often not the case in hospital. Women and birthing people at home are not restricted in where they labour and birth; therefore midwives should be prepared to facilitate in any number of locations in and around the birthing parents' home.

Practice Point:
Be creative when suggesting positions and mobility at home, and make the most of the space and environment that is available whilst considering the 'what ifs' – what if there is an emergency in a tight space such as a toilet? How will we manage that situation?

WHO WILL ATTEND?

When supporting home birth, a significant practical consideration is thinking about who within the care team should attend the birth (also see chapter *Antenatal Planning*). The benefits of continuity of care/carer are widely recognised (Sandall et al., 2016); therefore every effort should be made for the named midwife to attend. If this is not possible due to annual leave, days off, team sickness, and nights and weekends when on-call cover is utilised, are there any known midwives available? Within the author's team and in other teams providing homebirth services, we make an effort to ensure that a family planning a home birth has had the opportunity to meet all members of the team, and we share all our photos during home birth promotion events (with consent and prior agreement to ensure that at least our faces are recognised in the area). When to call a second midwife is also a key consideration. In most areas the second midwife or birth attendant (some areas use healthcare support workers) is usually called as the second stage approaches; however, a number of factors can influence this such as the progress of the birth, whether the woman or birthing person is birthing outside of guidelines, the support that the family need, the experience of both midwives, and the geography of the area to name but a few. The midwives supporting the birth will also be required to keep in touch regularly with the local unit, for both lone working and unit activity planning purposes. This should be reflected in local guidelines and standard operating procedures and feature in planning discussions with women and their families.

> **Practice Point:**
> Facilitate named or known midwives to attend home births wherever possible. Where appropriate, consider communicating with colleagues via confidential text message, providing the midwife coordinating the unit is in agreement and appropriate data protection and standard operating procedures allow. This might be less disruptive to the birthing space.

Continued periodic and dynamic risk assessment is a vital part of the care we provide as midwives, and this is no different when supporting a home birth. Depending on the local arrangements and guidelines, a risk assessment should take place for planned home birth no later than 36 weeks, whereby midwifery or obstetric-led care can be assessed and advice and recommendations for birth made. If obstetric-led care is planned, those birthing at home may be doing so outside of guidelines, requiring additional plans (see chapters *Antenatal Planning* and *Home Birth in the Presence of Complex Needs*). Risk assessment is undertaken continually whilst providing care at home. Guidelines and documents for supporting normal birth make it very easy to spot many deviations from normal, which supports midwives to think about whether they are in the safest place to provide ongoing care (Images 3 and 4).

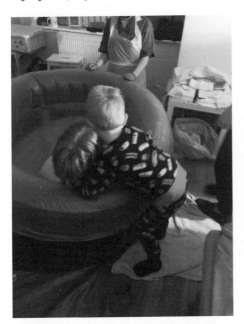

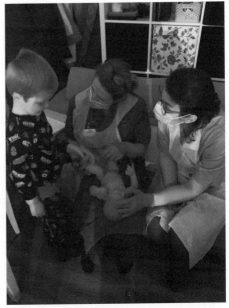

Image 3 Gabriel comes in just after his mum has given birth

Image 4 Gabriel meets his baby brother Isaac as he is checked by midwife Rhiannon and student midwife Izzy

THE SECOND STAGE OF LABOUR

The second stage of labour can be assumed when the cervix is found to be fully dilated, the baby is visible, or expulsive surges are present (NICE, 2017). It is recommended to offer a vaginal examination hourly during the active second stage of labour (NICE, 2017).

> **Practice Point:**
> When this stage of labour commences, the second midwife or birth attendant should be called if not already done so.

- Hourly blood pressure.
- Four hourly temperature.
- Half hourly documentation of frequency of surges.
- Intermittent auscultation of the fetal heart for at least 60 seconds immediately following a surge, at least every 5 minutes.
- Maternal pulse every 15 minutes, palpated during auscultation to differentiate between the two heartbeats.
- Offer vaginal examination hourly in the active second stage.

Fig. 6.1 Recommended observations in second stage of labour (NICE 2022b).

Practice Point:
Consider adjusting the temperature of the room and/or the birth pool at this stage (see chapter *Labour and Birth in Water*), and equipment may need moving to be close to hand; many women and birthing people find themselves birthing in a smaller space than originally intended, often the bathroom. Carpets, rugs, beds, and sofas should be covered with shower curtains, waterproof sheets, absorbent pads, towels etc. Observations including auscultation of the fetal heart should be increased in frequency in line with NICE (2022b) guidelines (Fig. 6.1). Continual risk assessment persists, to ensure that there are no deviations from normal.

As discussed, subtle differences may be observed between women and birthing people experiencing a second stage in hospital vs at home. Many midwives will report seeing far more 'text book' births at home when compared to a hospital setting. This is thought to be because women and birthing people are in their own environment, thus more calm, relaxed, and uninhibited, meaning that they experienced increased oxytocin which can lead to a quicker, more 'textbook' birth. This of course is a generalising statement, and by no means is this the case for every birth.

FEAR, TENSION, PAIN

It is thought that the 'fear tension pain' cycle, first discussed by Dick-Read in 1942 (Dick-Read, 2013), is seen less frequently at home. This could be for many reasons: a familiar environment, feeling more comfortable and relaxed, having more birth partners present than a hospital environment would permit, or feeling more in control. During this cycle, increased fear, for a variety of reasons, leads to an increase in muscle tension and activates the sympathetic nervous system's 'fight' response. This leads to an increased surge of adrenaline, as well as reducing the blood flow to the uterus, inhibiting the release of endorphins, the body's natural pain-relieving hormones. Furthermore, there is a decrease in the release of oxytocin, which can suppress surges and birth progress. An increased level of pain follows these changes, which creates increased fear, continuing this perpetuating cycle.

In contrast, the hormonal cycle commonly seen whilst supporting birth at home is that of the 3Cs. Calmness, confidence, and control suppress the release of adrenaline and ensure oxytocin is plentiful, resulting in more blood flow to the uterus and relaxed muscle fibres. This promotes comfort and enhances feelings of calm, confidence, and control. Many birth preparation classes will refer to this cycle, and methods such as hypnobirthing can aid in reducing fear of birth during the antenatal period.

Practice Point:
Reducing fear in labour by promoting a calm, relaxed, familiar birthing space with minimal disturbances, such as a home birth environment, can help to keep the fear tension pain cycle at bay.

MONITORING MATERNAL WELLBEING AND PROGRESS

Many families planning a home birth may be seeking a more 'hands-off' experience, and midwives skilled in supporting home birth are often highly experienced in supporting physiological birth for those with minimal complicating factors. As such, numerous techniques and observations can be used to determine both onset of the second stage of labour and progress to birth. Vaginal examinations are commonly used to 'diagnose' the onset of the second stage in both hospital and home setting, with NICE guidelines (2022b) recommending this. Many women and birthing people in a home setting decline vaginal examinations; therefore the skill of the midwife in observing and interpreting instinctive uninhibited behaviours displayed by women is fundamental in assessing the progress of labour in the absence of such intimate examinations (Images 5, 6 and 7).

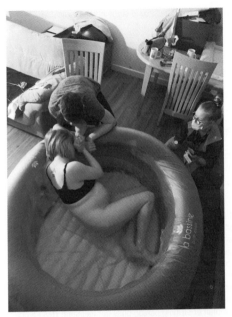

Image 5 Community midwife Lisa in labour at home, supported by her partner Graham, and midwife Hannah P

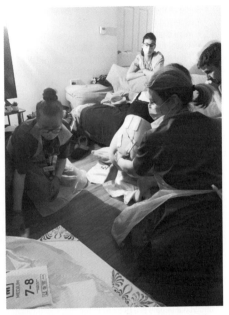

Image 6 Community midwife Lisa and her birth team, using the comfort of the sofa, and the tens machine for a break from the pool

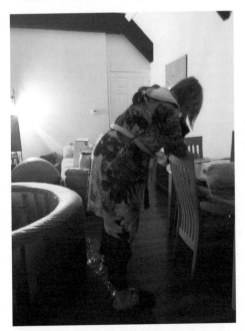

Image 7 Community midwife Lisa in early labour, utilising the table and chairs for support

Practice Point:
Vaginal examinations provide an indication of progress at the exact moment the examination is performed, and things can advance very rapidly at home births; it is important to be able to interpret other signs and indicators for this very reason. Vaginal examinations are also subjective.

Some of the commonly observed visual and behavioural indicators of the second stage of labour include:

- Opening the bowels
- Anal dilatation
- Vulval fullness or vaginal 'gaping'
- Spontaneous rupture of membranes (SROM)
- Change in maternal behaviours and sounds, such as grunting, a 'moo'-like sound, appearing and sounding to be bearing down
- Purple line in the cleft of the buttocks (Shepherd et al., 2010)
- Legs cold up to knee
- Involuntary pushing
- Requests for comfort measures, or expressing feelings of doubt/requesting analgesia/epidural
- Vomiting
- Vaginal show, which can appear as mucous-type discharge often stained with old blood
- Rhombus of Michaelis moving backwards and becoming visibly prominent (Sutton, 2000)
- Rising onto tip toes with surges
- A change in smell of the birth environment
- Presenting part visible

The use of these signs to detect the commencement of the second stage of labour very much adopts the 'watchful attendance' theory (De Jonge, Dahlen, & Downe, 2021), whereby midwives are observers and protectors of normal, physiological birth. Another way of describing this is 'being with' rather than 'doing to'. This fits with the fact that midwives are guests in the family's home, and in the absence of clinical concerns watchful attendance is often the most appropriate approach to providing care during a home birth.

Additionally, we must also consider the possibility of cervical recoil. As stated, vaginal examinations only indicate dilatation at the time of the examination, and it is widely recognised that dilatation can regress, or recoil (Wickham, 2014). This is thought to occur when women and birthing people feel interrupted or disturbed in the flow of their birth, or additional people are present in the room with whom the woman or birthing person does not feel safe. This theory likens us to the rest of the mammalian species, as we know that animals can halt the birthing process when predators are near, and until they can seek out a private, safe, dark birthing space. Other indicators of maternal wellbeing and progress are maternal sound and behaviours.

Practice Point:

Sounds and behaviours may change with the onset of the second stage of labour. Women and birthing people may require additional emotional support during this time, and midwives and birth attendants can aid in protecting the birth space. This can include fostering and facilitating a calm atmosphere. Often families have considered one type of music for their birth experience; however, a change that they have not prepared for may be desired. Knowing the names of a few different playlists can be invaluable for families who need a change of pace and atmosphere and has served many home birth midwives well. Consideration of comfort measures is also an important factor when discussing progress in the second stage of labour.

EXPULSIVE PHASE

When providing care at a home birth, unless there are clinical indicators otherwise, we can assume that there are minimal reasons why active pushing is necessary and therefore is rarely observed in a home setting. Some women and birthing people will actively push as this is instinctive to them, and this instinct should be gently encouraged. Coached pushing, or Valsalva pushing, can adversely affect urodynamic factors during the postnatal period (Prins et al., 2011) and therefore it is best avoided in the absence of complications or concerns. Alternative techniques such as coached active pushing may, however, be appropriate in situations such as a prolonged second stage or presence of other concerns, as it is proven to reduce the length of the second stage (Prins et al., 2011), and always accompanied by a clear plan for transfer to hospital.

Practice Point:

Women and birthing people should be encouraged to listen to their body during the second stage of labour, and involuntary pushing will often be observed. Those who have used hypnobirthing may adopt the practice of 'down breathing' (Graves, 2012), sometimes also referred to as 'J breathing', to gently breathe their baby down, visualising this as they exhale. Coached pushing can be used if concerns regarding timing arise.

Midwives and birth attendants providing care at home during the second stage of labour should be mindful of many of the same things as those providing care during birth in a hospital such as bladder care, maternal position, fetal wellbeing, and progress of the birth (Fig. 6.2). Of utmost importance is careful consideration of progress and any potential delays due to the necessity for transfer in such a situation and possible delay in obtaining obstetric and

- Assess progress by observing maternal behaviour, progress of pushing, and baby's position and station.
- Continue to consider maternal position, hydration, and comfort measures.
- Expect birth to occur within 3 hours for nulliparous women and people, and 2 hours for multiparous.
- Consider a potential delay in the second stage after 2 hours for primiparous women and people, and 1 hour for multiparous.

Fig. 6.2 Recommended care in the second stage of labour (NICE 2017) in addition to that outlined in Fig. 6.1.

neonatal support due to transfer delays. Many factors will need to be considered such as transfer method, ambulance availability and waiting time, activity levels in the receiving unit, and journey time (see also chapter *Antenatal Planning*). Midwives should therefore maintain a helicopter view of the entire clinical situation to remain objective in decision making (see also *duration of second stage* below).

During the expulsive phase, many signs of an imminent birth may be visible. In the absence of concerns and where constant verbal, physical, and emotional support is not required, quietly observing is often the best approach: holding space for the woman or birthing person to follow their instincts and listen to her body. Many will be fearful of opening their bowels during this stage of labour, even though we know this is regularly seen during the expulsive phase.

> **Practice Point:**
> Whilst clearing away any faecal matter can reduce potential embarrassment, it has been argued that this should not be done if it involves touching or wiping the vulva/buttock area, as this has been anecdotally observed to often cause the woman or birthing person to tense up, and disturb their birth space and flow.

As explained, many women and birthing people birthing at home will display truly instinctive and uninhibited behaviours. These are often sounds, position changes, or movements that will optimise physiology and aid with progress. One example can be seen during birth in a kneeling or all-fours position. It is common to see women bear lower down onto their heels shortly before the presenting part becomes visible. Whilst this may mean reduced visibility for attending staff, it should not be discouraged as this position opens the pelvic outlet, and women and birthing people will instinctively rise onto their knees again when baby is coming.

MIDWIFERY CARE

Another of the advantages of providing care at a home birth is that there are usually two midwives present, lacking the external disruptions and challenges of labour ward birth, for example, no phones or buzzers to answer, no shouts for the drug cupboard keys!

Many low-risk physiological labour pathways necessitate minimal long hand note keeping. This means the two midwives/birth attendants can be truly present and provide a higher level of holistic support.

> **Practice Point:**
> This could include massage, aromatherapy (where competent to do so), verbal encouragement, supporting other children and pets, making food and drinks for everyone, and even taking birth photos for families following discussion and with their consent (usually using the family's own phone or camera). A further consideration during the second stage of labour is the environment. Adjustments to music/lighting/position/location can provide women and birthing people with the optimum space that they need for the final stages of labour.

Those birthing at home usually feel more uninhibited and may therefore be more likely to listen to their body in terms of positions, behaviours, and sounds and will often ask for what they need from birth attendants more readily. Additionally, they are in their own environment and as such are more likely to adjust the lighting and music without prompting than in a hospital setting.

> **Practice Point:**
> A common anecdotal observation amongst midwives is that some women and birthing people who have used hypnobirthing techniques may benefit from a more significant change of environment during the second stage of labour, in order to energise and prepare for the expulsive phase. Often a change in genre of music does the trick; however, some midwives make use of cold compresses to further support this change of pace and dynamic.

As the birth of the baby draws closer, pets and other children who had previously been present may disappear. When considering older siblings, midwives and birth attendants should be guided by the wishes of the family and the behaviour of the children themselves. Some children will want to be very much involved and present, and some may choose to leave the room.

> **Practice Point:**
> It's always a good idea to encourage families to have a space set up with toys/books, and an additional person present in the house who doesn't mind not witnessing the birth if they plan on having a child present, just in case they change their mind last minute. Birth attendants should advise parents to be led by the children regarding whether they are in the room or not.

Many families planning home births hire birthing pools, and as previously stated it is important to adjust the water temperature in preparation for the baby's birth as well as frequency and types of observation. It is not uncommon for partners to be in the pool with women and birthing people, and this is something we cannot disallow (refer to chapter *Labour and Birth in Water*) (Images 8–12).

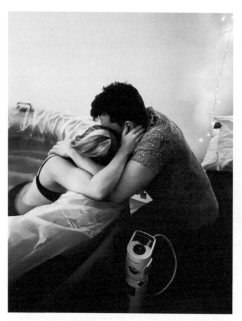

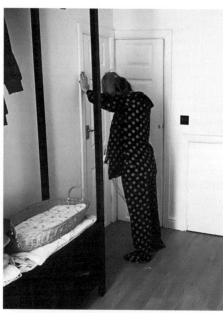

Image 8 Community Midwife Hannah J during her home birth, supported by husband Sion

Image 9 Community midwife Hannah J in early labour, in the corner of her birth space, using the wall for support

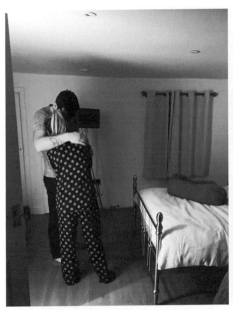

Image 10 Community midwife Hannah J supported by her husband Sion

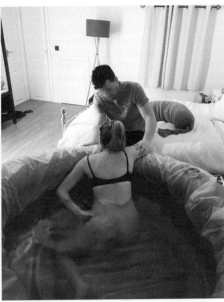

Image 11 Community midwife Hannah J instinctively performing a 'hip squeeze' on herself during the latter stages of her birth

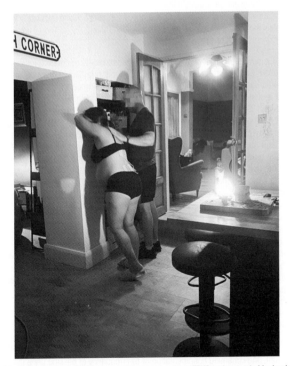

Image 12 Sophie moving instinctively round her home, using a TENS and supported by her husband.

MONITORING AND FETAL WELLBEING

Consideration of fetal wellbeing is especially important during the second stage of labour. If local guidelines refer to NICE 2022b, the frequency of intermittent auscultation (IA) increases from every 15 minutes to every 5 minutes (NICE, 2022b). In reality, this may be after every surge. Frequency of auscultation is increased as the second stage of labour demands more oxygen for the fetus. As with the first stage of labour, the technique of IA is utilised to ensure the early detection of any concerns or abnormalities in the fetal heart rate that could suggest a deterioration in fetal wellbeing and to enable timely consideration of potential transfer for continuous monitoring (Lewis & Downe, 2015).

Practice Point:

The fetal heart is auscultated directly after a surge in order to detect any decelerations and overshoots of the fetal heart rate from its baseline. The fetal heart is not auscultated during a surge as we know that physiological head compression can result in changes to the fetal heart during a surge; it is the heart rate after the surge that we want to hear, to detect how the fetus has recovered and to establish their wellbeing when the uterus is at rest (NICE, 2014). It is good practice to feel the maternal pulse whilst listening to the fetal heart, to establish a difference between the two.

Women and birthing people should be asked about their fetal movement pattern in the 24 hours preceding the onset of birth (NICE, 2022b). If fetal movements are reported during birth then auscultating the heart and detecting an acceleration can exclude hypoxia, although fetal movements are often reported less frequently during the second stage of labour.

Practice Point:

If fetal heart abnormalities are detected, provided there is no immediate concern for significant compromise, it is good practice to consider auscultating again after the next surge and reassess the clinical picture, including factors such as maternal temperature, pool temperature, progress of the birth, maternal position, presence of fetal movements (as these exclude hypoxia), maternal hydration, and comfort measures all whilst considering and implementation arrangements for transfer, particularly if there is likely to be a delay in ambulance attendance or transfer time. Fetal scalp stimulation via a vaginal examination is a good tool for use whilst supporting birth at home, as if accelerations are noted, then fetal hypoxia is very unlikely (NICE, 2022b).

Confirmation or serious suspicion of an ongoing fetal heart abnormality or concern indicates the need to advise a transfer to the nearest obstetric unit for continuous fetal heart monitoring. This requires a cardiotocograph (CTG) monitor and therefore cannot be performed at home. Continuous monitoring can support us to ascertain a truer picture of fetal wellbeing through assessment of variability, which is not possible with IA (NICE 2022a).

As previously mentioned, SROM may signify the commencement of the second stage of labour. Whilst meconium-stained liquor can be insignificant and is commonly seen after 40 weeks gestation, its presence can sometimes indicate fetal compromise (NICE, 2022b). Meconium staining is classified as significant or insignificant, depending on the colour and texture of the meconium, as well as the clinical picture (NICE, 2022b). Many areas across the UK have varying guidelines on meconium-stained liquor and home births. If local guidelines suggest transfer to an obstetric unit, this should always be considered and arrangements instigated, particularly if there is likely to be a delay in ambulance attendance or transfer time in relation to the stage of labour, fetal presentation, and whether birth is imminent.

Practice Point:

If an SROM has occurred in the second stage then an antenatal transfer may not be possible, and it may be safer to plan a postnatal transfer. Despite this, no delay in summoning help for transfer should be experienced; therefore the call should be made sooner rather than later. Some local guidelines suggest transfer to facilitate continuous fetal heart rate monitoring, and/or paediatric presence for birth, followed by observations of the newborn during the early postnatal period. (NICE, 2022b).

In addition to fetal heart auscultation, frequency of maternal observations increases once the second stage of labour is reached (see Fig. 6.1). National guidance recommends that frequency of surges should be assessed half-hourly, as well as hourly blood pressure, four-hourly temperature, hourly maternal pulse (although it is good practice to palpate this with each fetal heart auscultation), and continued documentation of the frequency of passing urine (NICE, 2022b). Local guidelines and policies may differ. Providing care during the second stage of labour at home provides a real opportunity to be 'with woman', not with machines or phones etc, and to observe and support the physiology of birth. Birth attendants should, however, always be mindful of any changes to the clinical picture that are presented through maternal and fetal observations and ensure maternal and fetal wellbeing is prioritised through timely enactment of transfer to hospital.

OPTIMAL POSITIONING AND MOBILITY

It is widely recognised that upright positions and mobility can reduce the length of labour. Supporting women and birthing people to be upright and mobile during the second stage of labour can reduce the length of the second stage, reduce the incidence of assisted birth, and result in fewer abnormal heart rate patterns (Gupta et al., 2017). As previously discussed, there are often more possibilities for different positions at home compared to in hospital, and women and birthing people tend to change position more freely in their own environment. They are also more prone to changing location when birthing at home, moving from room to room within their own familiar environment.

Birthing in the pool naturally lends itself to upright positions and frequent position changes, owing to the buoyancy that the water provides. Women and people who have been in the bath or pool may wish to exit the pool.

> **Practice Point:**
> Care should be taken to ensure they are dry and warm and that the floor is covered so that they don't slip. Midwives should encourage them to adopt upright positions wherever possible if they choose to exit the pool.

We also know that the diameters of the pelvis, and the relationship between the pelvis and the baby change as the woman or birthing person alters their posture and position. Whilst supporting a fellow midwife to birth at home, I observed her squeeze her hips with her hands during the second stage of labour. The baby was born shortly after. When we chatted after the birth, she stated she had no idea why she squeezed her hips and had not seen it before, but it felt like the right thing to do and was helping. Later that week she sent me a social media post demonstrating how hip squeezing can open the pelvic outlet. This is a true example of our bodies knowing just what to do, and birthing in a home environment usually strengthens this instinct. Another example of a position to widen the outlet is to keep the thighs and knees together but widen the calves and feet; whilst this feels counterintuitive to what we feel may expedite the birth, it in fact widens the outlet.

> **Practice Point:**
> Examples of upright positions to make use of at home are:
> - Sitting on or straddling the toilet or a dining chair
> - Crab walking (walking sideways) up and down the stairs
> - Kerb walking outside the house (one foot on the road and one on the pavement)

> - Leaning and swaying over the kitchen worktop
> - Standing using the support of the bannister to hang onto
> - Mobilising in the bath or shower
> - Walking outside in the garden

Another excellent consideration for home birth attendants is additional training in positions and manoeuvres to aid the progress of labour and correct malpositions. Courses such as Biomechanics for birth by Optimal Birth (O'Brien, 2022) will support birth workers to learn the benefits of positions such as side lying release and forward-leaning inversion, as well as the safe and effective use of rebozo (Wickham, 2017). It is important that additional training is undertaken in these techniques, as each has its own set of contraindications; however, it is widely reported that these methods are extremely beneficial, particularly in the incidence of a delay during birth.

NUTRITION/HYDRATION, ANALGESIA, AND COMFORT MEASURES

Wherever birth occurs, the midwife will need to be mindful of nutrition and hydration. The body works extremely hard during birth and therefore adequate fuel is required in order to sustain the work of the uterus and other bodily functions. If the body enters a ketotic state, then surges can reduce, and birth can stall. Urinalysis can be used to swiftly exclude this. If a woman or birthing person has ketones in their urine, or if their surges are spacing out, snacks and increasing hydration may help to resolve this. Dried fruit, sweets, isotonic drinks, or a spoonful of honey or jam are just a few suggestions. Care should be taken to avoid overhydration that may lead to hyponatraemia (Moen et al., 2009).

There are many different comfort measures commonly available at home: water, Transcutaneous Electrical nerve stimulation (TENS), massage, hypnobirthing, aromatherapy, and Entonox, to name a few. Hot water bottles may help with lower back pain, and the bath or shower can be used if the family has decided not to hire a birthing pool. Paracetamol can be taken; however women and birthing people should be advised that paracetamol can hinder prostaglandin production (Graham & Scott, 2005), which may in turn slow the progress of birth.

Some areas support the use of pethidine at home, either via the local unit or the GP (see *Antenatal Planning*). Others do not support its use due to the limited available neonatal support available at home and the logistics of transporting a controlled drug. Nevertheless, multiple comfort measures are available in the home setting and can be considered to aid maternal progress and relief during the second stage of labour. In some cases women may decide to transfer to hospital for analgesia not available at home. The birthplace study (Brocklehurst et al., 2011) identified that only 5.1% of women were transferred for epidural from home.

> **Practice Point:**
> Discuss comfort measures with women and birthing people whilst planning for home birth, as some of these may need to be prearranged. Advise families to shop for drinks and snacks for the birth.

DURATION OF THE SECOND STAGE OF LABOUR

A delay in the second stage of labour can be identified if the active second stage has lasted for 2 hours for nulliparous women and birthing people, and 1 hour for multiparous women and birthing people NICE 2022b. Within the Birthplace study, transfer to obstetric unit from home due to a delay in the first or second stage of labour occurred in 32.4% (Brocklehurst et al., 2011), with delays in transfer during labour identified as contributor factors to poor outcome within ESMiE confidential enquiry into midwifery-led settings (Rowe et al., 2020). Once a delay is suspected or confirmed, transfer to hospital should be offered and arranged for obstetric review, and for birth to be expedited according to clinical need. Clear and effective communication should also occur between the attending midwives and the local obstetric unit about the plan of care to ensure that they are ready to receive the transferred woman to the correct clinical area, that is, labour ward or theatres, and that appropriate clinicians such as obstetricians, anaesthetists, and neonatal team are available. If a delay in the second stage of labour is suspected at home, the considerations are similar to those in a hospital setting.

Many techniques are employed by midwives who regularly support home births when considering a delay, most considering ways to increase natural oxytocin levels. Birth attendants at home might need to be a little more creative in improving oxytocin levels to negate a delay in the second stage, or in the presence of such whilst awaiting transfer. They can employ a number of techniques that arguably could be used within a hospital environment also. Acting on a delay in birth would mean a transfer from home that would often involve an ambulance ride, which can be disruptive for all involved.

> **Practice Point:**
> Methods to try and expedite birth through increasing oxytocin production:
> - A change in maternal position
> - Nipple stimulation
> - Encouraging diet and hydration
> - Considering comfort measures
> - Altering the environment (lights, music, people present)
> - Mobilising around the house, stairs, and garden
> - Providing privacy for oxytocin stimulation
> - Encouraging laughter
> - Aromatherapy

Methods that are perhaps used a little more in a home setting include aromatherapy. Often hospitals and birth centres have guidelines in place about the use of essential oils and may not support the use of diffusers; however, in their own home setting, women and birthing people are able to use aromatherapy more readily and freely. Families who plan a home birth may have considered complementary therapies during their birth preparation and purchased some essential oils. Midwives require additional specialist training and competencies to be able to provide and advise on essential oils as part of the care they give (NMC, 2018); however, women and birthing people may choose to make use of specific oils in the case of a delay. Oils such as lavender support feelings of calm and control, which may inhibit the release of oxytocin, and clary sage can increase oxytocin and enhance surges.

Oxytocin can also be released through physical touch. Massage, stroking, and light touch, as well as providing privacy for women/birthing people and their partners to kiss and cuddle, can be hugely beneficial. Huge amounts of oxytocin are released during sexual pleasure and orgasm, and whilst this may not appeal to many during the second stage of labour, some may wish to explore this. Laughter can also be used to encourage oxytocin; therefore putting on a comedy show on television or telling a funny story might be considered.

THE BIRTH OF THE BABY

The actual birth of a baby at home in many ways is essentially the same as in any setting, although there is perhaps more flexibility with position options and less of an emphasis on birthing on a bed. At the point birth is imminent, consideration should be given to ensuring:
- Temperature of the birth environment supports optimum neonatal thermoregulation by closing windows and where possible doors to support this, as well as turning heaters/heating on if necessary

- Equipment and phones are immediately at hand in case a deviation from normal physiological processes occurs and additional help is needed
- Birth partners are encouraged to be as involved as they would like to be.

Midwives may become aware of the presenting part advancing either by visualising it themselves or by the woman or person informing them they can feel it if they are in a position that does not facilitate visualisation of the perineum (e.g. on all fours in the pool). Some midwives may wish to discreetly use a mirror and a small torch to support visualisation; however, some will feel comfortable listening to the woman or person.

> **Practice Point:**
> Provided all is well, it is important to continue facilitating a calm and dimly lit environment for the birth itself if this is what's desired. Therefore a torch, head torch, or another light source such as a lamp or fairy lights can be used to aid visibility if required.

> **Practice Point:**
> Consider encouraging the women to gently touch the head of the fetus as it either becomes visible or begins to crown. Some women may wish to, some not.

PERINEAL SUPPORT DURING BIRTH

The 'hands-on vs hands-poised' debate continues. A recent study showed that 38.6% prefer a hands-off or hands-poised approach (Stride et al., 2021). Current national guidance suggests that either is acceptable (NICE, 2022b); however, since the last published review, the Royal College of Obstetricians and Gynaecologists have implemented, with the endorsement of the Royal College of Midwives, the OASI (obstetric anal sphincter injury) care bundle project (RCOG, 2022) involving amongst four specific interventions, manual perineal protection by way of applying the Finnish grip where the perineum can be visualised. Results of one study showed a reduction of 0.3% in OASI amongst the 55,000 women that the project included (Gurol-Urganci et al., 2020); however, other studies have been unable to demonstrate the same reduction, and as such the debate surrounding the care bundle continues (Thornton & Dahlen, 2020). It is important that discussions regarding perineal management be undertaken with the woman/birthing person prior to labour and birth to discuss acceptability and preference in order that informed consent for any intervention be gained prior to and during labour. It is worth considering that the OASI method cannot be undertaken during water birth and may be difficult in standing or other more active positions and therefore may not always be readily utilised during home births. Robust evidence supporting the use of warm compresses exists and therefore is a widely recognised method to reduce severe perineal trauma (Magoga et al., 2019), and it is hypothesised that the warmth of the water in the birth pool is thought to achieve the same effect (see also chapter *Labour and Birth in Water*). Perineal trauma aside, those who birth at home commonly have a very hands-off experience throughout the first stage of labour, with minimal interruption and interference, and may wish for the second stage of their labour to be the same.

> **Practice Point:**
> Midwives and birth attendants should support women and people to birth in upright and mobile positions, encouraging them to consider options other than the bed. A pillow, cushion, or beanbag can be placed on the floor if the woman or person is birthing in a standing position. If the second birth attendant has not yet arrived, the midwife could consider phoning a colleague in the birth centre or obstetric unit should they wish support with noting times. Windows should be closed, fans turned off, pools topped up with hot water, and heating turned up to ensure a warm birth environment. Families may wish to 'catch' their own baby, which is more possible during water birth due to the very nature of the hands-off approach that it dictates. Catching babies is also very possible during land births too; however, midwives may need to be closer by to provide support if needed.

THE THIRD STAGE OF LABOUR

The third stage of labour refers to the time between the birth of the baby and the birth of the placenta and membranes (NICE, 2017). A discussion should have taken place before the birth as to whether the woman or birthing person wishes for a physiological or an active third stage. This discussion may have been supported or informed by risk assessment tools such as 'OBS Cymru', which is a postpartum haemorrhage tool that is used across Wales or recommendations from NICE (2017) taking into account a dynamic risk assessment. If they wish for a physiological third stage, and blood loss is minimal, there is little to be done straight away.

During these initial moments, skin to skin can be facilitated unless there are neonatal concerns or the woman or birthing person does not wish this. Skin to skin is the most effective way to keep a baby warm after birth, provided baby is full-term and healthy. Undisturbed skin to skin during an undisturbed 'golden hour' regulates baby's breathing, heart rate, temperature, and blood glucose, as well as encourages instinctive feeding behaviours and promotes comfort and calmness. Furthermore, breastfeeding during this hour can reduce excessive blood loss, expedite the birth of the placenta, promote bonding, and prolong the period of the overall breastfeeding journey.

> **Practice Point:**
> The 'golden hour' should be observed where possible, which entails minimal separation and disturbance during the first hour of baby's life. In the absence of clinical concerns the focus should be on the family, discovering the sex of the baby, taking photos, and welcoming their new arrival. Siblings and pets may reappear once they can hear that the baby has been born.

Optimal cord clamping should be observed as the benefits for baby are widely acknowledged; if the woman is in a birthing pool, this can often be left until they wish to get out and the cord has stopped pulsating, or even until after the placenta is birthed. It is recommended to wait at least 60 seconds to cut the cord (NICE, 2022b). The 'Wait for White' campaign led by midwife Amanda Burleigh (2022) shared the benefits of delayed cord clamping, such as reduced anaemia and increased stem cell provision.

The use of hats can avoided in the absence of concerns, as research has shown that women and birthing people smelling their babies' heads after birth supports bonding and increases oxytocin (Lundstrom et al., 2013). Providing a hat can interrupt this, along with baby's instinctive feeding behaviours and breast crawling (Ashworth, 2020). Despite this, hats should always be available and in the case of preterm or unwell babies used as part of the escalation of concerns. It is important to ensure that skin to skin is undertaken safely and that baby's head is upright, neck is straight, and the face can always be visualised. Breastfeeding during third stage of labour is an effective way to expedite the birth of the placenta, due to the surges of oxytocin that this encourages. Furthermore, families wishing to artificially feed should be encouraged to do this in skin to skin during the golden hour to promote bonding and close loving relationships.

> **Practice Points:**
> Consider whether a baby hat is necessary in skin to skin, and encourage early feeding in order to benefit both the woman/birthing person and the baby.

Whilst facilitating the golden hour and family bonding, midwives and birth attendants should be keeping a close watchful eye on the woman or birthing person and their blood loss. This is relatively simple and easy to visualise in the pool, as the colour of the water can be observed. A separation bleed is often seen as a large 'gush' into the pool but should quickly settle. If the water continues to rapidly darken this may be a sign to encourage exiting the pool (also see *Managing Emergencies at Home*).

> **Practice Point:**
> Discussion about third-stage preferences should have taken place before the birth. In the case of a rhesus-negative blood group that requires cord bloods to be taken, these can be done before the cord is clamped and cut, and whilst the woman or birthing person is in the pool.

As most women and birthing people birthing at home will have a low chance of extensive bleeding (Nove, Berrington, & Matthews, 2012), a physiological third stage might be requested due to its hands-off and drug-free nature. Some women may prefer an active third stage, and individual plans can be made for those with complex factors or predisposing factors for postpartum haemorrhage.

If they wish for an active third stage, an oxytocic should be given, and this can be in the deltoid if the woman or birthing person is in the pool (All Wales Midwife Led Care Guidance, 2022; NICE, 2022b), and then time can be given for this to take effect. As with any active third stage, clear signs of placental separation should be observed prior to commencing controlled cord traction; however, consideration should be given at this point as to where this is going to be performed safely – a sofa, bed, or even the floor can be used but be mindful of the potential for blood spills! Whilst an oxytocic can be given to commence an active third stage with the woman or birthing person remaining in the pool, exiting the pool is suggested for controlled cord traction to help birth the placenta. This is due to a theoretical chance of water embolism from deploying traction on the cord and then letting it go (Odent, 1983), plus the difficulty in guarding the uterus due to the logistics of being in the pool.

- Monitoring blood loss.
- General physical condition (colour, and how they feel).
- Check blood pressure, heart rate, respiration rate, and temperature following the birth of the placenta, or before this if a delay is suspected.

Fig. 6.3 Observations during the third stage of labour (NICE, 2022b).

Physiological third stages, however, commonly and unintentionally occur in the water or as the woman exits the pool. Remaining in the pool, having skin-to-skin contact with baby, and breastfeeding can support oxytocin release during this time. Exiting the pool, unless clinically indicated or with maternal preference, may disrupt the birthing space and atmosphere.

During the third stage of labour, maternal wellbeing should be assessed, as stated in Fig. 6.3.

Again, the midwife should be mindful of time during the third stage, without putting undue pressure on the woman. The third stage should be complete within 30 minutes for an active third stage, and active management should be offered if the placenta is not born within 60 minutes for a physiological third stage (NICE, 2022b).

> **Practice Point:**
> If there is a delay (and even when there isn't) with a physiological third stage, a change of position can help encourage the birth of the placenta by maternal effort alone. Sitting on the toilet can be a great position (be sure to put a pad or bowl in the toilet so that you don't have to fish the placenta out!). Other positions that may be useful are squatting, swaying, and kneeling, anything upright where gravity can aid. Additionally, emptying the bladder should always be considered.

> **Practice Point:**
> After cutting the cord, removing the clamp from the placenta and allowing the blood to drain from the placenta can aid in the completion of the third stage, as well as creating downwards pressure, which can be done by encouraging coughing or asking the woman or birthing person to blow into a plastic bottle, a practice commonly utilised across Africa (Otoo, Habib, & Ankomah, 2015).

Guidance for the third stage of labour and ongoing risk assessment suggests that any and all blood loss be weighed rather than estimated where possible (Bell et al., 2021). The use of absorbent or incontinence (inco) pads when on land aid in this significantly. In hospital the dry weights of towels, sheets etc are largely known; however, at home this wouldn't be the case unless the midwife weighs the family's linen before the birth.

Setting up scales is undertaken in anticipation of the neonatal weight being taken; therefore the same equipment can be used to weigh blood loss, enabling an accurate assessment of blood loss and facilitating timely transfer in the event of escalating concerns. Of course, blood loss cannot be weighed in the pool; however there are numerous methods for estimating blood loss in the pool, some relating to the colour of the water, some relating to the visibility of the bottom of the pool, and some in relation to the colour of the water compared with different wines (Garland, 2017). Some areas choose to simply define blood loss as either less than or more than 500 mL for water births owing to the difficulty in estimating an exact figure (Goodman, 2015) (see chapter *Labour and Birth in Water*).

> **Practice Point:**
> Have the scales set up ready to weigh any measurable blood loss, and if possible, record a dry weight before the birth for any pads or towels the woman has in her home.

In the absence of excessive bleeding other factors might be considered during the third stage of labour. Some families may plan a lotus birth, whereby the placenta and cord are left intact and attached to the baby, until the cord dries and separates naturally (Monaghan, 2022). Whilst this practice is not commonly observed, it can promote skin to skin and more effective establishment of feeding as the baby is more difficult to dress (Monaghan, 2022). It has been argued that this practice can increase the likelihood of infection and jaundice (Ittleman et al., 2019); however, little evidence to support this exists. The informed choice of lotus birth should be respected and supported, and practices such as washing and preparing the placenta should be facilitated.

> **Practice Point:**
> The family should always be asked whether they have any specific wishes or requests regarding their placenta. Many wish to see it, and some wish to keep it. To many families, the placenta is an important organ which has grown their baby, and having its structure and different parts explained to them is fascinating. Some families wish to photograph or take art from their placenta, such as placenta prints which uncannily resemble a tree. A handy addition to a home birth midwives' kit is a few sheets of A3 paper to be able to offer this to families who may not have considered it.

Following the birth of the placenta, the midwife usually assesses the perineum and vagina for any damage or injury (see chapter *Postnatal Care at Home*). This can be done in many locations; sofa, bed, floor, and skin to skin can be continued during this time. Lighting is important, and many midwives carry head torches for this reason. If suturing is required, this can again be done in many places.

> **Practice Point:**
> For more significant tears, a great position that mimics lithotomy as best as possible makes use of two dining chairs. Ask the woman or birthing person to position themselves on the edge of the bed or sofa, and place their feet on the dining chairs. Skin to skin can absolutely be continued during suturing and can reduce pain and discomfort for women and birthing people during the procedure (Zou et al., 2021).

TRANSFER CONSIDERATIONS FOR HANDOVER WELLBEING, HANDING OVER TO TEAMS

Whilst transfer is considered in other chapters of this book, it is important to briefly discuss arrangements for such in the event of either intrapartum or postnatal transfer. Transfer from a home to hospital setting occurs for 45% of nulliparous women and birthing people and 12% of multiparous women and birthing people (Brocklehurst et al., 2011). There are numerous reasons why a transfer may be indicated during the second and third stage of labour, which can include:

- A delay in the first or second stage 32.4% (Brocklehurst et al., 2011)
- Fetal heart abnormalities 7.0% (Brocklehurst et al., 2011)
- Requests for additional comfort measures
- Meconium-stained liquor 12.2% (Brocklehurst et al., 2011)
- Prolonged third stage/retained placenta 7.0% (Brocklehurst et al., 2011)
- Excessive bleeding
- For assessment and/or repair of perineal trauma 10.9% (Brocklehurst et al., 2011)
- For ongoing observations or care of the woman/birthing person or baby (5.1% neonatal [Brocklehurst et al., 2011])

> **Practice Point:**
> The whole clinical picture should be assessed when considering a transfer, as well as additional factors such as potential transfer time and distance to the nearest obstetric unit. Stage of labour should also be considered; there may be concerns that would indicate transfer; however, if birth is imminent, it may be safer to remain in situ and call for help if further concerns are anticipated. When birth attendants advise that a transfer is indicated before the birth, or for maternal reasons after the birth, the decision ultimately resides with the woman or birthing person.

Once the decision for transfer has been made by the family and birth attendants, there are a number of things to do whilst continuing support of the family and documenting care that is given. These include:

- Communicating with and offering reassurance to the woman/birthing person and partner
- Arranging transport (this is often ambulance but may differ among geographical areas)
- Informing the receiving obstetric unit using a recognised handover method, that is, SBAR
- Packing up the midwife's birth kit and equipment
- Ensuring bags are packed and ready
- Supporting the woman/birthing person to prepare for transfer (getting dressed or covered to maintain dignity, going to the toilet)
- Documentation of conversations with other professionals

A midwife will usually accompany the woman or birthing person on the transfer; however, this decision will be made usually by the paramedic team. Whilst most transfers do not involve providing active care during the duration of the journey, it's imperative to ensure the necessary equipment is to hand should things change, for example, the birth becoming imminent, excessive bleeding, and the need for neonatal resuscitation.

> **Practice Point:**
> It is important to either take a full kit on the transfer or to take the elements of the kit that the ambulance does not carry (this is often just oxytocic drugs and neonatal resuscitation equipment but will differ between areas).

Safety is paramount during transfer; therefore passengers (including the midwife) will be encouraged to be seated and belted wherever possible, and the woman or birthing person will also have a seatbelt on the stretcher. Paramedics will have Entonox available and are able to carry out routine maternal observations during the transfer if necessary. Please also see chapter *Transfer and Multidisciplinary Team Working*.

> **Practice Point:**
> It's worth noting that the lights in the back of the ambulance can be dimmed on request, the radio can be played in the back, and the windows can be opened for fresh air. The stretcher can be adjusted between sitting and lying, giving options for positions. If the transfer is during or after the third stage, many paramedics will be happy to transfer in skin to skin, provided there is a partner to take the baby or a car seat should the clinical picture change. The ambulance crew will have blankets available to facilitate this; also bear in mind the weather and the time of day, and remember to bring clothes for the baby.

As stated, minimal care is provided during the transfer, with the exception of emergency treatment. The fetal heart can be auscultated upon entry to the ambulance and then on entry to the obstetric unit, bearing in mind that any fetal heart information will not usually change the management of the transfer unless, for example, a blue light response is needed. There is therefore little reason to auscultate during the active transfer and whilst the ambulance is in motion. In the absence of extreme fetal heart concerns during the second stage, active pushing is usually discouraged to make the transfer more comfortable and to reduce the likelihood of a birth. Documentation usually consists of time transfer initiated and fetal heart before leaving, and then arrival to the unit, unless any care has been provided en route.

> **Practice Point:**
> Phoning and pre-alerting the obstetric unit when arrival is imminent can enable staff to open doors, stop lifts, and direct you to the prepared room to help a smooth entry into the unit. If appropriate, staff can also be asked to prepare the environment in the room, low lights, and music. Although the transferring midwife usually hands over care at this point, many may stay to provide support for the woman or birthing person and their partner, as the receiving midwife is usually busy with arranging reviews and care, and documentation. Some guidelines require that the transferring midwife remain with the woman and will be dictated by local arrangement. This enables consistency and advocacy in support and regarding birth wishes and preferences. It's also important to consider that the family will have come from their home with just two staff present, to an unfamiliar environment where multiple staff may now be present including additional midwives, obstetricians, neonatologists, and anaesthetists. As such it's important to ensure only those who really need to be present are there and to always preserve dignity and privacy.

The second midwife or birth attendant usually follows behind in a car and can then bring the transferring midwife back to their car once care has been safely handed over.

> **Practice Point:**
> As partners usually accompany women and birthing people on transfer, the house is likely to be locked when the midwives return for the car, so it's important for the second midwife to ensure all their kit/equipment/diaries/belongings have been returned to the car up before following the ambulance.

REFERENCES

All Wales Midwife Led Care Guidance, 2022 (still in draft at time of writing but due to be published later this year).

Ashworth E. 2020. Baby hats: Wasted wool? Retrieved from: https://www.therealbirthcompanyltd.com/2020/12/09/baby-hats/

Bell, S., Collis, R., Pallman, P., Bailey, C., James, K., John, M., Kelly, K., Kitchen, T., Scarr, C., Watkins, A., Edey, T., Macgillivray, E., Greaves, K., Volikas, I., Tozer, J., Sengupta, N., Roberts, I., Francis, C., Collins, P. 2021. Reduction in massive postpartum haemorrhage and red blood cell transfusion during a national quality improvement project, Obstetric Bleeding Strategy for Wales, OBS Cymru: An observational study. BMC Pregnancy and Childbirth. 21:377.

Brocklehurst, P., Hardy, P., Hollowell, J., Linsell, L., Macfarlane, A., McCourt, C., Marlow, N., Miller, A., Newburn, M., Petrou, S., Puddicombe, D., Redshaw, M., Rowe, R., Sandall, J., Silverton, L., Stewart, M. 2011. Perinatal and maternal outcomes by planned place of birth for healthy women with low risk pregnancies: The Birthplace in England national prospective cohort study. British Medical Journal. Retrieved from: https://www.bmj.com/content/bmj/343/bmj.d7400.full.pdf

Burleigh, A. 2023. Wait for White. Retrieved from: https://waitforwhite.com

De Jonge, A., Dahlen, H., Downe, S. 2021. 'Watchful attendance' during labour and birth. Sexual and Reproductive Healthcare. 28: p1-2.

Dick-Read, G. 2013. Childbirth without fear. London: Pinter and Martin Ltd

Garland, D. 2017. Revisiting waterbirth. (2nd edn). London: Palgrave.

Goodman, A. 2015. Pictorial estimation of blood loss in a birthing pool: An aide memoire. The Practising Midwife. 18(4).

Graham, G., Scott, K. 2005. Mechanism of action of paracetamol. American Journal of Therapeutics. 12(1):46–55.

Graves, K. 2012. The hypnobirthing book. Wiltshire: Katharine publishing.

Gupta, J., Shood, A., Hofmeyr, G., Vogel, J. 2017. Position in the second stage of labour for women without epidural anaesthesia (Review). Cochrane Database of Systematic Reviews.

Gurol-Urganci, I., Bidwell, P., Sevdalis, N., Silverton, L., Novis, V., Freeman, R., Hellyer, A., van der Meulen, J., Thakar, R. 2020. Impact of a quality improvement project to reduce the rate of obstetric anal sphincter injury: A multicentre study with a stepped-wedge design. BJOG. 128(3):584–592.

Ittleman, B., German, K., Scott, E., Walker, V., Flaherman, V., Szabo, J., Beavers, B. 2019. Umbilical cord nonseverance and adverse neonatal outcomes. Clinical Paediatrics. 58(2):238–240.

Lewis, D., Downe, S. 2015. FIGO consensus guidelines on intrapartum fetal monitoring: Intermittent auscultation. Retrieved from: https://obgyn.onlinelibrary.wiley.com/doi/10.1016/j.ijgo.2015.06.019

Lundstrom, J., Mathem A., Schaal, B., Frasnelli, J., Nitzche, K., Gerber, J., Hummer, T. 2013. Maternal status regulates cortical responses to the body odor of newborns. Frontiers in Psychology. https://doi.org/10.3389/fpsyg.2013.00597

Magoga, G., Saccone, G., Al-Kouatly, H., Akbarzadeh, M., Ozcan, T., Berghella, V. 2019. War, perineal compresses during the second stage of labor for reducing perineal trauma: A meta-analysis. European Journal of Obstetrics & Gynecology and Reproductive Biology. https://doi.org/10.1016/j.ejogrb.2019.06.011

Moen, V., Brudin, L., Rundgren, M., Irestedt, L. 2009. Hyponatraemia complicating labour – Rare or unrecognised? A prospective observational study. BJOG. 116(4):552–561.

Monaghan, A. 2023. Factsheet – lotus birth. Retrieved from: https://www.all4birth.com/lotus-birth/

National Institute for Health and Care Excellence. 2014. Intelligent auscultation – 'Listen' for fetal wellbeing. Retrieved from: https://www.nice.org.uk/sharedlearning/intelligent-auscultation-listen-for-fetal-wellbeing

National Institute for Health and Care Excellence. 2022a. Fetal monitoring in labour. Retrieved from: https://www.nice.org.uk/guidance/ng229/resources/fetal-monitoring-in-labour-pdf-66143844065221

National Institute for Health and Care Excellence. 2022b. Intrapartum care for healthy women and babies. Retrieved from: https://www.nice.org.uk/guidance/cg190/resources/intrapartum-care-for-healthy-women-and-babies-pdf-35109866447557

NMC. 2018. The Code: Professional standards of practice and behaviour for nurses, midwives and nursing associates. Nursing and Midwifery Council.

Nove, A., Berrington, A., Matthews, Z. 2012. Comparing the odds of postpartum haemorrhage in planned home birth against planned hospital birth: Results of an observational study of over 500,000 maternities in the UK. BMC Pregnancy and Childbirth. 12:130.

O'Brien, M. 2022. Biomechanics for birth online. Retrieved from: https://www.optimalbirth.co.uk/index.php/courses-and-availability/biomechanics-for-birth-online

Odent, M. 1983. Birth under water. Lancet. 2:8365–8366.

Otoo, P., Habib, H., Ankoman, A. 2015. Food prohibitions and other traditional practices in pregnancy: A qualitative study in western region of Ghana. Advances in Reproductive Sciences. 3:41–49.

Prins, M., Boxem, J., Lucas, C., Hutton, E. 2011. Effects of spontaneous pushing versus Valsalva pushing in the second stage of labour on mother and fetus: A systematic review of randomised trials. BJOG. 118(6):662–670.

RCOG. 2022. OASI Care Bundle Project. Retrieved from: https://www.rcog.org.uk/oasicarebundle

Resuscitation Council UK. 2021. Equipment used in homebirth. Retrieved from: https://www.resus.org.uk/library/quality-standards-cpr/equipment-used-homebirth

Rowe, R. et al. 2020. Intrapartum-related perinatal deaths in births planned in midwifery-led settings in Great Britain: Findings and recommendations from the ESMiE confidential enquiry. BJOG. 127(13):1665–1675. https://doi.org/10.1111/1471-0528.16327.

Royal College of Obstetricians and Gynaecologists and Royal College of Midwives. 2017. Care bundle project. Retrieved from: https://www.rcog.org.uk/OASICareBundle

Sandall, J. et al. 2016. Midwife-led continuity models versus other models of care for childbearing women. Cochrane Database of Systematic Reviews [Preprint]. 4. Retrieved from: https://doi.org/10.1002/14651858.CD004667.pub5

Shepherd, A., Cheyne, H., Kennedy, S., McIntosh, C., Styles, M., Niven, C. 2010. The purple line as a measure of labour progress: A longitudinal study. BMC Pregnancy and Childbirth. 10(54) Pages 1–7.

Stride, S., Hundley, V., Way, S., Sheppard, Z. 2021. Identifying the factors that influence midwives' perineal practice at the time of birth in the United Kingdom. Midwifery. 102. https://doi.org/10.1016/j.midw.2021.103077

Sutton, J. 2000. Birth without active pushing and a physiological second stage of labour. TPM. 3(4):32–34.

Thornton, J. & Dahlen, H. 2020. The UK Obstetric Anal Sphincter Injury (OASI) care bundle: A critical review. Midwifery. 2020(90).

Wales Maternity and Neonatal Network. (2022). All Wales Midwifery-Led Care Guidelines 6th Edition. Retrieved from: https://wisdom.nhs.wales/all-wales-guidelines/all-wales-guidelines/all-wales-midwifery-led-care-guideline-2022/

Wickham, S. 2014. What is cervical recoil? Retrieved from: https://www.sarawickham.com/original-articles/exploring-cervical-recoil/

Wickham, S. 2017. The evidence for rebozos – Part 2. Retrieved from https://www.sarawickham.com/articles-2/the-evidence-for-rebozos-part-2/

Zou, Y., Li, Y., Jiang, M., Liu, X. 2021. Early skin-to-skin contact after vaginal delivery on pain during perineal wound suturing: A randomized controlled trial. Journal of Obstetrics and Gynaecology Research. https://doi.org/10.1111/jog.15120

CHAPTER 7

CONSIDERATIONS FOR LABOUR AND BIRTH IN WATER AT HOME

Dr Claire Feeley, Dr Ethel Burns, Anna Madeley

INTRODUCTION

Choosing to labour and/or give birth in water is an increasingly popular pain relief option in all birth settings, including homebirth. While using a shower or a bath at home can be very relaxing, a birth pool (in any birth place setting) is preferable because it is larger, enables greater buoyancy and ease of movement. It is also safer because it is less shallow. This chapter focusses on birth pool use in the home setting.

EVIDENCE FOR WATER IMMERSION

There is strong evidence in favour of planned homebirths with skilled midwifery birth attendance for healthy women who experience a straightforward pregnancy and have a spontaneous labour (Hutton, Reitsma et al. 2009; Reitsma, Simioni et al. 2020). Below highlights the key research findings regarding labouring and giving birth in water in any birth setting, but it is worth noting that the benefits of labouring and giving birth in a birth pool are particularly strong for healthy nullipara, and especially those who choose to have their baby at home or in a freestanding midwifery unit (Burns et al. 2012):

- Buoyancy enhances mobility, freedom of movement, and positional changes that facilitate physiological labour and birth outcomes (Burns, Ethel et al. 2022; Feeley, Cooper et al. 2021).
- Pain perception: release of endogenous endorphins/analgesic properties (Benfield, Hortobágyi et al. 2010; Maude 2004) can enhance confidence during labour (Feeley, Cooper et al. 2021) and increase control. The birth pool provides a natural personal space (Maude & Foureur 2007; Hall & Holloway 1998).
- Reduces epidural use (Burns, Feeley et al. 2022) (and risks associated with epidurals [Jones, Othman et al. 2012]) and injected opioid use (Burns, Feeley et al. 2022).
- Reduces the likelihood of requirement for labour augmentation (Burns, Feeley et al. 2022).
- Increases the likelihood of giving birth spontaneously, particularly in the community setting (freestanding midwifery units and women's home) (Burns et al. 2012; Carpenter, Burns et al. 2022).
- Reduces transfer likelihood from home/freestanding midwifery-led units (Lukasse, Rowe et al. 2014).
- Increases the likelihood of having an intact perineum (no tear).
- Does not increase the chance of an obstetric anal sphincter injury (OASI) (Burns, Feeley et al. 2022).
- Reduces likelihood of episiotomy (Burns, Feeley et al. 2022).
- Reduced likelihood of primary postpartum haemorrhage (Burns, Feeley et al. 2022).
- Improves satisfaction (Burns, Feeley et al. 2022).
- Enhances feelings of safety, protection, and privacy (Feeley, Cooper et al. 2021).
- Facilitates (for some) a positive state of altered consciousness during labour (Feeley, Cooper et al. 2021).
- Facilitates easier pushing experience (as reported by women) (Feeley, Cooper et al. 2021).
- Enables positive birth experiences with positive implications for postnatal mental-emotional health and wellbeing (Feeley, Cooper et al. 2021).

> **Women's Voices**
>
> *It's just being able to move and not be clumsy. Because in the end, I mean of the pregnancy, you are pretty heavy. So, I was really happy to be able to twist and turn and relax and the warmth. That is really nice and you can feel it in your whole body, so it was...and that is the greatest advantage...that you can move as you want to.*
> –Interview #12 (Ulfsdottir, Saltvedt et al. 2018)
>
> *Another world...it was like by the ocean, and then you come back to land and you are in another country...They call it 'labourland'... It really was another world, and you think about the journey that you make from being pregnant to becoming a mother... An incredible journey.*
> –Rosa (Sprague 2004)

Giving birth in water has not been shown to present a risk for baby. A large meta-analysis reported no difference in neonatal condition at birth (particularly Apgar score ≤7 at 5 minutes), requirement for resuscitation measures, respiratory difficulty, or neonatal death (Burns, Feeley et al. 2022). Other studies have not found any increased rates of admission to the neonatal intensive care unit (Sidebottom, Vacquier et al. 2020; Lanier, Wiegand et al., 2021; Aughey, Jardine et al., 2021). However, one factor that research has found is an increased likelihood of umbilical cord avulsion during waterbirth (Burns, Feeley et al. 2022). This is likely to occur when baby is helped to the surface, which may exert undue tension on the cord, causing it to snap. If identified and remedied by immediate cord clamping. The absolute risk of adverse outcome is rare (Burns, Feeley et al., 2022).

Practice Point: Avoiding Cord Avulsion

When supporting the baby's head out of the water and check there is no undue traction on the umbilical cord.

HOME BIRTH SPECIFIC CONSIDERATIONS: PRACTICALITIES

Preparing for a water labour and birth at home presents few additional requirements and considerations from those conducted within an institutional environment.

ANTENATAL PREPARATION

Many women will know if they are planning to labour and birth in water; however, for some, they may not realise that this is an option for them at home. When discussing options for birth at home, therefore, you should be able to effectively provide information for women and their families regarding both the evidence base (as above) and practical considerations. NICE (2017) states that women should be offered the chance to labour in water for its pain-relieving properties and this is no different for birth at home. It would be useful to have a list printed to give to the woman to source equipment. This may include:

- Where to source a pool and associated equipment without directly recommending a particular source (also see useful contacts and organisations at the end of this book) and/or information from the maternity service, should birthing pools be provided.
- When to obtain the pool (usually after 36 weeks for 6-week duration).
- Suggested equipment required to be provided by the woman (Fig 7.1).
- Location considerations for siting the pool.
- Recommendations for a 'dry run' prior to labour to prevent delays once labour commences. This might include cleaning the equipment ready for the actual day.
- Ensuring everyone who attends the birth knows their role in inflating and filling the pool.

BIRTH POOL LOCATION

The location of the pool should be discussed early to assist the woman to choose the size and capacity of the pool they obtain. Information about the combined weight of the pool and water can be obtained from providers and taken into consideration when, for example, the pool is to be sited on anything other than the ground floor or in a flat. Whilst very unlikely to cause a problem, this will almost certainly be an important consideration on a houseboat/barge. The type of flooring that the pool is to be sited on will need to be solid and preferably with no damage, that is, wooden floor with rotten joists/boards. If the house in which the pool is to be sited is old or there are questions over loading, it may be necessary to have the floors inspected. If the floors are hard, consider laying a soft layer (blanket, towels, or

- Pool*.
- Disposable pool liner*.
- Nontoxic food grade hose pipe*.
- Tap connectors*.
- Submersible pump*.
- Mirror*.
- Thermometer* (if not being brought by midwives).
- Pool cover (optional).
- Step/foot stool (optional).
- Tarpaulin or another floor covering, preferably wipe clean.
- Additional towels (bath sheets are very good post birth).
- Bucket.
- Jug.
- Sieve* (preferably one that can be disposed of/washed and recycled post birth).
- Absorbent pads to place around the pool.
- Puncture repair kit*.

*May be provided as part of pool hire, check with provider.

Fig. 7.1 Suggested equipment provided by woman.

matting) under/over the waterproof layer upon which it is sited. This will also be useful if the pool does not have a padded bottom to support the knees of the labourer.

The pool should be located where it can be filled easily, either by running the hose or buckets (noting that this method takes a long time!). Advise the woman to check the tap connector to make sure they fit where the hose will run from to avoid having to repeatedly boil the kettle! Additionally, consider how the pool is to be emptied – will the hose reach a toilet, sink, or outside window?

Key Points
- Aim for access to all sides of the pool for the midwives and the woman. Entry is usually by stepping in and out of the pool (a step may help here) or sitting on the side of the pool (if firm enough) and swinging legs in and out. For some pools with chambers, the top chamber can be slightly deflated to assist entry for women of shorter stature.
- If in the unlikely event of having to assist in evacuation of the pool for collapse, access to all sides may help in swift exit.
- Make sure that electrical equipment and sockets are not within splashing distance.
- Avoid puncturing the pool by making sure the floor is prepared (swept, vacuumed, soft layer before the pool is inflated).
- When the pool arrives and you are ready to inflate it, follow manufacturer's instructions. Take the pool out of any box/bag and allow it to warm up to room temperature if it has been kept in a car or garage. This ensures that when unfolding and inflating it does not force creases to rip to tear.
- Some women may choose to place their pool in a conservatory. Consider privacy and dignity during labour and birth, also ability to keep the room warm.
- Advise pool safety if filling in advance, for example, keeping small children and pets away from the pool.

EQUIPMENT AND FILLING THE POOL

Equipment considerations can be seen in Figs. 7.1 and 7.2. Advising when to start filling the pool will be dependent on a variety of factors such as water pressure, whether the water is supplied through gas-fired water heating or an immersion heater, and where you are filling from (kitchen or bathroom). Generally, though, concerns can be allayed by suggesting a trial run to time how long it takes and get used to assembling everything at short notice (and draining!). Once the pool is filled, advise women and their families to be aware of drowning risk with children and animals. When topping up with hot water to maintain the temperature, be careful not to pour anywhere near the woman in the pool and be mindful of removing the same amount of cold water. Birthing pools can take 20–30 minutes to fill, and sometimes women labour too quickly to access; therefore it is helpful to start running the pool sooner rather than later.

WHEN TO ENTER A BIRTH POOL

Clinical guidance can influence when women access a birthing pool. For example, some local maternity guidelines advocate that a woman's cervix be at least 4 cm dilated before she can enter a birth pool. However, there is no evidence to support this recommendation. Furthermore, cervical dilatation in itself is a subjective, limited measurement and does not account for effacement, cervical application to the presenting part of the fetus, its position or descent in the women's pelvis; a women's cervix might be 1–2 cm dilated, but fully effaced and well applied to the presenting part, and the uterine contractions good, whilst conversely, a woman's cervix could be ≥5 cm dilated, uneffaced, and she not be not in established labour. In the context of homebirth women may choose to enter the pool before the midwife's arrival; therefore women should be supported to use the pool as and when they prefer and should not be contingent on cervical dilatation. It is not unusual for contractions to slow down shortly after entering a birth pool. As with any change during labour, contractions can ease off for a while, for example, staff shift change or intrusion. Likewise, water immersion can also exert a transient physiological (Benfield, Hortobágyi et al. 2010).

Practice Point:
There is no research to support exerting a cervical dilatation caveat before birth pool entry.

- Water thermometer.
- Waterproof doppler for fetal heart auscultation.
- Birth mirror (If not disposable, should be autoclavable or able to be cleaned and sterilised).
- Additional clinical waste bags/absorbent sheets.
- Gloves for pool use. Some trusts utilise the disposable long arm-length gloves or plastic aprons with gloves.

Fig. 7.2 Additional equipment for midwives.

BIRTH POOL TEMPERATURE

The water temperature should not exceed normal body temperature, that is, 37°C. It is advisable to suggest that the woman immerse in a cooler than her usual bath temperature. This is important because a hot labouring person will compromise a fetus whose temperature is physiologically up to a degree hotter (Asakura 2004). A labouring person is usually warm, even hot, and being too hot may affect the benefit of immersion and thus equilibrium. Raised maternal temperature is a key risk factor with epidural analgesia and negative impact on the fetus (Sharpe & Arendt 2017).

Key Points for Labour Care
- Pool has enough water to submerge the woman's abdomen and bottom.
- Pool is big enough to enable a woman to flip over and adopt different positions with ease.
- Usual observations apply including hourly water temperature checks.
- Intermittent auscultation with a waterproof sonic aid.
- Vaginal examinations, if required, can be performed in or outside the pool.
- If concerned by labour dystocia, exiting the pool temporarily and adopting positions such as pelvic rocking and sitting on the Toilet to empty the bladder may assist progress. Similarly, walking around for a while or lateral resting.

TRANSITION/SECOND STAGE OF LABOUR CARE

Transition characteristics such as anal pouting and a visible rhombus of Michaelis and/or the purple line along with maternal behaviour in conjunction with the switch to a rush of catecholamines will present in water, as on land. It is advisable that any woman in labour is supported to push as and when she has an urge to do so, and waterbirth is no different (Haseeb, Alkunaizi et al. 2014; Wright, Nassar et al. 2021). Fatigue is more likely if a woman is instructed to engage in direct pushing, irrespective of whether she gives birth in water or on land. Sustained breath holding can inhibit perineal stretching and the accompanying reduced placental perfusion may also compromise the fetus (Haseeb, Alkunaizi et al. 2014). Some midwives prefer to use a torch and mirror to observe progress, while others find it unnecessary. While the midwife should be hands off during a waterbirth, some women will reach down to touch the baby's head, which should be unhindered. Depending on the woman's position and preferences she may wish to 'catch' the baby; this should be supported where possible. Of importance, once the fetal head is born, it remains underwater. Should a woman raise her bottom out of the water at this point, the rest of the birth should be facilitated out of the water and must not be re-submerged – to avoid any risk of water inhalation. Additionally, it is important to avoid cord traction (Burns 2012; Burns et al. 2022).

Retrospective research expressed concern that waterbirth may predispose women to sustaining an extensive perineal tear involving the anal sphincter (OASI) (Cortes, Basra et al. 2011); however, prospectively collected data analysis found no such association (Burns, Feeley et al. 2022). When a midwife assists a woman to give birth in water, typically she adopts a hands-off approach, a practice that is currently not recommended for women giving birth on land. The advent of the OASI 'bundle' has exerted a drive to encourage midwives to routinely adopt a hands-on approach to birth; however, the evidence supporting this intervention is less than robust and being challenged (Thornton & Dahlen 2020). Unfortunately, some maternity units have set the OASI bundle as a mandate, which may present a confidence and skills issue for midwives regarding water and land birth.

Key Points for Waterbirth:
- Follow the woman's instinctive pushing cues.
- Continue with usual observations and signs of progression.
- Adopt a hands-off approach.
- Support the woman to remain submerged during the birth; otherwise, avoid re-submersion of baby's head.
- Avoid traction on the cord as baby is lifted gently out of the water.

Practice Point:
It is sufficient to just have baby's head out of the water. Should a cord avulsion occur, clamp the cord immediately, assess baby's condition, and act accordingly.

THIRD-STAGE CARE

Various hospital guidelines recommend leaving the pool for placental birth (whether active or physiologically managed); however, this is not necessary and may interfere with the high release of oxytocin that occurs following birth (Fry 2013). This release of oxytocin facilitates the detachment and expulsion of the placenta; therefore interfering (e.g. turning lights on, talking loudly, moving the mother out of the pool) may increase bleeding and/or haemorrhage. Therefore the warmth of the pool, maintaining ambient lighting, and minimising distractions and stimulation will reduce the release of catecholamines and facilitate safe physiological placental birth in the pool (Fahy, Hastie et al. 2010). Furthermore, the vast neonatal benefits from delayed cord clamping, which means enabling the woman to remain in the pool to birth her placenta followed by cord clamping, should not present a problem. It is easy to revert to active management in the event of concern.

CONCERN ABOUT ESTIMATING BLOOD LOSS IN A BIRTH POOL

Visual blood loss estimates are only ever an educated guess during spontaneous or operative vaginal birth. Aids in the form of photographs of different blood volumes in a standard-size, plumbed-in birth pool with reference points to rose/red wine have been developed to guide midwives in their estimation. However, regarding waterbirth, anxiety lingers in this area even though the blood loss one sees is married to the women's condition and factors such as the length of her labour and past history. Worry around possibly not identifying excessive blood loss in a timely manner may be making some midwives ask that women leave the pool for the third stage of labour, disrupting the mother-baby crucial skin-to-skin contact. estiMATE is an online tool developed to improve visual blood loss estimations during waterbirth showed promise in estimates and midwives' confidence (Burns, Hunter et al. 2019).[1] A large-scale evaluation conducted during 2019 will soon be ready to submit for publication. This tool involves simulations using live models and involving a range of different blood volumes using expired blood filmed in real time will hopefully assist in resolving this worry and result in less third-stage disturbance in the absence of a problem.

> **Key Points for Placental Birth:**
> - Keep an ambient environment avoiding disturbing the mother-baby dyad.
> - Support/encourage uninterrupted skin-to-skin contact and/or initiation of breastfeeding.
> - Observe for signs of placental detachment (cord lengthening, small acute blood loss, cramping) and gently encourage woman to work with those cramps to expel the placenta.
> - Observe for excessive blood loss in the pool, and if required, support the woman to exit the pool and revert to active management (if consented).

> **Practice Point:**
> Most of the research regarding water immersion outcomes has involved healthy women and has been undertaken in the obstetric unit setting, with further research upcoming/ongoing for those who may have a risk factor, for example, a previous caesarean section, or a BMI >30. Across the UK, many women deemed 'out of guidelines' have experienced successful waterbirths. While the physiology of birth does not change (!), our empirical knowledge of specific conditions during pregnancy and whether they affect water immersion outcomes remains a work in progress.
>
> A limitation found in the research is that the majority of women using a birth pool are white and from higher socio-economic backgrounds. (Aughey et al. 2021). This raises concerns that birthing pool access is inequitable, therefore, the onus is on maternity professionals to ensure all women are provided with meaningful, evidence-based information to reduce such inequities.

ORGANISATIONAL MIDWIFERY CARE AND EMERGENCY PREPAREDNESS

As with any care provided at a home birth, midwives attending should ensure that their safety is treated as a priority. The risk assessment undertaken during preparation for labour and birth (including the ongoing dynamic assessment in labour and birth) should include consideration of their own safety, for example, manual handling implications (also refer to chapter *Planning for Homebirth: Organisational Considerations*). From an organisational perspective, community-based study days to raise awareness and knowledge of physiological labour and birth in water and to troubleshoot concerns should feature in any mandatory training (also see chapter *Planning for Homebirth: Organisational Considerations*).

> **Key Points for Organisational Midwifery Care and Emergency Preparedness**
> - Ensure that you are comfortable with supporting women in water at home, or if you are planning services, ensure that arrangements are in place to upskill and improve competence and confidence.
> - As an attending midwife, if you have anxieties around any aspect of supporting waterbirth either institutionally or at home, seek support to develop skills, competence, and confidence.
> - Consider using a buddy system to familiarise inexperienced midwives and preceptors with facilitating water birth at home.
> - Ensure that where possible student midwives are exposed to immersion and birth in water at home.
> - As with any home birth, upon arrival, ensure that a neonatal station is set up early. This should be close enough to be able to manage any unanticipated neonatal concerns but outside the eye line of the labouring woman if possible.
> - Ensure that there is space for the woman to exit the pool if she wishes to come out or if needed in the event of an emergency.
> - In a room with a warm pool and windows closed it can be easy to neglect our own wellbeing. Ensure that you stay hydrated.

[1]To keep up to date with latest research and information, particularly regarding the eSTiMATE tool please see https://www.brookes.ac.uk/research/units/hls/groups/maternity-and-childbirth-oxmater and/or Twitter @OxMateR.

> **Practice Point: Addressing the Myth of 'Slashing the Sides'**
> An urban myth that seems to have grown across birthing communities is that in the event of having to evacuate a birthing pool quickly, midwives will slash the sides. This is not supported practice and despite anecdotal accounts of this occurring, practically, it would add little value (and in fact will cause many more problems) in a potentially challenging situation. Slashing the sides of the pool is likely to flood the immediate area, create hazards with electrical equipment, and release floating debris in the water and there will be no control over how the water escapes. A safer method would be to, in the event of a collapse, support the woman's head to remain above the water line (some midwives or birth pool packs carry neck flotation devices) and manage removal in a safe and controlled manner. Emergency skills and drills for home birth attending midwives and paramedics should include safe emergency evacuation of the pool.

WHEN TO ADVISE LEAVING THE POOL

It is important that, as with any labour and birth, any deviations from normal physiological processes or concerns regarding maternal or fetal wellbeing be immediately addressed and escalated. Such concerns might include (list non-exhaustive):

- Fetal distress or heart rate concerns
- Any concerns about maternal wellbeing
- Concerns about progress of labour in first or second stage
- Any request for opioid or epidural analgesia/request to leave pool
- Any vaginal bleeding
- Maternal pyrexia - where leaving the pool may correct overheating caused by the water being too hot. However, also take into consideration recommendations for escalation if pyrexial on two separate occasions 30 minutes apart (NICE, 2017)
- Maternal hypertension or tachycardia
- Meconium-stained liquor
- Any obstetric emergency

Emergency care at home has been discussed elsewhere in this book. These arrangements remain appropriate for emergency care in water at home unless discussed here specially. Principles of identifying evolving deterioration should be closely followed including maintaining situational awareness, appropriate staffing, and equipment; as well, ongoing dynamic risk assessment will ensure that concerns are identified in a timely manner and escalated. Where possible women should be asked to remove themselves from the pool; however, if the woman is unable to move herself, immediate assistance should be summoned. It may be necessary to stabilise the woman and then move after; clinical judgement in this case should prevail.

CONCLUSION

Water immersion during labour and waterbirth is a low-tech intervention that optimises the normal physiological processes of labour and birth. We call for midwives and maternity professionals to familiarise themselves with labour and birth care in a birthing pool to ensure more women have access to its benefits. Pain management is a key element of respectful and dignified maternity care, in which we advocate birthing pools should be as available as pharmacological options and be encouraged, where possible, for those planning a homebirth. Fundamentally, clinical care for women who choose to labour and birth at home in water differs little from physiological birth on dry land. This chapter has discussed some of the additional considerations from an organisational perspective and attending midwives to support respectful and safe care for birthing pool use at home.

REFERENCES

Asakura, H., 2004. Fetal and neonatal thermoregulation. Journal of Nippon Medical School, 71(6), pp. 360–370.

Aughey, H., Jardine, J., Moitt, N. et al, 2021. Waterbirth: a national retrospective cohort study of factors associated with its use among women in England. BMC Pregnancy Childbirth, 21, p. 256. https://doi.org/10.1186/s12884-021-03724-6

Benfield, R., Hortobágyi, T., Tanner, C., Swanson, M., Heitkemper, M. and Newton, E., 2010. The effects of hydrotherapy on anxiety, pain, neuroendocrine responses, and contraction dynamics during labor. Biological Research for Nursing, 12(1), pp. 28–36.

Burns, E., Boulton, M., Cluett, E., Cornelius, V. and Smith, L., 2012. Characteristics, interventions, and outcomes of women who used a birthing pool: a prospective observational study. Birth, 39(3), pp. 192–202.

Burns, E., Feeley, C., Hall, P.J. and Vanderlaan, J., 2022. Systematic review and meta-analysis to examine intrapartum interventions, and maternal and neonatal outcomes following immersion in water during labour and waterbirth. BMJ Open, 12(7), p. e056517.

Burns, E., Hunter, L., Rodd, Z., Macleod, M. and Smith, L., 2019. Developing and evaluating an online learning tool to improve midwives' accuracy of visual estimation of blood loss during waterbirth: an experimental study. Midwifery, 68, pp. 65–73.

Carpenter, J., Burns, E. and Smith, L., 2022. Factors associated with normal physiologic birth for women who labor in water: a secondary analysis of a prospective observational study. Journal of Midwifery & Women's Health, 67(1), pp. 13–20.

Cortes, E., Basra, R. and Kelleher, C., 2011. Waterbirth and pelvic floor injury: a retrospective study and postal survey using ICIQ modular long form questionnaires. European Journal of Obstetrics, Gynecology, and Reproductive Biology, 155(1), pp. 27–30.

Fahy, K., Hastie, C., Bisits, A., Marsh, C., Smith, L. and Saxton, A., 2010. Holistic physiological care compared with active management of the third stage of labour for women at low risk of postpartum haemorrhage: a cohort study. Women and Birth: Journal of the Australian College of Midwives, 23(4), pp. 146–152.

Feeley, C., Cooper, M. and Burns, E., 2021. A systematic meta-thematic synthesis to examine the views and experiences of women following water immersion during labour and waterbirth. Journal of Advanced Nursing, 77(7), pp. 2942–2956.

Fry, J., 2013. Physiological third stage of labour: support it or lose it. British Journal of Midwifery, 15(11), pp. 693–695.

Hall, S. and Holloway, I., 1998. Staying in control: women's experiences of labour in water. Midwifery, 14(1), pp. 30–36.

Haseeb, Y., Alkunaizi, A., Al Turki, H., Aljama, F. and Sobhy, S., 2014. The impact of Valsalva's versus spontaneous pushing techniques during second stage of labor on postpartum maternal fatigue and neonatal outcome. Saudi Journal of Medicine & Medical Sciences, 2(2), pp. 101–105.

Hutton, E.K., Reitsma, A.H. and Kaufman, K., 2009. Outcomes associated with planned home and planned hospital births in low-risk women attended by midwives in Ontario, Canada, 2003–2006: a retrospective cohort study. Birth, 36(3), pp. 180–189.

Jones L, Othman M, Dowswell T, Alfirevic Z, Gates S, Newburn M, Jordan S, Lavender T, Neilson JP. Pain management for women in labour: an overview of systematic reviews. Cochrane Database of Systematic Reviews 2012, Issue 3. Art. No.: CD009234. DOI: 10.1002/14651858.CD009234.pub2.

Lanier, A. L., Wiegand, S. L., Fennig, K., Snow, E. K., Maxwell, R. A., & McKenna, D. (2021). Neonatal Outcomes After Delivery in Water. Obstetrics and gynecology, 138(4), 622–626. https://doi.org/10.1097/AOG.0000000000004545

Lukasse, M., Rowe, R., Townend, J., Knight, M. and Hollowell, J., 2014. Immersion in water for pain relief and the risk of intrapartum transfer among low risk nulliparous women: secondary analysis of the Birthplace national prospective cohort study. BMC Pregnancy and Childbirth, 14, pp. 60.

Maude, R., 2004. Using water for labour and birth – fiction, evidence and stories, New Zealand College of Midwives 8th Biennial National Conference, 16–18 September 2004, Wellington Convention Centre, Wellington, New Zealand.

Maude, R. and Foureur, M., 2007. It's beyond water: stories of women's experience of using water for labour and birth. Woman and Birth, 20(1), pp. 17–24.

NICE, 2017. Intrapartum care for healthy women and babies, https://www.nice.org.uk/guidance/cg190

Reitsma, A., Simioni, J., Brunton, G., Kaufman, K. and Hutton, E.K., 2020. Maternal outcomes and birth interventions among women who begin labour intending to give birth at home compared to women of low obstetrical risk who intend to give birth in hospital: a systematic review and meta-analyses. The Lancet, 21, 100319.

Sharpe, E. and Arendt, K., 2017. Epidural labor analgesia and maternal fever. Clinical Obstetrics and Gynecology, 60(2), pp. 365–374.

Sidebottom, A. C., Vacquier, M., Simon, K., Wunderlich, W., Fontaine, P., Dahlgren-Roemmich, D., Steinbring, S., Hyer, B., & Saul, L. (2020). Maternal and Neonatal Outcomes in Hospital-Based Deliveries With Water Immersion. Obstetrics and gynecology, 136(4), 707–715. https://doi.org/10.1097/AOG.0000000000003956

Sprague, A., 2004. The outcomes and experiences of deep water immersion during childbirth, Master's Thesis: Australian Catholic University St Patrick's Campus Melbourne, Victoria.

Thornton, J. and Dahlen, H., 2020. The UK Obstetric Anal Sphincter Injury (OASI) Care Bundle: a critical review. Midwifery, 90, p. 102801.

Ulfsdottir, H., Saltvedt, S., Ekborn, M. and Georgsson, S., 2018. Like an empowering micro-home: a qualitative study of women's experience of giving birth in water. Midwifery, 67, pp. 26–31.

Wright, A., Nassar, A.H., Visser, G., Ramasauskaite, D. and Theron, G., 2021. FIGO good clinical practice paper: management of the second stage of labor. International Journal of Gynecology & Obstetrics, 152(2), pp. 172–181.

CHAPTER 8

PHYSIOLOGICAL BREECH BIRTH AT HOME

Dr Shawn Walker, Amy Meadowcroft, Emma Spillane

BACKGROUND

This chapter covers vaginal breech births that occur in the woman's home. The approach described in this chapter is informed by research concerning physiological breech birth (Walker et al, 2016a; Walker et al, 2016b) and the Opti-Breech Care Trial (https://optibreech.uk) (Walker, 2022). Physiological breech birth training has been fully evaluated within the UK (Walker, 2017) including the only evaluation to include clinical outcome data (Mattiolo et al, 2021).

A completely spontaneous vaginal breech birth, needing no assistance, is a dance between mother and baby. Our goal as midwives is to create the potential – hold the space – for that to occur while recognising the times when an equally beautiful and empowering outcome is best achieved with swift assistance from skilled hands.

INDIVIDUALISED CARE PLANNING

BREECH PRESENTATION DIAGNOSED IN LABOUR

The most reliable way to detect breech presentation in the third trimester is by routine ultrasound scan (Salim et al, 2021). Increasingly, these are done by midwives in hospital and community settings using handheld scanning devices (Keable et al, 2018; Barnfield et al, 2019). This approach is clinically effective and economically efficient (Wastlund et al, 2019) and avoids the increase in interventions associated with routine third trimester biometric scans (Bricker et al, 2015). Home birth teams may wish to consider implementing routine presentation scanning.

Without routine ultrasound, the rate of breech presentation diagnosed in labour is 20–30% (Walker, 2013; Walker and Cochrane, 2015). Almost all of these will be low-risk women who have no other indications for a third trimester scan, and approximately one-third of these will remain undiagnosed despite multiple examinations in labour. This is because the anterior buttock leads in normal breech mechanisms and is often mistaken for a head with 'sutures not felt', and the anal cleft is not palpable on vaginal examination until the cervix is dilated to 6 cm or more.

For most women, regardless of the outcome, diagnosis of breech presentation in labour is a fearful and traumatic event (Lightfoot, 2018). Midwives have a pivotal role in ensuring women feel in control, which has a significant impact on their psychological adjustment to the events of their birth (Walker and Cochrane, 2015; Lightfoot, 2018; Cook and Loomis, 2012). A breech presentation diagnosed in labour at home should be escalated to enable the option of a swift transfer to a hospital setting. If the birth is progressing quickly, it may be safer to remain at home as the baby emerges. If the woman is fully dilated, do not attempt to interfere with descent. The risk of cord compression increases as the baby descends in the pelvis and attempting to stop this progress until arrival at the hospital could introduce a risk of hypoxia. If any part of the baby is visible, prepare for a birth at home, unless this is a foot and you have confirmed that the cervix is not yet completely dilated.

If you are transferring care and there is likely to be time to offer the woman a caesarean birth, you should begin to offer her basic counselling about this option, using the current Royal College of Obstetricians and Gynaecologists (RCOG) (Impey et al, 2017) and your employer's guideline as a reference. Make sure the person knows whether you or a member of your team can offer them continuing support for a vaginal breech birth if that is their preference. Midwives may find it helpful to consider in advance their own level of experience in reference to available competency frameworks (Walker et al, 2016a) and whom they could call for support should this situation occur.

PLANNED BREECH BIRTH AT HOME

Giving birth to a breech baby at home is likely to have the same benefits as planning a cephalic home birth, such as a quicker labour, reduced need for pharmacological pain relief, and less risk of intervention (Birthplace in England Collaborative Group, 2011). But the potential risks of a vaginal breech birth are different from cephalic birth, no matter what the setting (Impey et al, 2017). Studies in multiple settings have demonstrated that when breech births become complicated at home, a severe adverse outcome is more likely to result (Symon et al, 2010; Cheyney et al, 2014; Bastian et al, 2014). Because of this, most healthcare providers will recommend birth in a hospital setting. In centralised settings there is easy access to obstetric services, in case an emergency caesarean birth is needed, and neonatal services, in case immediate neonatal care is required.

When a home breech birth is planned, documentation should cover discussion of these risks, the offer of a physiological breech birth in a hospital setting if possible, and availability of experienced attendants. Evidence indicates that some women choose to give birth at home because they feel they will not be supported to plan a physiological breech birth with minimal disturbance in a hospital-based setting (Symon et al, 2010; Dhalen, 2014; Kotaska, 2011). We all have a duty to address the alienation some women feel that prevents them from accessing care that would benefit them.

If breech birth at home is planned, you should have a low threshold for transfer into hospital if all is not progressing straightforwardly. Indications include but are not limited to meconium-stained liquor at any point during the *first* stage of labour, active pushing of over an hour, and any other variations from normal. The availability and response time of an ambulance and the potential transfer time to the nearest maternity unit should also be considered and discussed when planning care.

Further information to inform counselling for mode of birth is available from the RCOG *Management of Breech Presentation* guideline (Impey et al, 2017).

BREECH BIRTH IN WATER

Many women who plan for a homebirth opt to have a birthing pool. There is no contraindication to using water for pain relief in the first stage of labour. And there is no evidence that breech birth in water carries any greater risk than with cephalic birth. However, facilitating a birth in water adds additional complexity to what is likely to be a new or unfamiliar skill for many midwives, managing a vaginal breech birth. Therefore, especially for unplanned events where there is time, we recommend giving birth out of water, where visualisation, monitoring, and manoeuvres are all easier. However, if an undiagnosed breech emerges in water and is progressing rapidly, there may be little benefit of moving the woman at that point. Instead, consider getting out of the pool your first manoeuvre if you perceive any delay.

VARIATIONS OF BREECH PRESENTATION

Breech babies can assume a variety of positions:

Extended/frank: Fetal sacrum presenting, legs extended, feet up by head.

Flexed/complete: Fetal sacrum +/− feet presenting, hips flexed, knees flexed. Feet may be just below sacrum but legs are not extended.

Semi-flexed/incomplete: Sacrum +/− one foot presenting, both hips flexed, one knee flexed, one knee extended up or down.

Kneeling: Hips are extended and one or both knees present before the sacrum.

Standing/footling: Hips are extended and foot or feet present with the fetal sacrum not in maternal pelvis.

The type of breech presentation at diagnosis may also be different during the birth as the baby continues to move and flex its limbs (Russell, 1969). All variations of breech presentation can be delivered vaginally and will follow the same principles of the normal mechanism, but the risk of cord prolapse differs. Cord prolapse is just as unlikely as cephalic presentation with the fetus in extended breech position (0.5%, 1:200) with the fetal sacrum engaged in maternal pelvis. For a flexed/semi-flexed breech, the risk is 5% (1:20) (Ghesquière et al, 2020; Broche et al, 2005). Very little data is available about the outcomes of kneeling and standing breech presentations at term, but it can be assumed to be higher due to the irregularity of the presenting parts. Outcomes following cord prolapse for a breech are generally good, but a delay in transfer to the hospital could compromise the baby (Ghesquière et al, 2020; Broche et al, 2005).

FLEXED BREECH PRESENTATION AND THE 'DROPPED FOOT'

With any variation of flexed legs, one or both feet will almost always be felt on vaginal examination. This should not be considered an indication for a caesarean birth, provided progression and well-being parameters are normal. As labour progresses one limb will often slip down, a 'dropped foot' baby. Contrary to popular belief, this variation is not at higher risk than an extended breech presentation at term (Ghesquière et al, 2020; Broche et al, 2005). A 'dropped foot' usually occurs at advanced dilation and descent, when there is increased room under the sacrum, and can be viewed as a positive sign of progress. Nothing needs to be done with the limb; it is especially important that it is not pulled or pushed, which could potentially interfere with the normal mechanism and therefore cause complications. Limbs which are born prior to the birth can often be bruised and swollen; this is not harmful to the baby and you can reassure parents that the bruising will resolve within the first few weeks.

NORMAL BREECH PHYSIOLOGY

MATERNAL BIRTH POSITION

We have written the remainder of this chapter with the assumption that most women giving birth to a breech baby at home will be in an upright position. This is commonly a kneeling position, leaning slightly forward with forearms rested on a bed, couch, chair, or lap, which enables the birthing person to squat back easily onto their heels. The available evidence indicates that where attendants have appropriate training, both women and healthcare professionals prefer this upright position as a default.[5,26] Use of upright positioning in vaginal breech births reduces the length of second stage, interventions required, and maternal and neonatal injuries (Mattiolo et al. 2021; Louwen et al, 2017; Bogner et al. 2015).

But upright positioning is a tool and not a rule of physiological breech birth (Walker et al, 2016b). All manoeuvres follow the same principles as those used in supine birth, focussing on rotation and/or flexion rather than traction.

OPTIMAL TIME INTERVALS

When Mary Cronk encouraged birth attendants to keep their 'Hands off the Breech!' (Cronk, 1998) she was responding to a dangerous tendency to intervene, especially by pulling, even in births that were progressing normally. Unfortunately, there has been an equally dangerous tendency to avoid intervening, coupled with minimal education about how to recognise abnormality. Many previous recommendations focussed only on delay following birth of the pelvis or umbilicus, but we now know that breech babies are also at increased risk of asphyxia due to cord compression at later stages of descent in the maternal pelvis. Having an overall sense of 'normal' time intervals helps to determine when intervention is likely to be of more benefit than risk.

The available evidence (Spillane et al. 2022; Reitter et al. 2020) indicates that, in most births with good outcomes that require no interventions, the birth is complete within 5 minutes of 'rumping' – that is, +3 station, when both buttocks and the anus are visible between contractions. Most births with good outcomes that require no interventions are complete within 3 minutes of the birth of the fetal pelvis, and within about a minute of when the umbilicus and/or arms are born. This does not mean that a spontaneous birth outside of these parameters is not possible. But the reality of vaginal breech birth is that some heads require 4 or more minutes to be born, even with assistance, and it is difficult to predict which ones will prove trickier than others.

For this reason, our safest expectation is one of continuous progress following rumping. The woman should feel the urge to push continuously as the fetus is emerging regardless of contractions (Walker et al. 2022). This should not be interrupted and should be encouraged, if necessary, to achieve a swift birth. **DO NOT instruct a woman to wait for the next contraction following the birth of the body.** There is nothing in the uterus at this point and the next contraction, which may be after some time, will begin the process of placental separation. If a delay in progress of 30 seconds occurs, or if there is a deviation from the normal mechanism such as lack of rotation, encourage maternal movement and effort – 'wiggle and push' – as a first-line intervention. If this is unsuccessful, suggested interventions are summarised below and in the Physiological Breech Birth Algorithm (Fig. 8.1A).

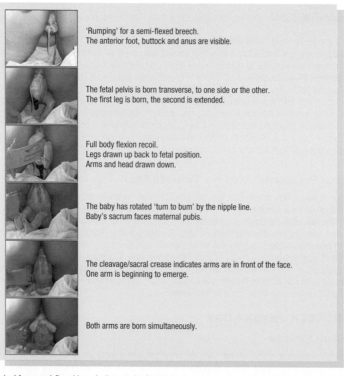

'Rumping' for a semi-flexed breech.
The anterior foot, buttock and anus are visible.

The fetal pelvis is born transverse, to one side or the other.
The first leg is born, the second is extended.

Full body flexion recoil.
Legs drawn up back to fetal position.
Arms and head drawn down.

The baby has rotated 'tum to bum' by the nipple line.
Baby's sacrum faces maternal pubis.

The cleavage/sacral crease indicates arms are in front of the face.
One arm is beginning to emerge.

Both arms are born simultaneously.

Fig. 8.1 A. 'Rumping' for a semi-flexed breech; the anterior foot, buttock, and anus are visible. The fetal pelvis is born transverse, to one side or the other; the first leg is born, and the second is extended. Full body flexion recoil; legs drawn up back to fetal position; arms and head drawn down. The baby has rotated 'tum to bum' by the nipple line; baby's sacrum faces maternal pubis. The cleavage/sacral crease indicates that arms are in front of the face; one arm is beginning to emerge. Both arms are born simultaneously. Baby makes a second attempt at flexion; tone is less than before and chin does not become visible. Checking to confirm the chin is low, head is at the pelvic outlet. Simple shoulder press; fingers across the chest, just below the clavicle; push straight back between maternal thighs; pubic bone pushes occiput forward as the face sweeps down across the perineum. Baby remains face-down for the first 10–15 seconds after birth to allow fluids to drain from air passages. Baby is ready to react. (Picture source Shawn Walker, c. 2013.) **B.** 'Wiggle and push'. (Illustration: Merlin Strangeway.)

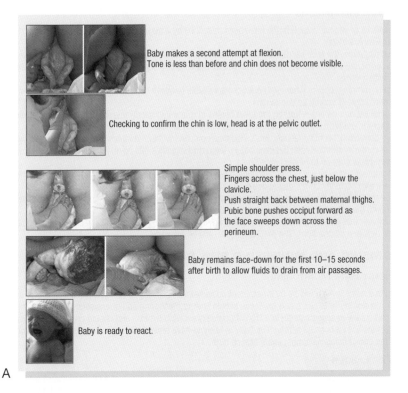

Baby makes a second attempt at flexion.
Tone is less than before and chin does not become visible.

Checking to confirm the chin is low, head is at the pelvic outlet.

Simple shoulder press.
Fingers across the chest, just below the clavicle.
Push straight back between maternal thighs.
Pubic bone pushes occiput forward as the face sweeps down across the perineum.

Baby remains face-down for the first 10–15 seconds after birth to allow fluids to drain from air passages.

Baby is ready to react.

A

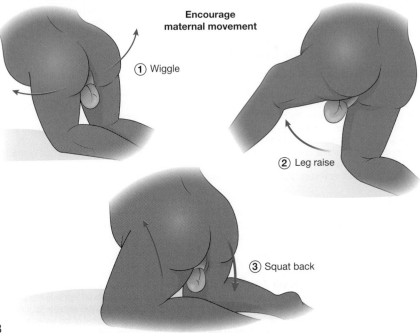

Encourage maternal movement

① Wiggle

② Leg raise

③ Squat back

B

Fig. 8.1, cont'd

THE NORMAL MECHANISMS

The mechanisms of vaginal breech births have been described by a number of authors (Louwen et al. 2017; Reitter et al. 2020; Evans, 2012a).

1. After full dilatation, the fetal sacrum descends into the birth canal. The anterior buttock leads and is seen first. The fetus is facing the mother's side, sacrum transverse. Buttocks will advance with a contraction and retract between, just as with a vertex.
2. Eventually 'rumping' occurs when both buttocks are visible between contractions. At this point, the 7-minute clock starts, and progress should be continuous.
3. As the fetal sacrum emerges further, the fetus begins to rotate into sacro-anterior or 'tum to bum'. Following birth of the sacrum, the birth should be complete in less than 5 minutes.
4. Legs are born almost simultaneously. Birth should be complete within 3 minutes following delivery of the umbilicus – a loop of cord can often be seen between baby's legs which signifies this point. Rotation should be complete by the time the fetus is born up to nipple line/scapula.
5. An uncompromised baby will usually exhibit a full-body flexion reflex 'tummy crunch' to bring down the arms, which are also normally born simultaneously, and to aid flexion of the head.
6. The face then sweeps the perineum as the occiput rotates around the pubic arch and birth is complete. In an upright birth the baby falls forward, helping to drain fluids from the air passage.

In the event that a foot/leg/both legs are delivered first, the 7-minute clock will still start when the buttocks are both visible between contractions. The mechanism will still be the same.

RECOGNISING AND MINIMISING RISK DURING LABOUR

FETAL HEART RATE MONITORING

Monitoring in a home setting will be by intermittent auscultation. Following rumping, it will become very difficult to accurately monitor the fetal heart, and the focus should shift to monitoring and/or assisting progress. A high or rising baseline, particularly in second stage, is a sign of gradually evolving hypoxia and should prompt consideration of immediate transfer to a hospital setting. The baby is likely to have fewer reserves to cope with the cord occlusion that occurs at the end of labour in almost every breech birth.

LENGTH OF LABOUR

The progress of labour, dilation, and descent, are the most predictive indicators of a straightforward breech birth (Walker et al, 2016 b). Passive second stages, even in women without epidural pain relief, are not uncommon (Goffinet et al. 2006). Descent should still occur during this period, and the RCOG guideline suggests that active pushing should not be encouraged until the buttocks are visible on the perineum (Impey et al, 2017). There is an association between active second stages of longer than 20–40 minutes and adverse neonatal outcomes (Azria et al. 2012; Su et al. 2003; MacHarey et al. 2017). This should be considered in light of transfer distances required if help is needed.

RELIEVING OBSTRUCTED LABOUR

MINIMISING DELAY ON THE PERINEUM

In cephalic birth a midwife may observe the vertex long before the birth of the baby. With a baby in a head-down position, it is still easy to auscultate the fetal heart at this point in the second stage and there is no cord compression as the body is in the uterus and not in the maternal pelvis. With a breech baby however, when the sacrum is on the perineum, the fetal body is in maternal pelvis and cord compression is likely; it will also likely be impossible to auscultate the fetal heart at this point. Therefore birth needs to occur swiftly to optimise fetal outcome.

If both buttocks are visible between contractions (rumping) but the pelvis is not born with the next contraction, intervention needs to be taken. This can include:

- Encouraging maternal movement, change of position, and/or pushing
- Buttock lift
- Perineal sweep
- Episiotomy, which can be performed with the woman in an upright position

You should expect the pelvis to be born with the next maternal effort after an episiotomy. If any further delay occurs, consider transfer and/or expect the need for neonatal resuscitation (Fig. 8.1B).

MINIMISING DELAY DURING EMERGENCE

Should delay occur following the birth of the pelvis, the first intervention is to encourage maternal movement, such as shaking or wiggling her bottom side to side (Evans, 2012 b). Getting her to lift her leg into a 'lunge' or 'running start' position – lifting the leg on the side the baby is facing – increases the space in the pelvis on that side and progress may resume. If these interventions do not result in progress, delivering the legs can help you evaluate your next steps. This can be done by placing your thumbs or forefingers between the baby's legs at the level of the knees and drawing them to the sides of baby's body – the legs will bend at the knee like a frog and flop out.

If you need to intervene to assist the birth at any point, you should carry on assisting. In physiological breech birth you are only intervening because you have recognised a delay that maternal movement and effort alone have not resolved. It may also be that the initial problem occurs due to a complication at the next stage of birth. For example, if the legs are not born spontaneously at roughly the same time, this could be due to a complication with the arms as they are navigating the inlet of the pelvis. Similarly, delay with the arms may be the result of delayed engagement of the aftercoming head. With any complication, you should also expect to provide respiratory support to the infant at birth, maintaining an intact umbilicus ideally until spontaneous respiration begins.[1]

RESOLVING ARM COMPLICATIONS

Partial Rotation

If rotation has started but the full 90-degree turn has not completed and a delay occurs, this usually indicates that the pubic arm is stuck at the pelvic outlet on the ischial spine (Reitter et al. 2020). Maternal movement or 'running start' may resolve this issue (Walker, 2017). If not, the arm can be swept down by inserting two fingers behind the pubic shoulder and sweeping the arm down across the baby's face and chest. The rotation will then be complete and the sacral arm should spontaneously deliver. If not, it can be swept down using your other hand, sweeping the arm across the baby's face and chest. You should then assist delivery of the head immediately.

No Rotation

If there is no rotation at all as the baby descends – the baby is still facing to one side completely – this may indicate an obstruction of the pubic arm on the symphysis pubis. The baby has their arm up beside or behind their head, preventing descent into the pelvis, known as a 'nuchal arm'. Using flat hands on the baby's chest and back, as far up as you can reach, use finger pressure along the shoulder girdle to rotate the baby to face the arm that is caught – face-to-pubes (Walker et al. 2020). The pubic arm will then be felt in front of the baby and can be gently drawn down across the body using your fingers. Keeping your hands in place, rotate the baby back (tum-to-bum) to restore the mechanism. The sacral arm should spontaneously deliver when you rotate the baby back, but if not, it can be swept down. If the rotations are difficult and the arm(s) feel impacted, push the baby back up to a higher station, and attempt rotation again. You should proceed to assist delivery of the head immediately (Fig. 8.2).

VARIATIONS OF HEAD ENTRAPMENT

Head entrapment is arguably the clinician's greatest fear with breech birth. For term breech babies, the likelihood of the diameter of the head being greater than the diameter of the fetal pelvis combined with fetal legs is very small. A more likely situation is that the head is not flexed in the ideal manner through the baby's efforts alone. A well-oxygenated, neurologically intact fetus will assist in their own birth (Walker et al, 2016 b). Once the legs are born, they will exhibit a full-body flexion reflex (Reitter et al. 2020; Evans, 2012b). The baby attempts to return to their normal fetal position, pulling legs up and arms and head down towards the abdomen. When a baby becomes compromised due to hypoxia, they will not do this, and more active assistance will be required.

When the aftercoming head is not born spontaneously, attendants' greatest advantage is understanding what is happening.

Obstruction at the Pelvic Outlet or Mid-Pelvis

This is the most common occurrence and can be unpredictable. In this situation your goal is to elevate the occiput, pushing it back up into the pelvis as much as possible to give the head room to flex. You can do this manually, with

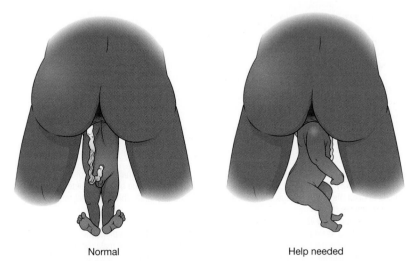

Normal   Help needed

Fig. 8.2 Lack of rotation by the nipple line, rotational manoeuvres needed. (Image: Merlin Strangeway.)

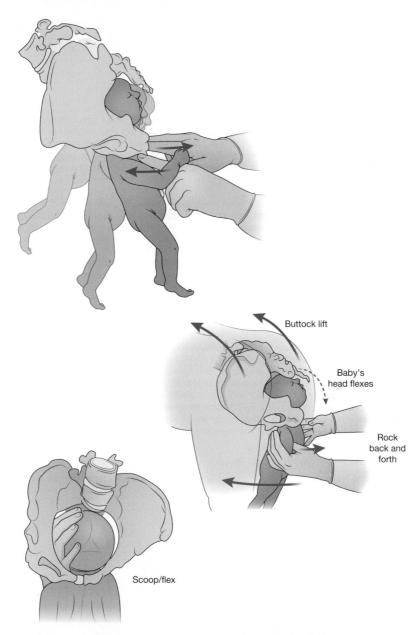

Fig. 8.3 The principles of shoulder press. (Image: Merlin Strangeway.)

the fingers of one hand, while the fingers of the other hand press down on the malar bones of the fetal face to flex the head. You can also do it by performing a shoulder press manoeuvre, gripping the baby's shoulder girdle and moving the whole body through the maternal legs, straight back towards the abdomen. This uses fetal reflexes and the maternal pubic bone to flex the head.

The same principles apply when the head is stuck mid-pelvis (Fig. 8.3).

If the head is aligned, facing the sacrum, elevate the occiput, pushing it back up into the pelvis. Bring the chin and face down, using either shoulder press or your fingers. Fingers can be placed on the malar bones, or the entire hand can be scooped in alongside the head until the fingers are over the forehead/sinciput, face-to-palm. Flex the face down.

When there is a tight fit, be patient and keep repeating the actions to flex the head. An assistant can help by lifting the maternal buttocks up and away from the perineum, which lifts the sacrum slightly and helps the perineum sweep over the forehead. An assistant can also scoop-and-flex the head internally at the same time as shoulder press is attempted (Fig. 8.4).

Obstruction at the Pelvic Inlet

The head can also become trapped because it is extended at the pelvic inlet. You will recognise this by running a finger up along the baby's neck. If the chin is felt just within the introitus, the head is engaged in the pelvis. If the head is extended and unengaged, you will have to run your finger quite high, until you reach only the bottom of the chin. The shoulders will be tight against the perineum, and the chest usually puffed out. If this happens, attempt to fold the shoulders akin to the shoulder press, pushing, push the whole baby back up so that the head lifts off the pelvic inlet. You can then use flat hands to rotate the baby to oblique or transverse to assist engagement of the head. If the head is impacted, it may help to use your fingers alongside the occiput to push it into oblique to release (Fig. 8.5).

MISALIGNMENT

Once in the pelvis, sometimes the head needs assistance to align, occiput-anterior, face-to-sacrum, in order to be born. You may feel an ear instead of the baby's chin when you run your finger up. When this happens, you can use your whole hand on the pubic side of the face to scoop and flex the forehead into alignment.

CERVICAL HEAD ENTRAPMENT

A false cervical head entrapment can occur if the uterus is slightly prolapsed, low in the pelvis, and remains around the baby's face as it descends. This occurs with some multiparous women, but the cervix remains loose and can be pushed back over the face, which can then be flexed to deliver.

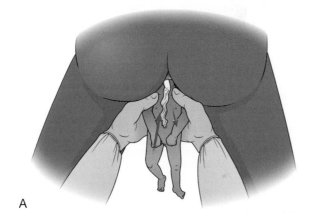

A

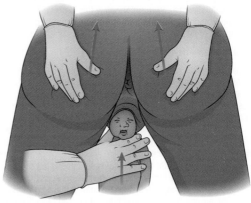

B

Fig. 8.4 A. Thumb position for shoulder girdle grip. B. Buttock lift. (Image: Merlin Strangeway.)

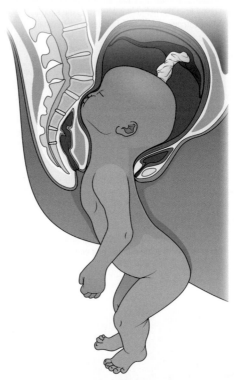

Fig. 8.5 Head entrapment at the pelvic inlet. (Reproduced by kind permission of the Breech Birth Network)

True cervical head entrapment for a term baby is rare, as the diameter of the pelvis is roughly equivalent to the head (10 cm). But it can occur if there is delay in recognising head extension at the inlet. This is because with the head at the inlet and the shoulders born, nothing is holding the cervix open. It can retract, much like following the birth of a first twin. For this reason, we recognise that if the chin is not visible and/or the mother's anus is not dilated following birth of the arms, the attendant should determine if the head is in the pelvis and assist it swiftly if not.

REVERSE FACE PRESENTATION

This is uncommon, but it does happen. If, on investigation, you feel no chin and no ear, the occiput may have engaged first, in a reverse face presentation. When this occurs, chin will be posterior and occiput anterior. If the birth is progressing with maternal effort, simply allow this to occur. If not, you may need to gently move the baby's body towards the maternal abdomen, tummy to tummy. In extreme circumstances the fetal head may need to be displaced upwards, over the inlet of the maternal pelvis, so that it can re-engage face-first (Fig. 8.6).

OPTIMISING NEONATAL OUTCOMES

Midwives attending a breech birth at home should have their resuscitation equipment laid out, close to the birthing mother, ready in case it is required. It can be covered with a towel so as not to cause anxiety for the woman or birth partners. Breech babies are commonly born appearing stunned, and you should expect this. If you need to handle, assess, or stimulate the baby, do this with the baby facing down or to the side for the first 10–15 seconds to allow fluids to drain from the baby's mouth.

If ventilation support is needed, it is particularly important for breech babies that this occur with the umbilicus intact until the onset of spontaneous respirations. Acute hypoxia due to cord occlusion is the most common cause of reduced Apgars in the first minute of life after a breech birth. Preserving the umbilical connection to the placenta is the quickest way to ensure oxygenated blood immediately reaches the baby. This can be confirmed by auscultating the neonate's heart; the rate will rise audibly even without ventilation as the occlusion is released.

Neonatal physiology research has identified that cord clamping prior to the establishment of respiration in mildly hypoxic infants may initiate a reflex bradycardia and reduction in cardiac output, due to sudden cessation of blood flow returning to the heart. Such an ischemic insult may exacerbate any asphyxic insult (Kluckow and Hooper, 2015; Hooper at al. 2015). Initiation of ventilation with an intact umbilicus has the potential to reduce the need for extensive

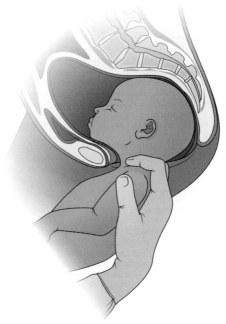

Fig. 8.6 Reverse face presentation. Moving baby's body to maternal body.

resuscitation, neonatal intensive care admissions, and long-term adverse outcomes related to hypoxic-ischemic encephalopathy, including birth-related cerebral palsy (Kluckow and Hooper, 2015; Hooper at al. 2015).

SUMMARY

When breech births occur at home, the principles of physiological breech birth can help achieve a safe-as-possible outcome. Enable the woman to be upright and active. Encourage her to 'wiggle and push' if you suspect delay once both buttocks are visible on the perineum. Assist if strong maternal effort does not result in significant descent. And be prepared to assist neonatal transition with the umbilicus intact.

REFERENCES

Azria, E., le Meaux, J.P., Khoshnood, B., Alexander, S., Subtil, D. and Goffinet, F. (2012) Factors associated with adverse perinatal outcomes for term breech fetuses with planned vaginal delivery, American Journal of Obstetrics and Gynecology; 207(4): 285.e1–9. doi:10.1016/j.ajog.2012.08.027

Barnfield, L., Bamfo, J. and Norman, L. (2019) Should midwives learn to scan for presentation? Findings from a large survey of midwives in the UK, British Journal of Midwifery; 27(5): 305–311. doi:10.12968/bjom.2019.27.5.305

Bastian, H., Keirse, M.J. and Lancaster, P.A. (1998) Perinatal death associated with planned home birth in Australia: Population based study, BMJ; 317(7155): 384–388.

Birthplace in England Collaborative Group. (2011) Perinatal and maternal outcomes by planned place of birth for healthy women with low risk pregnancies: The Birthplace in England national prospective cohort study, BMJ; 343: d7400. doi:10.1136/bmj.d7400

Bricker, L., Medley, N. and Pratt, J. (2015) Routine ultrasound in late pregnancy (after 24 weeks' gestation), Cochrane Database of Systematic Reviews; (6): CD001451. doi:10.1002/14651858.CD001451.pub4

Broche, D.E., Riethmuller, D., Vidal, C., Sautière, J.L., Schaal, J.P. and Maillet, R. (2005)[AK1] Obstetric and perinatal outcomes of a disreputable presentation: The nonfrank breech, Journal de Gynecologie, Obstetrique et Biologie de la Reproduction; 34(8): 781–788. Accessed September 26 2022. Available at: http://www.ncbi.nlm.nih.gov/pubmed/16319769

Bogner, G., Strobl, M., Schausberger, C., Fischer, T., Reisenberger, K. and Jacobs, V.R. (2015) Breech delivery in the all fours position: a prospective observational comparative study with classic assistance, Journal of Perinatal Medicine; 43(6): 707–713. doi:10.1515/jpm-2014-0048

Cheyney, M., Bovbjerg, M., Everson, C., Gordon, W., Hannibal, D. and Vedam, S. (2014) Outcomes of care for 16,924 planned home births in the United States: The Midwives Alliance of North America Statistics Project, 2004 to 2009, Journal of Midwifery & Women's Health; 59(1): 17–27. doi:10.1111/JMWH.12172

Cook, K. and Loomis, C. (2012) The impact of choice and control on women's childbirth experiences, Journal of Perinatal Education; 21(3): 158–168. doi:10.1891/1058-1243.21.3.158

Cronk, M. (1998) Hands off the breech, Practising Midwife; 1(6): 13–15.

Dahlen, H. (2014) Undone by fear? Deluded by trust? Midwifery; Published online September 2014. doi:10.1016/j.midw.2014.09.004

Evans, J. (2012a) Understanding physiological breech birth, Essentially MIDIRS; 3(2): 17–21.

Evans, J. (2012b) The final piece of the breech birth jigsaw? Essentially MIDIRS; 3(3): 46–49. Available at: http://search.ebscohost.com/login.aspx?direct=true&db=jlh&AN=2011522453&site=ehost-live

Evans, J. (2014) Undiagnosed breech-part of midwifery practice, Practising Midwife; 17(11): 27–29. Accessed February 2, 2015. Available at: http://0-www.ingentaconnect.com.wam.city.ac.uk/content/mesl/tpm/2014/00000017/00000011/art00009

Ghesquière, L., Demetz, J., Dufour, P., Depret, S., Garabedian, C. and Subtil, D. (2020) Type of breech presentation and prognosis for delivery, Journal of Gynecology Obstetrics and Human Reproduction; 49(9): 101832. doi:10.1016/j.jogoh.2020.101832

Goffinet, F., Carayol, M., Foidart, J.M., et al. (2006) Is planned vaginal delivery for breech presentation at term still an option? Results of an observational prospective survey in France and Belgium, American Journal of Obstetrics and Gynecology; 194(4): 1002–1011. doi:10.1016/j.ajog.2005.10.817

Hooper, S.B., Te Pas, A.B., Lang, J., et al. (2015) Cardiovascular transition at birth: A physiological sequence, Pediatric Research; 77(5): 608–614. doi:10.1038/pr.2015.21

Impey, L., Murphy, D., Griffiths, M., Penna, L. and on behalf of the Royal College of Obstetricians and Gynaecologists. (2017) Management of breech presentation, BJOG; 124(7): e151–e177. doi:10.1111/1471-0528.14465

Keable, J. and Crozier, K. (2018) Detection of breech presentation: Abdominal palpation and hand-held scanning by midwives, British Journal of Midwifery; 26(6): 371–376. doi:10.12968/bjom.2018.26.6.371

Kluckow, M. and Hooper, S. B. (2015) Using physiology to guide time to cord clamping, Seminars in Fetal and Neonatal Medicine; 20(4): 225–231. doi:10.1016/J.SINY.2015.03.002

Kotaska, A. (2011) Commentary: Routine caesarean section for breech: the unmeasured cost, Birth; 38(2): 162–164. doi:10.1111/j.1523-536X.2011.00468.x

Lightfoot, K. (2018) Women's Experiences of Undiagnosed Breech Birth and the Effects on Future Childbirth Decisions and Expectations. DHealthPsych. University of the West of England. Available at: http://eprints.uwe.ac.uk/33278

Louwen, F., Daviss, B., Johnson, K.C. and Reitter, A. (2017) Does breech delivery in an upright position instead of on the back improve outcomes and avoid caesareans? International Journal of Gynecology & Obstetrics; 136(2): 151–161. doi:10.1002/ijgo.12033

MacHarey, G., Ulander, V.M., Heinonen, S., Kostev, K., Nuutila, M. and Vaïsänen-Tommiska, M. (2017) Risk factors and outcomes in "well-selected" vaginal breech deliveries: A retrospective observational study, Journal of Perinatal Medicine; 45(3): 291–297. doi:10.1515/jpm-2015-0342

Mattiolo, S., Spillane, E. and Walker, S. (2021) Physiological breech birth training: An evaluation of clinical practice changes after a one day training program, Birth; 48(4): 558–565. doi:10.1111/birt.12562

Reitter, A., Halliday, A. and Walker, S. (2020) Practical insight into upright breech birth from birth videos: A structured analysis, Birth; 47(2): 211–219. doi:10.1111/birt.12480

Russell, J.G. (1969) The position of the lower limbs in breech presentations, Journal of Obstetrics and Gynaecology of The British Commonwealth; 76(4): 351–353.

Salim, I., Staines-Urias, E., Mathewlynn, S., Drukker, L., Vatish, M. and Impey, L. (2021) The impact of a routine late third trimester growth scan on the incidence, diagnosis, and management of breech presentation in Oxfordshire, UK: A cohort study, PLoS Medicine; 18(1): e1003503. doi:10.1371/journal.pmed.1003503

Spillane, E., Walker, S. and McCourt, C. (2022) Optimal time intervals for vaginal breech births: a case-control study, NIHR Open Research; 2: 45. doi:10.3310/nihropenres.13297.2

Su, M., McLeod, L., Ross, S., et al. (2003) Factors associated with adverse perinatal outcome in the Term Breech Trial, American Journal of Obstetrics and Gynecology; 189(3): 740–745. doi:10.1067/S0002-9378(03)00822-6

Symon, A., Winter, C., Donnan, P.T. and Kirkham, M. (2010) Examining autonomy's boundaries: A follow-up review of perinatal mortality cases in UK Independent midwifery, Birth (Berkeley, Calif.); 37(4): 280–287. http://ovidsp.ovid.com/ovidweb.cgi?T=JS&CSC=Y&NEWS=N&PAGE=fulltext&D=psyc6&AN=2010-24172-003. Accessed September 26 2022.

Walker, S. (2013) Undiagnosed breech: Towards a woman-centred approach, British Journal of Midwifery; 21(5): 316–322. Accessed March 7, 2014. Available at: http://www.intermid.co.uk/cgi-bin/go.pl/library/article.cgi?uid=98340;article=BJM_21_5_316_322

Walker, S. (2017) Running Start. The Midwife, the mother and the breech blog. Available Running start-Breech Birth Network. Accessed September 26 2022.

Walker, S. and Cochrane, V. (2015) Unexpected breech: what can midwives do? Practising Midwife; 18(10): 26–29.

Walker, S., Das, S., Meadowcroft, A. and Spillane, E. (2022) Continuous Cyclic Pushing: A Non-Invasive Approach to Optimising Descent in Vaginal Breech Births. The OptiBreech Project. Accessed June 28, 2022. Available at: https://optibreech.uk/2022/04/03/continuous-cyclic-pushing

Walker, S., Dasgupta, T., Hunter, S., et al. (2022) Preparing for the OptiBreech Trial: A mixed methods implementation and feasibility study, BJOG; 129(S1): 70. doi:10.1111/1471-0528.10_17178

Walker, S., Reading, C., Siverwood-Cope, O. and Cochrane, V. (2017) Physiological breech birth: Evaluation of a training programme for birth professionals, Practising Midwife; 20(2): 25–28.

Walker, S., Scamell, M. and Parker, P. (2016a) Standards for maternity care professionals attending planned upright breech births: A Delphi study, Midwifery; 34: 7–14. doi:10.1016/j.midw.2016.01.007

Walker, S., Scamell, M. and Parker, P. (2016b) Principles of physiological breech birth practice: A Delphi study, Midwifery; 43(0): 1–6. doi:10.1016/j.midw.2016.09.003

Walker, S. and Spillane, E. (2020) Face-to-pubes rotational maneuver for bilateral nuchal arms in a vaginal breech birth, resolved in an upright maternal position: A case report. Birth; 47(2): 246–252. doi:10.1111/birt.12486

Wastlund, D., Moraitis, A.A., Dacey, A., Sovio, U., Wilson, E.C.F. and Smith, G.C.S. (2019) Screening for breech presentation using universal late-pregnancy ultrasonography: A prospective cohort study and cost effectiveness analysis, PLoS Medicine; 16(4): e1002778. doi:10.1371/journal.pmed.1002778

CHAPTER 9

POSTNATAL CARE AT HOME

Anna Madeley

Perhaps one of the most appealing benefits of birth at home for women and birthing people is the prospect of an un-hurried period immediately following the birth of the baby and placenta, without the need to arrange transfer from the labour ward to home or to the postnatal ward for ongoing care.

Postnatal care at home in principle varies little from the care delivered in a hospital setting; however, there are some important practical considerations that involve early detection of problems, timely transfer of care, and logistical factors for attending midwives. This chapter therefore assumes a level of knowledge of both standard recommendations for general postnatal care outlined by national guidance (NICE, 2021) and local guidelines and aims to build upon this by exploring homebirth-specific considerations for the period between birth of the neonate and placenta and until the midwives leave.

PRINCIPLES OF POSTNATAL CARE FOLLOWING HOMEBIRTH

Fundamentally, the principles of postnatal care differ little from that of any other location for birth. Previous discussions with the woman or birthing person and their birth partner should inform the needs, wants, and preferences for postnatal and neonatal care. This may include wishes for skin-to-skin, cord cutting preferences (or not in the case of a lotus birth), who wishes to observe the sex of the neonate and initial and ongoing feeding preferences. NICE (2021, p. 87) recommends early assessment of a woman or birthing person's response to labour and birth and assessment of emotional and psychological condition. Some women may wish to immediately discuss their birth experience, and some may wish to do this after some time. Where birth at home has been unexpected, such as a born before arrival (BBA), this may have been a traumatic or frightening experience; therefore an opportunity to debrief or access support should be invited. All information provided needs to follow the principles of personalised care and therefore should be in a format that is easy to understand, supportive, respectful, evidence based, and consistently presented between clinicians. Information should consider language needs and remain culturally sensitive.

IMMEDIATE CARE OF THE POSTNATAL WOMAN

Provided that the birth has been uneventful and, for the neonate, transfer to extrauterine life has occurred as expected, there is no immediate rush to separate the neonate from their parent to begin immediate postnatal and neonatal checks (see below, *immediate care of the neonate*); however, a continual visual assessment of both should be made to ensure any deterioration is identified early and acted upon. In the meantime, the following can be completed:

- Encourage skin-to-skin and breast- or chestfeeding where appropriate, guided by the parent's wishes.
- If the woman or birthing person wishes to leave the pool, support them to do so.
- You might encourage them to pass urine if possible. Observe volume.
- Respect and support the woman/birthing person's right to cultural or spiritual practices such as lotus birth or the Adhan (Gatrad and Sheikh, 2001; Dennis et al., 2007).
- Arrange for refreshments for the family (and midwives!). Taking a break at this point provided the woman and neonate are stable allows you to plan the next steps and maintain a helicopter view.
- Inform the labour ward coordinator of the birth (see chapter *Antenatal Planning - Organisational Considerations* for discussions of lone working) and to make any arrangements for non-emergency transfer if indicated.
- If placenta has birthed, use this time to examine the placenta, cord, and membranes for completeness. Respect the wishes of the woman/birthing person regarding disposal of the placenta. If the placenta is being disposed of on behalf of the family, bag or box the organ (dependent on local guidelines) and set aside for transport.
- Clear up any rubbish and refuse (keeping blood loss/pads/incontinence pads separate for weighing and in case of a postpartum haemorrhage).
- Take this opportunity to start documentation!

When ready, offer your first set of physiological observations and document on maternal early warning chart and notes (Fig. 9.1). This will assist in identifying any deterioration and allow prompt escalation.

Make sure adequate postnatal analgesia is available and taken by the woman or birthing person. This should have been discussed antenatally and be available – simple analgesia such as paracetamol or ibuprofen can be self-administered by the woman or birthing person.

- Observation and appearance of the woman/birthing person.
- Ask how they are feeling and listen to their response.
- Pain score and location of pain.
- Blood pressure.
- Heart rate.
- Temperature.
- Respirations.
- Neurological response (AVPU- Alert, Verbal/Voice, Pain, Unresponsive).
- Lochia.
- Involution of the uterus (palpated).
- Oxygen saturations (if equipment available).
- Examination of the perineum.

Fig. 9.1 Immediate physiological observations post birth.

Practice Point: Ensure That Clinical Deterioration and Illness Is Identified in All Ethnicities
MBRRACE-UK reports on maternal and perinatal mortality since 2019 (Knight et al., 2019) have highlighted that women or birthing people and babies from some minority ethnic backgrounds have an increased likelihood of death. Subsequent reports into black and minority ethnic maternal experiences (Birthrights, 2022; Peter et al., 2022) have highlighted how amongst other serious issues related to racism, stereotyping, and discrimination, deterioration and illness in women and babies are missed because of not being listened to and clinical presentation of cyanosis, paleness, and jaundice not recognised in brown or black skin. It is vital that when assessing both women and neonates postnatally that the white body is not held as the norm or default and that variations in clinical presentation in specific ethnic groups is recognised.

PERINEAL CARE AND SUTURING

Approximately 85% of women will experience perineal trauma during a vaginal birth and of this number, around 70% will require some degree of repair (Kettle and Tohill, 2008). As discussed in the chapter *Homebirth – The Evidence*, Reitsma et al. (2020) suggested that perineal outcomes for women and birthing people who begin labour intending to birth at home were favourable with a significant reduction in likelihood of sustaining a third- or fourth-degree tear (obstetric anal sphincter injury or OASI). In the UK the incidence of OASI sits at 2.9%, with incidence variation in primigravida and multigravida women (6.1% and 1.7%, respectively) (Thiagamoorthy et al., 2014; RCOG, 2015).

Grade	Description of Injury
First-degree tear	Involves perineal skin and or vaginal mucosa
Second-degree tear	Involves perineal muscles, NOT involving anal sphincter
Third-degree tear	Involves perineum AND anal sphincter. Subdivided into:
	• 3a <50% of external anal sphincter
	• 3b >50% of external anal sphincter
	• 3c Both external and internal anal sphincter
Fourth-degree tear	Involves perineum, anal sphincter complex, and anorectal mucosa

Based on Sultan (1999); RCOG (2015); NICE (2017).

It is vital that the degree of perineal trauma sustained is properly identified and appropriate repair is undertaken. Incorrect identification or inappropriate repair can lead to potentially serious issues for the woman or birthing person including sexual dysfunction, incontinence, rectovaginal fistula, psychological injury, and trauma (Roper, Sultan, and Thakar, 2020). For women or birthing people suspected of sustaining an OASI, therefore, this should only ever be undertaken by an obstetrician and therefore will necessitate transfer to hospital and subsequently theatres for repair under a spinal or general anaesthetic.

Provided that there is no excessive per-vaginum bleeding, examination can be undertaken whenever the woman or birthing person feels they are ready so as not to interfere with bonding (NICE, 2017). Before assessing, ensure that full, unbiased information is provided in order to facilitate informed consent to both an examination and any repair offered (NICE, 2017). Once consent is gained, select a suitable location for examination. This should be done with a good light source, maintaining the woman or birthing person's dignity and privacy, always following an aseptic technique with sterile gloved hands. Many midwives carry head torches for this purpose. Consider having the woman or birthing person lying comfortably at the edge of a bed or sofa, with legs propped up with chairs and you sitting on the floor, cushion, or stool, or you may also be able to assess sitting aside the woman or birthing person on the bed. In any case positioning should be comfortable for the woman or birthing person and ensure that the external genitalia can be seen clearly (NICE, 2017). You should advise them that the examination is likely to be painful and/or uncomfortable and therefore offer analgesia/pain relief such as Entonox during the examination and maintain an aseptic field where swabs and instruments are to be located. Ensure that if they ask you to stop that you do this immediately and do not recommence until such time as you have gained full consent again.

The examination should follow local guidelines for a systematic approach to ensure that OASI and complicated tears such as 'buttonhole' tears are identified (Roper, Sultan, and Thakar, 2020):

- Firstly, visually observe the external genitalia, taking note of obvious sites of bleeding or trauma.
- Part the labia gently and examine the vagina, visualising the apex of the tear and identifying the full extent of vaginal injury.
- Offer a rectal examination to exclude damage and injury to the anal sphincter and anorectal mucosa.
- If there are *any* concerns, you are unsure of the extent of the injury, or you are not confident that the repair can be safely undertaken at home, consider transfer to an obstetric unit for assessment and/or repair (NICE, 2017).
- If you identify any trauma that can be safely and competently repaired at home, discuss with the woman and birthing person your recommendations for repair and gain informed consent prior to repair. Once identified, and with consent, this should be undertaken as soon as possible to reduce the risk of both infection and bleeding.
- ALWAYS use appropriate levels of local anaesthetic. If at any point you are unable to complete a repair due to inadequate pain relief, consider transfer to hospital for more effective methods.

Procedures for completing perineal repair are outside the scope of this book due to the constantly evolving nature of evidence-based guidelines; therefore when undertaking the repair, follow all local and national advice. Advice regarding ongoing perineal care should be provided including regular analgesia such as paracetamol and ibuprofen (if indicated), hygiene advice for changing pads, bathing/showering, and pelvic floor exercises. Finally, as part of routine postnatal advice, reassurance can be provided alongside pathways for obtaining help and assistance where they have any concerns over pain levels, infection, or feeling unwell.

Practice Point: Equipment Checks and Disposal

Given the constraints of setting up equipment at home it is vital that all procedures for counting swabs and sharps be fully adhered to prevent them from being left behind. Check all equipment, count swabs and sharps before and after a repair, then fully document. When transporting these and clinical waste from home to hospital for disposal, ensure that these are safely stowed and stored.

IMMEDIATE CARE OF THE NEONATE

Most neonates (approximately 85%) will not require any assistance to transition from intra- to extrauterine life and will independently establish regular respirations. An additional 10% will require minimal intervention such as drying, stimulation, and opening of the airway (RCUK, 2021). Close observation of this process should be undertaken therefore immediately post birth to identify any deviations and commence appropriate measures where transition is slow or absent including an early call for assistance and potential transfer. As with any birth, an Apgar score can help to assess this transition, noting that neonates born underwater are sometimes slightly slower to transition but still within normal parameters. When documenting neonatal observations, it might be useful to complete this on a scoring system such as a validated Newborn Early Warning System (NEWS). Not only will this help identify illness or potential deterioration over the entire postnatal period, but NICE (2021) suggests that this can support communication with parents in identifying newborn condition. Neonatal observations (Fig. 9.2) should be completed as soon after the first hour

- Weight.
- Head circumference.
- Temperature.
- Activity, movement, and tone.
- Appearance (colour).
- Maintain thermoregulation.
- Initiate feed and discretely observe, helping if required.

Fig. 9.2 Immediate neonatal care and observations.

Parents expressing concern over condition of newborn	Non-blanching rash
Needing any cardiopulmonary resuscitation	Bulging or sunken fontanelle
Looking unwell or ill	Abnormal movements
Unresponsive or difficult to rouse	Obvious or suspected seizure including focal
Cyanosis, pale, ashen, or mottled skin (signs of hypoxia)	Not passing or reduced quantities of urine or meconium
Abnormal breathing such as grunting, chest recession, nasal flaring, raised respiratory rate, tachypnoea (>60/min)	Feeding difficulties, intolerances such as vomiting, abdominal distension, or gastric aspirates
Abnormal heart rate (high or low)	Signs of clinical shock
High or low temperature (<26°C/>38°C) not linked to environment	Suspected infection in woman or birthing person
Cry appears high pitched, weak, or continuous	Jaundice within 24 hours of birth
Apnoeic episode	Jittering or signs of hypoglycaemia
Abnormal tone or floppiness	Projectile or bilious vomiting
Meconium liquor	Oxygen saturation below 95% or according to age (RCUK, 2021)

Fig. 9.3 Summary of signs and symptoms of an unwell or deteriorating newborn that indicates immediate referral for neonatal review.

following birth; however, routine care should avoid separation and disruption of the mother-infant dyad (NICE, 2017), taking into account the clinical presentation of both.

Signs and symptoms of an unwell neonate are discussed in depth in the chapter *Additional Neonatal Considerations* (summarised here in Fig 9.3) and management of newborn resuscitation in the chapter *Managing Emergencies at Home*. If at any point, however, there is a concern about the neonate (transitioning to extrauterine life, requiring newborn resuscitation, abnormal observations, or identified issues during the initial examination of the newborn), especially in the presence of maternal red flag risk factors for early-onset neonatal infection, immediate escalation and transfer for review should be instigated.

FEEDING SUPPORT

It would be easy to dedicate a whole chapter to supporting feeding after any birth. This is a fundamental element of postnatal care and discussing this in detail is outside the scope of this text. There are however pertinent considerations that need to be addressed before leaving the home.

Discussions and support around feeding choices should remain respectful and be guided by the needs, wants, and preferences of the woman or birthing person. Regardless of how a woman or birthing person chooses to feed their baby, all advice and support should remain evidence based and follow a personalised, tailored approach. In any case all advice should be documented and remain consistent whilst ensuring the family are aware of:

- Whom to contact and how in the event of any type of feeding concerns once you have left the house.
- Providing written information to support and supplement verbal, one-to-one discussion.
- Signs of effective and ineffective feeding
- Responsive feeding
- If formula feeding, safely making up and administering feeds.

Before leaving the house, you should ensure that the neonate has fed at least once, a feeding plan is in place and agreed upon with the woman or birthing person, and, if breastfeeding, you offer to observe and support a feed. Additionally signs and symptoms of an unwell baby including signs of jaundice should be discussed in the context of feeding and contact details for parents to escalate to 24 hours a day if they are concerned. Local feeding guidelines and protocols should be followed by healthcare professionals and details of support networks and groups signposted.

INDICATIONS FOR TRANSFER

As with the antenatal and intrapartum period, there are various indications to suggest transfer from home to hospital for obstetric review. The following lists some of these indications for the woman or birthing person (non-exhaustive):

Maternal Request	Tachycardia
Excessive bleeding or postpartum haemorrhage	Pyrexia (temperature >38°C once, or >37.5°C on two consecutive readings 1 hour apart)
Any signs of sepsis or infection (see chapter *Managing Emergencies at Home*)	Suturing is unable to complete at home OR if suspected obstetric anal sphincter injury (OASI)
Pain management	Chest pain or breathing difficulties
Hypertension	Persistent or severe headache
Unable to void bladder	Offensive lochia
Incomplete placenta and membranes	Any obstetric or medical emergency

Indications for transfer, also refer to chapter *Managing Emergencies at Home* for specific actions to take.

Practice Point: Practical Postnatal Transfer Considerations (also see chapters *Paramedic Transfer and Multidisciplinary Working With Ambulance Services* and *Managing Emergencies at Home*)

When arranging and managing a transfer to hospital, consider the following:

- Always discuss and gain informed consent from the woman or birthing person. Discuss reasons, rationale, how the transfer is to happen, and how long it will take. Always respect their wishes.
- Provide opportunity to answer questions.
- Always ensure the woman or birthing person's dignity is respected, and wrap or cover in a blanket or support them to get dressed, ensuring they are as comfortable as possible.
- Work with emergency attenders/paramedics to support the woman or birthing person to choose what position to adopt in transfer, taking into consideration the emergency positions discussed here.
- Where possible and in consultation with the paramedics, a midwife should travel with the woman or birthing persons for continuity and to hand over care. Make sure that arrangements for the partner to either travel alongside or in their own transport are discussed.
- Where possible and in consultation with the paramedics, try to ensure that the woman or birthing person and neonate (if born) are not separated.
- Ensure that neonatal thermoregulation is not compromised by transfer
- Don't forget to take bags!

LEAVING THE HOUSE

Deciding when to leave the house following a homebirth is a decision that you make in consultation with your colleagues and the woman or birthing person. If the birth has gone smoothly and there are no concerns, usually you will be able to leave the house within 2–3 hours of the birth. There are no hard-and-fast rules to follow; however, there are some key considerations, observations, and information that should be shared before leaving to restock equipment, complete paperwork and notifications, and return clinical waste. These are:

- You should be satisfied that the woman or birthing person is physiologically well. Observations (discussed previously) should all be within normal limits and documented.
- Encourage the woman to pass urine at least once (more if possible) and document approximate (or exact if possible) volume.
- You should be satisfied that the woman or birthing person's uterus is well contracted with no signs of excessive blood loss. Discuss with the woman or birthing person normal physiological blood loss post birth to enable them to identify abnormal bleeding and potential postpartum haemorrhage. This should include providing advice about lochia, changes in colour and texture of lochia, size and quantity of clots, offensive odour etc.
- You should be satisfied that the neonate is physiologically well having undertaken a full top-to-toe examination, documented a full set of neonatal observations (see Fig. 9.2), provided feeding advice, and observed a feed. Check that where the cord is clamped or tied it is secure.
- A discussion of signs and symptoms of an unwell neonate and how to escalate/whom and how to call for help should be conducted. This includes advising that if meconium has not been passed within 24 hours, they seek help and support.
- If rhesus negative and consent has been given for a Klaihauer-Betke test, both cord bloods and maternal bloods should be properly labelled, checked, and transported in accordance with local guidelines. This should be documented and flagged for follow-up when handing over care.

- Ensure that the woman or birthing person and their family have details of when and how to call for assistance in the event of concerns or questions. This should include when to call an ambulance for serious concerns, discussion of signs and symptoms of an unwell neonate, or deterioration of the woman or birthing person. Documentation detailing and supporting this advice should be left in a format that is easy to understand including telephone numbers and emergency advice.
- Ensure discussion of safe sleeping advice, ongoing perineal health, normal bowel and bladder function, breast care, normal blood loss, analgesia, and mental health. Signs and symptoms of infection, anaemia, and thromboembolism should be fully discussed and document clearly.
- Ensure that postnatal and neonatal notes are left with the family (unless electronic records).
- Details of when subsequent postnatal visits should be expected, a description of the ongoing care plan, and whom to contact outside of these visits. This should include a discussion of arrangements for the complete examination of the newborn (if not done already) and newborn hearing screening.

Once all agree that all is well and you leave the house, ensure that you have all equipment, instruments, and clinical waste. Notify the designated person you are leaving (labour ward coordinator etc) following your local guidelines for lone working and personal safety.

CONCLUSION

This chapter has discussed some key considerations for safe and respectful postnatal care unique to homebirth. It is hoped that by building upon existing knowledge of postnatal care, the practical advice offered here will reinforce the fundamentals of midwifery care at home whilst improving confidence in how and when to escalate deviations from normal physiology. Postnatal care is often described as the Cinderella service; however, with good planning, robust knowledge, and skills, midwives are expertly placed to facilitate a calm transition from pregnancy to parenthood, providing the best start for all.

REFERENCES

Birthrights, 2022. Systemic racism, not broken bodies. Birthrights, London.

Dennis, C.-L. et al. (2007) 'Traditional postpartum practices and rituals: A qualitative systematic review', *Women's Health*, 3(4), pp. 487–502. Available at: https://doi.org/10.2217/17455057.3.4.487.

Gatrad, A.R. and Sheikh, A. (2001) 'Muslim birth customs', *Archives of Disease in Childhood – Fetal and Neonatal Edition*, 84(1), p. F6. Available at: https://doi.org/10.1136/fn.84.1.F6.

Kettle, C. and Tohill, S. (2008) 'Perineal care', *BMJ Clinical Evidence*, 2008, p. 1401.

Knight, M., Bunch, K., Tuffnell, D., Shakespeare, J., Kotnis, R., Kenyon, S., Kurinczuk, J., 2019. Saving Lives, Improving Mothers Care - Lessons learned to inform maternity care from the UK and Ireland Confidentia Enquiries into Maternal Death and Morbidity 2015-2017. National Perinatal Epidemiology Unit, University of Oxford, Oxford.

NICE (2017) 'Intrapartum care for healthy women and babies'. National Institute for Health and Care Excellence. Available at: https://www.nice.org.uk/guidance/cg190/chapter/recommendations#pain-relief-in-labour-nonregional (Accessed 29 January 2021).

NICE (2021) 'Postnatal care'. National Institute for Health and Care Excellence. Available at: https://www.nice.org.uk/guidance/ng194/chapter/Recommendations#organisation-and-delivery-of-postnatal-care (Accessed 31st October 2022).

Peter, M., Wheeler, R., Awe, T., Abe, C., 2022. The Black Maternity Experiences Survey: A Nationwide Study of Black Womens Experiences of Maternity Services in teh United Kingdom. FiveXMore.

RCOG (2015) 'Management of third and fourth degree perineal tears'. Royal College of Obstetricians and Gynaecologists. Available at: https://www.rcog.org.uk/globalassets/ documents/ guidelines/gtg-29.pdf (Accessed 31 October 2022).

RCUK (2021) 'Newborn resuscitation and support of the transition of infants at birth Guidlines'. Resuscitation Council UK.

Reitsma, A. et al. (2020) 'Maternal outcomes and birth interventions among women who begin labour intending to give birth at home compared to women of low obstetrical risk who intend to give birth in hospital: A systematic review and meta-analyses', *EClinicalMedicine*, 21, pp. 100319–100319. Available at: https://doi.org/10.1016/j.eclinm.2020.100319.

Roper, J., Sultan, A. and Thakar, R. (2020) 'Diagnosis of perineal trauma: Getting it right first time', *British Journal of Midwifery*, 28(10), pp. 710–715.

Sultan, A. (1999) 'Obstetric perineal injury and anal incontinence', *Clinical Risk*, 5, pp. 193–6.

Thiagamoorthy, G. et al. (2014) 'National survey of perineal trauma and its subsequent management in the United Kingdom', *International Urogynecology Journal*, 25(12), pp. 1621–1627. Available at: https://doi.org/10.1007/s00192-014-2406-x.

CHAPTER 10

NEONATAL CONSIDERATIONS FOR HOMEBIRTH

Katy Powis and Lesley Kilby

INTRODUCTION

Most decisions to home birth will be for low-risk pregnancies and will be made in line with recommended guidance. *Better Births Maternity Review* (NHS, 2016) advocates for the freedom of choice when deciding on birthing plan; however, at times women's choices may go against guidelines and recommendations. Typically, newborns deemed as 'high risk' would be cared for in the hospital setting with dedicated specialist teams to facilitate immediate care and formulate management plans as required; however, a woman, birthing person, and their partners that choose to birth outside of guidance need to be considered in relation to increased health risks and co-morbidities as a result of fetal, maternal, or placental factors (Mirzakhani et al., 2020). The importance of guidance is in order to preserve the safety and wellbeing of infants in the reduction of adverse events and serious incidents. These must be taken into account when discussing place of birth in relation to neonatal care. Nursing and midwifery professionals have a duty to work within their scope of practice, have an understanding of professional accountability, vicarious liability and adhere to all professional standards and codes (NMC, 2018).

It is important to remember that in UK law, until a baby is born and has separate existence from its mother, their legal human rights are superseded by the maternal rights (United Kingdom: Human Rights Act, 1998). Once born, the right of the child entitles them to access the highest attainable standard of health and also the elimination of preventable child mortalities and morbidities (UNGA CRC, 2013) (see chapters *The Evidence for Homebirth* and *Managing Emergencies at Home*).

THE CORNERSTONES OF NEONATAL MANAGEMENT AT HOME

As neonatal professionals, we expect certain fundamentals to be done well with the ethos of prevention. These cornerstones are paramount in achieving safe care and positive outcomes in whichever setting the baby is born in. While the broad principles discussed here apply to all assessment and neonatal management following birth at home, the following focuses on care which might be necessary outside that of routine postnatal and antenatal care.

An airway, breathing, and circulation (ABC) approach is always the priority in the assessment and management of any patient and it is no less important in the neonate, especially when sudden collapse is usually respiratory in nature. This very special patient group is unique in that it is making the transition into extrauterine life and taking its first breaths. This transition may need to be supported in some cases, especially where risk factors are identified. Fetal risk factors include prematurity, being small for gestational age, multiple pregnancy, oligo/polyhydramnios, and some congenital abnormalities. Other risk factors may also include gestational diabetes, or high maternal BMI, (UK, 2021). *Professionals attending home deliveries where risk factors have been identified should be trained in Newborn Life Support and adhere to a robust protocol for transfer of care into hospital should adverse events be anticipated or occur* (BAPM, 2022b; RCUK, 2021). This includes the presence of meconium-stained liquor, which should always prompt immediate transfer to a secondary care setting (further details on Newborn Life Support can be found in chapter *Managing Emergencies at Home*).

THERMOREGULATION

Keeping a baby warm after birth is an essential element of early management of any newborn, as initial temperature is seen as strong predictor for outcomes across all gestations (McCall et al., 2018). Newborn babies are at risk of hypothermia due to physiological immaturity and a large surface area to mass ratio. Some infants are, however, at further risk and will require a proactive approach to the maintenance of normal temperature. These babies include, but are not limited to, babies born before 37 weeks gestation, small for gestational age babies, pathologically growth-restricted babies, and any baby that has an additional energy requirement (e.g. sepsis, hypoglycaemia, hypoxia).

The World Health Organization (WHO) defines neonatal hypothermia as an axillary temperature below 36.5°C and is stratified as either mild (36–36.4°C), moderate (32–35.9°C), or severe hypothermia (<32°C) with the severity scale carrying prognostic implications (WHO, 1997). The practical management in the maintenance of normothermia relies on an understanding of the four methods of heat loss: convection, evaporation, conduction, and radiation. With these in mind, prevention strategies include:

- Ensuring the delivery area is draught free and maintaining an environmental temperature of between 23 and 25°C
- Drying and wrapping the baby immediately after birth and applying a hat
- Placing the baby skin to skin and covering

> **Practice point:**
> It is important to assess maternal temperature when considering skin to skin as if she is cool to touch and/or her temperature is lower than that of the baby's, skin to skin may not but appropriate as this could have a cooling effect.

Transfer to hospital is indicated if unable to maintain a temperature above 36.5°C despite the above actions.

AVOIDING HYPOGLYCAEMIA

A key strategy in the support of transitioning to extrauterine life is to establish successful feeding in line with the choice of the mother. It is recommended that babies are breastfed within the first hour of life and then exclusively for the first 6 months of life (WHO, 2022). There is significant evidence that breastfeeding improves infant health, maternal health, and relationship building in the mother-baby dyad and reduces financial burden on the health service. In the short term the establishment of early feeding is to support the glycaemic transition from intra- to extrauterine life. Newborns experience a period of physiological hypoglycaemia following the cessation of maternal glucose supply when the umbilical cord is cut. For most babies, this will naturally resolve with early feeding. If any risk factors for neonatal hypoglycaemia are identified in the antenatal or postnatal period, careful assessment of the neonate for signs of hypoglycaemia (see Table 10.1 for signs of hypoglycaemia) is required to ensure a safe blood glucose is maintained (see Table 10.2 for risk factors). The evaluation of attachment and positioning is required to ensure the transfer of milk if breastfeeding or a sufficient amount of artificial milk is taken by bottle (aim for 60 mL/kg/day). Frequent feeds of 8–12 times in 24 hours are recommended (UNICEF BFI, n.d.) and review of the frequency and quality of urine and stool output will provide data in the overall assessment of the success of infant feeding.

> **Practice point:**
> Babies born at 34^{+0} to 36^{+6} or at low birthweight have reduced capacity to moderate temperature, normoglycaemia, and initiation of feeding and therefore the following settings are recommended for their ongoing care:
>
> | | | |
> |---|---|---|
> | 34^{+0} to 35^{+6} | ≤1600 g | Neonatal Unit |
> | 34^{+0} to 35^{+6} | >1600 g | Neonatal Transitional Care or Neonatal Unit |
> | 36^{+0} to 36^{+6} | 1600–2000 g | Neonatal Transition Care |
> | 36^{+0} to 36^{+6} | >2000 g | Universal care with enhanced monitoring (temperature, feeding, blood sugar) |
>
> Consider what you would accept as a minimum blood sugar before referring to a paediatrician for ongoing management in the moderate-to-late preterm infant.

(BAPM, 2023)

Table 10.1 Signs of Hypoglycaemia

Appears unwell	Altered level of consciousness	Reluctance to feed
Apnoea	Cyanosis	Hypothermia
Seizures	Jitteriness	Respiratory distress
Poor tone	Pallor	Lethargy

Signs of Hypoglycaemia

Table 10.2 Risk Factors for Hypoglycaemia

Maternal diabetes	Hypothermia
Intrauterine growth restriction	Feeding issues
Maternal treatment for hypertension (beta-blockers)	Small for gestational age
Preterm	Suspected sepsis
Intrapartum hypoxia	Family history of metabolic disorders

Risk factors for Hypoglycaemia

Table 10.3 Unexpected Problems

UNEXPECTED PROBLEMS	SIGNS AND SYMPTOMS	ACTIONS
Sepsis This can present with varied and non-specific symptoms.	Unstable temperature, both hypo/hyperthermia, that continues despite skin to skin, dressing, and hat and taking environmental factors into consideration. Poor suck reflex Hypotonia Hypoglycaemia Abnormal movements such as jittery movements or seizures Altered level of consciousness Bradycardia/tachycardia Respiratory distress/apnoea Pallor	Arrange for transfer to hospital for ongoing evaluation and intravenous antibiotics. Advise parents of potential stay in hospital, minimal period may be 48 hours. (NICE, 2021)
Cardiac abnormality	Cyanosis noted on lips, skin, nail beds Pounding heart Weak pulses Tachypnoea with or without other signs of recession or grunting Lethargy Poor feeding Pre- and post-ductal saturation difference of greater than or equal to 3%. *Congenital cardiac abnormalities cannot be diagnosed without further detailed investigation such as an echocardiogram.* *Some congenital abnormalities rely on the patent ductus arteriosus (PDA) remaining patent in order to ensure circulation of blood. This requires prompt treatment with IV Prostin to ensure PDA remains patent.*	Arrange urgent transfer to nearest Neonatal Unit (NNU). If possible utilise ambulance pulse oximeter; the adult finger clip can be used on neonate's foot. Advise parents that there may be admission to the neonatal unit. (McCarthy & Hoover, 2020)
Respiratory distress	Tachypnoea >60 breaths/min Bradypnoea <30 breaths/min Recession Grunting Nasal flaring Cyanosis	Arrange for transfer to nearest NNU. Advise parents of the potential need for admission, some respiratory support, and treatment for sepsis.
Ambiguous genitalia	An enlarged clitoris which may resemble a penis. Closed labia, or labia that includes folds and resembles a scrotum. Lumps that feel like testes in the enclosed labia. An abnormally small penis with urethral opening closer to the scrotum. Undescended testes and an empty scrotum that has appearance of labia with or without micropenis.	Arrange transfer to nearest NNU for further investigation and support. Advise parents of the potential for admission. Ambiguous genitalia may be an indication of congenital adrenal hyperplasia which can result in profound hypoglycaemia and hyponatraemia, which will require treatment and ongoing monitoring and investigation. (Lee, Strobel & Chu, 2021)

Continued

Table 10.3 Unexpected Problems—cont'd

UNEXPECTED PROBLEMS	SIGNS AND SYMPTOMS	ACTIONS
Cleft palate	Bilateral or unilateral cleft in lip Visible cleft in palate Bifid uvula Submucosal cleft palate Most cleft lips and palates are detected on antennal Ultrasound Scan (USS) or identified as part of the Newborn and Infant Physical Examination (NIPE) or equivalent.	If identified on USS contact will be made with the local cleft team and a plan devised. Ensure that plan is available prior to home delivery so that the team is aware of expected actions. If not identified prior to delivery arrange for transfer to postnatal ward. It is vital that the cleft team is informed urgently due to immediate need for feeding support and assessment. (CLAPA, 2022)
Imperforate anus	Absence of anus Anus in abnormal position, i.e. closer to scrotum or vagina than normal Faeces passed from penis or around the vagina Vomiting Distended abdomen	Arrange for transfer to nearest NNU. Advise parents of potential admission. Discontinue feeding.

SYSTEMATIC ASSESSMENT

Following the birth of a baby, a thorough assessment is required to establish that the ex-utero transitioning process has successfully occurred, or if there are any anomalies/abnormalities that require further evaluation. When carrying out this assessment, it is important to follow a systematic approach in order to assimilate clinical information accurately and determine the most appropriate course of action where concerns are identified. Whilst carrying out this assessment, the practitioner must have an open dialogue with the parent/caregiver and offer time for them to express any concerns and ask any questions. The following tables provide an outline of any expected and unexpected signs and/or symptoms that may be present upon assessment, with recommended actions. These lists are not exhaustive (see table 10.3 and 10.5). If the emergency transfer to hospital of a baby is required, call the emergency services.

Some congenital abnormalities may not be identified antenatally; they may be detected on the NIPE examination. It is important to understand that in the presence of one abnormality there is the assumption that there may be others. For example, in anorectal malformations there may also be other midline defects such as some heart defects. Extra digits either on feet or hands and other such non-urgent abnormalities can be documented and assessed with the NIPE and relevant referrals made.

SEPSIS

Sepsis can have devastating consequences for the neonate and the family; therefore it is important that Midwives are aware of identified risk factors for early onset sepsis as set out by National Institute for Health and Care Excellence (NICE, 2021). In the presence of either one red flag risk factor/clinical indicator or two other risk factors/clinical indicators (see Tables 10.4a and 10.4b), screening and treatment are strongly recommended and therefore any suspicion of sepsis should indicate an immediate transfer.

Table 10.4a Risk Factors for Early-Onset Neonatal Infection

RED FLAG RISK FACTOR	SUSPECTED OR CONFIRMED INFECTION IN THE CASE OF A MULTIPLE PREGNANCY
Other risk factors	Preterm birth following spontaneous labour before 37 weeks gestation
	Invasive group B streptococcal infection in a previous baby or maternal group B streptococcal colonisation, bacteriuria, or infection in the current pregnancy
	Confirmed pre-labour rupture of membranes at term for more than 24 hours before the onset of labour
	Confirmed rupture of membranes for more than 18 hours before a preterm birth
	Intrapartum fever higher than 38°C if there is suspected or confirmed bacterial infection
	Clinical diagnosis of chorioamnionitis

Table 10.4b Clinical Indicators of Possible Early-Onset Neonatal Infection (Observation and Events in the Baby)

RED FLAG CLINICAL INDICATORS	Apnoea (temporary stopping of breathing)
	Seizures
	Need for cardiopulmonary resuscitation
	Need for mechanical ventilation
	Signs of shock
Other risk factors	Altered behaviour or responses
	Altered muscle tone (e.g. floppiness)
	Feeding difficulties (e.g. feed refusal)
	Feed intolerance, including vomiting, excessive gastric aspirates, and abdominal distension
	Abnormal heart rate (bradycardia or tachycardia)
	Hypoxia (e.g. central cyanosis or reduced oxygen saturation level)
	Persistent pulmonary hypertension of newborns
	Jaundice within 24 hours of birth
	Signs of neonatal encephalopathy
	Temperature abnormality ($<36°C$ or $>38°C$) unexplained by environmental factors
	Unexplained excessive bleeding, thrombocytopenia, or abnormal coagulation
	Altered glucose homeostasis (hypoglycaemia or hyperglycaemia)
	Metabolic acidosis (base deficit of 10 mmol/L or greater)
	(modified from NICE, 2021)

Table 10.5 Anticipated Problems

ANTICIPATED PROBLEMS	POTENTIAL SIGNS AND SYMPTOMS	ACTION
Maternal hypothyroidism that is well controlled and NO previous treatment or history of hyperthyroidism or maternal Graves disease	Not commonly noted in the immediate postnatal period, they can include: Jaundice Poor feeding Sleeping more than usual Constipation Poor tone Large tongue Poor muscle tone Poor growth	Ensure that on days 5–8 blood spot screening is obtained as this will screen for congenital hypothyroidism.
Hyperthyroidism and maternal Graves disease. This can be caused by high levels of TSH receptor antibodies (TRAb) which cross the placenta and cause hyperthyroidism in the neonate	Intrauterine Growth Restriction (IUGR) Tachycardia Irritability Microcephaly Hypertension Flushing Sweating Diarrhoea Vomiting Enlarged spleen Jaundice Poor feeding and growth Bruising and petechiae	At birth – Cord blood taken for maternal TRAb levels. Arrange visit to postnatal ward for assessment. If well, can be discharged with advice to monitor heart rate, respirations, and temperature. Monitor feeding. Advise parents that on days 3–5 a further neonatal review is required and Thyroid Function Tests (TFTs), and if not already known, TRAb levels should also taken. If TRAbs are negative, no further follow-up required. If positive or unknown with normal TFTs repeat blood tests will be required on days 10–14. (Davis, Deamer & Andrews, 2020)

Continued

Table 10.5 Anticipated Problems—cont'd

ANTICIPATED PROBLEMS	POTENTIAL SIGNS AND SYMPTOMS	ACTION
Small for gestational age (SGA)	Birthweight <10th centile for gestation Hypothermia Hypoglycaemia Polycythaemia Signs of withdrawal if linked to substance misuse: if this is the cause, observation and management of withdrawal should take place in a hospital setting.	Optimise thermoregulation. Close monitoring of feeding. SGA newborns are at greater risk of hypoglycaemia due to the pathophysiological causes of SGA. If symptomatic for hypoglycaemia or hypothermia, arrange for urgent transfer to postnatal ward for assessment. (Kilby et al., 2020)
Infant of diabetic mother (IDM)	Large for gestational age SGA Hypothermia Hypoglycaemia Polycythaemia Respiratory distress	Hypoglycaemia is a significant risk for these infants and therefore will require initial blood sugar screening within the hospital setting. IDMs may have impaired surfactant production due to potential hyperinsulinism and therefore are at risk of respiratory distress syndrome and will require medical review. (BFI, 2013)
Substance misuse	Misuse of non-prescribed drugs of addiction during pregnancy Prescribed medications such as antidepressants and opioid pain relief Alcohol *Signs of withdrawal:* High-pitched cry Irritability and restlessness Sneezing Tremors Feeding difficulties Sleeping difficulties Diarrhoea Pyrexia/sweating Skin excoriation on buttocks In rare circumstances seizures can occur. In this situation call emergency services.	If identified antenatally a baby alert will be present with a plan of care set out. If not identified observe for signs of withdrawal and advise parents that observation and management of potential withdrawal symptoms will be required in a hospital setting and any safeguarding issues reviewed. (LODN, 2017)
HIV/Hep B	Maternal exposure to HIV and hep B will be confirmed within antenatal serology and maternal history. If identified in the antenatal period a postnatal plan will be documented in the records.	Follow local trust policy and postnatal plan as treatment is time critical. Advise the parents that in the case of HIV a blood test will be required prior to starting appropriate therapy as well as a hep B vaccine.
Haemolytic disease of the newborn	This can be caused by incompatibility in blood groups and rhesus status and results in increased breakdown in the newborn's RBC. This can result in anaemia and early onset jaundice in <24 hours, resulting in drowsiness and reluctance to feed. If left untreated in severe cases this can result in Kernicterus, a serious irreversible neurological condition. In some cases if undetected in the mother, a baby may be born unexpectedly hydropic and must be immediately transferred to hospital.	If mother is O negative, obtain cord blood for maternal group and antibody status. If there are antibodies present, then advise parents that their baby will require blood tests in hospital and if jaundice is present will require admission and phototherapy treatment. (RCOG, 2014)

TRANSPORTING A BABY TO HOSPITAL

Transfer of the neonate for a clinical emergency from home is a rare occurrence (BAPM, 2022b); however, clinical needs identified as requiring urgent transfer of a baby to the nearest hospital are less rare. It should be noted that delay in transfer and poor communication have been identified as key risk factors for poor outcomes in the context of home birth (Rowe et al., 2020). In this event, call must be made for transfer through the emergency 999 system with clear conveyance of urgency of clinical situation to call handler made. They will, through their triage system, evaluate the need of both baby and mother and dispatch clinicians and vehicles accordingly (see chapters *Paramedic transfer and multidisciplinary working with ambulance services* and *Managing Emergencies at Home*). The decision regarding how the baby and mother are transported lies legally with the paramedic team; therefore, this may mean that in some cases mother and baby are transported separately if necessary. The role of the attending practitioner includes ensuring that the ambulance is pre-warmed, the appropriate monitoring is in situ, vital signs are recorded throughout the journey, and the parents are fully informed of the indication for transfer. It is important to note that a newborn must not be transported skin to skin or on an adult's lap under any circumstances. They must always be secured in an appropriate child restraint system in accordance with local guidelines. Refer to chapters *Antenatal planning-organisational considerations* and *Managing Emergencies at Home* for suggested equipment.

OPTIMAL CORD MANAGEMENT

Optimal cord management (OCM) (clamping and cutting of the umbilical cord more than 60 seconds after birth, WHO, 2014) is widely accepted as the optimal management in the third stage of labour in both preterm and term infants. The benefits of allowing the physiological placental transfusion include the reduction in incidence of iron deficiency and anaemia and improvements in neurodevelopmental outcomes and various haemodynamic parameters. The deferring of cord clamping in some babies, including growth-restricted infants and monochorionic twins, may be potentially harmful and also where the cord or placenta are compromised, so it is not currently advised (Bruckner, Katheria & Schmölzer, 2021). There are suggestions that OCC may be even more beneficial in the non-vigorous or asphyxiated baby. These infants may not, however, enjoy any benefits of deferring clamping if this leads to a delay in offering respiratory support; therefore, the cord must be clamped and cut in the community setting if the baby appears compromised. There are suggestions that milking the cord may be an effective and quick way to ensure placental transfusion occurs in these depressed infants; however, there is no standardised procedure for this, so further research is required before this can be written into practice (Basile et al., 2019). (See also Chapter *Second and Thirds Stage of Labour at Home*.)

REFERENCES

Basile, S., Pinelli, S., Micelli, E., Caretto, M. & Panici, P.B. (2019) 'Milking of the umbilical cord in term and late preterm infants' *BioMed Research International*. 2019: 9185059; 9 pages. https://doi.org/10.1155/2019/9185059

British Association for Perinatal Medicine (2023) *Early postnatal care of the moderate-late preterm infant: A draft BAPM framework for practice*. Available at: https://www.bapm.org/resources/framework-early-postnatal-care-of-the-moderate-late-preterm-infant

British Association for Perinatal Medicine (BAPM) (2022) 'Neonatal support for freestanding midwifery led units and home births A framework for practice'. British Association of Perinatal Medicine. Available at: https://www.bapm.org/resources/framework-neonatal-support-for-stand-alone-mlu-and-home-births

Bruckner, M., Katheria, A.C. & Schmölzer, G.M. (2021) 'Delayed cord clamping in healthy term infants: More harm or good?' *Seminars in Fetal and Neonatal Medicine*. 26(2). https://doi.org/10.1016/j.siny.2021.101221

Cleft Lip and Palate Association (CLAPA) (2022) *Feeding*. Available at: https://www.clapa.com/treatment/feeding/

Davis, J., Deamer, S., & Andrews, E. (2020) 'The management of neonates born to mothers with thyroid disease'. Wessex Paediatric Endocrinology Network. Available at: https://www.piernetwork.org/hyperthyroidism.html

Kilby, L., Everrett, E., Powis, K. & Kyte, E. (2020) 'The preterm and low birthweight infant'. In Boxwell, G., Petty, J. & Kaiser, L. (eds) *Neonatal Intensive Care Nursing*. London: Routledge, pp. 46–49.

Lee, R.B., Strobel, M.K. & Chu, A. (2021) 'The neonate with ambiguous genitalia' Neoreviews. 22(4): e241–e249. https://doi.org/10.1542/neo.22-4-e241

London Operational Delivery Network (LODN) (2017) *Pan London peri-natal mental health: Guidance for newborn assessment*. Available at: https://www.londonneonatalnetwork.org.uk/wp-content/uploads/2016/10/FinalNeodoc-v4.pdf

McCall, E.M., Alderdice, F., Halliday, H.L., Vohra, S. & Johnston, L. (2018) 'Interventions to prevent hypothermia at birth in preterm and/or low birth weight infants' *The Cochrane Database of Systematic Reviews*. 2(2): CD004210. https://doi.org/10.1002/14651858.CD004210.pub5

McCarthy, N. & Hoover, K. (2020) 'Management of cardiovascular disorders'. In Boxwell, G., Petty, J. & Kaiser, L. (eds) *Neonatal Intensive Care Nursing*. London: Routledge, pp. 334–339.

Mirzakhani, K., Ebadi, A., Faridhosseini, F. & Khadivzadeh, T. (2020) 'Well-being in high-risk pregnancy: An integrative review' *BMC Pregnancy Childbirth*. 20(1): 526. https://doi.org/10.1186/s12884-020-03190-6

NHS (2016) *National maternity review: Better births; improving outcomes of maternity services in England. A five year forward view for maternity care*. Available at: https://www.england.nhs.uk/wp-content/uploads/2016/02/national-maternity-review-report.pdf

NICE (2021) *Neonatal infection: Antibiotics for prevention and treatment (NG195)*. Available at: https://www.nice.org.uk/guidance/ng195

Nursing and Midwifery Council (2018) *The code: Professional standards of practice and behaviour for nurses, midwives and nursing associates*. Available at: http://www.nmc.org.uk/globalassets/sitedocuments/nmc-publications/revised-new-nmc-code.pdf

Resus Council UK (2021) *Newborn resuscitation and support of transition of infants at birth guideline*. Available at: https://www.resus.org.uk

Royal College of Obstetricians and Gynaecologists (RCOG) (2014) *The management of women with red cell antibodies during pregnancy: Green-top Guideline No 65.* Available at: https://www.rcog.org.uk/guidance/browse-all-guidance/green-top-guidelines/the-management-of-women-with-red-cell-antibodies-during-pregnancy-green-top-guideline-no-65/

Rowe, R., et al. (2020) 'Intrapartum-related perinatal deaths in births planned in midwifery-led settings in Great Britain: Findings and recommendations from the ESMiE confidential enquiry' *BJOG.* 127(13): 1665–1675. https://doi.org/10.1111/1471-0528.16327

UNICEF Baby Friendly Initiative (UNICEF BFI) (2013) *Guidelines on the development of policies and guidelines for the prevention and management of hypoglycaemia of the newborn.* Available at: https://www.unicef.org.uk/babyfriendly/wp-content/uploads/sites/2/2010/10/hypo_policy.pdf

UNICEF Baby Friendly Initiative (UNICEF BFI) (n.d.) *Breastfeeding assessment tools.* Available at: https://www.unicef.org.uk/babyfriendly/

United Kingdom: Human Rights Act 1998 c. 42. Available at: https://www.legislation.gov.uk/ukpga/1998/42/contents

United Nations General Assembly Committee on the Rights of the Child (UNGA CRC) (2013) *General comment No. 15 (2013) on the right of the child to the enjoyment of the highest attainable standard of health (art. 24).* Available at: refworld.org/docid/51ef9e134.html

World Health Organization (1997) *Thermal protection of the newborn: A practical guide.* Available at: https://www.who.int/publications/i/item/WHO_RHT_MSM_97.2

World Health Organization (2014) *Guideline: Delayed umbilical cord clamping for improved maternal and infant health and nutrition outcomes.* Available at: https://apps.who.int/nutrition/publications/guidelines/cord_clamping/en/index.html

World Health Organization (2022) *Breastfeeding: Recommendations.* Available at: https://www.who.int/health-topics/breastfeeding

CHAPTER 11

MANAGING EMERGENCIES AT HOME

Carla Jayne Avery and Anna Madeley

INTRODUCTION

For homebirth to remain a safe place of birth, consideration should be given to the environment and caregivers, in this case midwives, to ensure they have the knowledge, confidence, and skills to facilitate both physiological birth but also emergencies and complications when they arise. Working in the home environment can present a number of challenges, and if prepared for those challenges, then outcomes might be improved. The purpose of this chapter is to outline the arrangements for managing emergencies and complications in the homebirth setting, with an emphasis on anticipating any issues that may arise.

- Thinking that one step ahead: What happens if...?
- How will I manage this...?
- How can I prepare for that...?

Always considering the potential issues without compromising the care that you are providing, and not compromising the environment, which in turn could compromise the hormonal response of the woman and her family.

The chapter complements the *Antenatal Planning – Organisational Considerations* chapter, which discusses considerations and preparation for birth at home, and during these scenarios, management will assume that midwives will carry all essential equipment. It is acknowledged that this is not always the case in some NHS Trusts, and we acknowledge that local guidelines might also need to be taken into consideration. The equipment lists illustrated; below will complement those provided in the *Antenatal Planning – Organisational Considerations* chapter and provide a checklist for each scenario, in turn also acknowledging that the list is not exhaustive, and that a risk assessment for the woman and their circumstances will need to also guide additional equipment and other considerations.

Key to the management of all the following scenarios is early recognition and appropriate escalations. If any doubt exists about the emergence of an emergency or that there is an imminent issue, this should be immediately escalated and transfer arranged alongside appropriate communication with the woman and her family.

The author also acknowledges that the words woman or women have been used for the purposes of the chapter; however, it is intended that this includes those people whose gender identity does not correspond with their birth sex or who may have non-binary identity.

Through utilising evidence based algorithms clear management, and accessing vignettes or case studies, you will feel more confident in your management of obstetric emergencies in the home environment.

HUMAN FACTORS

Reports such as the Ockenden report and the ESMiE independent enquiry into improving the safety of midwifery-led births (Ockenden, 2021; Rowe et al., 2020) provide recommendations for human factors training within healthcare settings to improve outcomes and experiences of people accessing the services. Human factors consider the impact on safety that organisations and individuals can influence through behaviours and circumstances. In the clinical setting this means lives can be at risk if human factors are not taken into consideration when planning care, or specifically providing care during an emergency situation (CHFG, 2021).

Within the homebirth environment, there are factors that can impact the outcome for women, newborns, and families, and as such, consideration of team training, including human factor training, is crucial in reducing poor outcomes, as evidenced in the literature (Timmons et al., 2015). Throughout this chapter, we will consider some of those challenges and how you can overcome them whilst minimising the impact.

Communication within the team and within that environment is crucial to ensure that mistakes do not happen and human error is minimised. In any circumstance emergencies will be accompanied by adrenaline, fear, and the unknown, however within the home environment with less access to equipment, less access to other members of the MDT, and the physical challenges that some home environments can pose, it is even more important that midwives are equipped with the knowledge, confidence, and skills to ensure that poor outcomes are minimised. It is also crucial that during the period of risk assessment with the woman that any issues around time to transfer to hospital, availability of emergency services, and limitations of practice for those midwives attending may influence potential outcomes. Anticipating problems or additional needs early will enable midwives to feel confident in the care they are providing, and being prepared for any eventuality and knowing how to manage is where this chapter comes in. Having a guide, a reference to the skills you already possess, will ensure that during those moments, you can be confident of your skills to manage them.

Practice Point:

In all of the following emergencies there are common considerations in relation to communication. Consider:

- Who is taking the lead in the emergency? This can be briefly discussed during handover between the paramedic crews and the midwives in attendance. Acknowledging that a paramedic crew may be more experienced with certain conditions such as an adult collapse, compromised airway etc.
- How have you communicated with the receiving obstetric unit and have you used a closed-loop feedback system?
- Communication with the family and partner is critical in ensuring cooperation. How can this be facilitated and what are the barriers to this? This should be considered as part of antenatal planning for the birth.
- Do clinicians know the capacity and capabilities of each other? What are you asking the paramedic crew to manage and what do they expect of midwives?
- Avoid using confusing abbreviations that may not be understood between teams and professionals.
- Local arrangements for handover and methods for such should be agreed upon in advance and planned multi-disciplinary training used to familiarise this. The use of an SBAR approach is common.
- The use of proformas can be useful in ensuring a systematic approach to emergencies as well as supporting record keeping.

Practice Point: Transfer Considerations

When arranging and managing a transfer to hospital, consider the following:

- Always discuss and gain consent from the woman or birthing person. Discuss reasons, rationale, how the transfer is to happen, and how long it will take. Always respect their wishes.
- Provide opportunity to answer questions
- Always ensure the woman's or birthing person's dignity is respected and wrap or cover in a blanket or support them to get dressed, ensuring they are as comfortable as possible.
- Work with emergency attenders/paramedics to support the woman or birthing person to choose what position to adopt in transfer, taking into consideration the emergency positions discussed here.
- Where possible and in consultation with the paramedics, a midwife should travel with the woman or birthing persons for continuity and to hand over care. Make sure that arrangements for the partner to either travel alongside or in their own transport are discussed.
- Where possible and in consultation with the paramedics, try to ensure that the woman or birthing person and neonate (if born) are not separated.

MATERNAL DETERIORATION AND COLLAPSE

RECOGNITION

One of the key messages in various enquiries into maternal mortality and morbidity over the last 2 decades has been to recognise and respond appropriately to both deterioration and collapse of a woman. The causes of these are wide and multifaceted. In the 2021 MBRRACE report venous thromboembolism (VTE) continued to be the leading cause of direct deaths occurring within 42 days of the end of pregnancy, despite a reduction overall in previous reports (Knight et al., 2021). Sepsis and obstetric haemorrhage were also noted to remain a significant cause of mortality, with sepsis-related death rates slowly increasing since the 2012/14 MBRRACE report. Deaths related to pre-eclampsia and eclampsia are non-statistically higher than their lowest recorded rate in 2012/14. Cardiac disease as an indirect cause of mortality leads with neurological causes, the second most common indirect cause of mortality (Knight et al., 2021, p. 11). Whilst most of the emergencies described in this chapter are focussed on the immediate intrapartum period (as is the nature of attendance of birth at home), however, it is entirely possible that a woman with deteriorating health or collapse might present at any gestation in the pre-hospital setting. A fundamental element in managing such a situation is the swift identification of deterioration and appropriate and immediate escalation.

Prevention of out of hospital cardiac arrest and deterioration is fundamental. Any persistent symptoms in pregnancy such as fainting (especially during exercise, sitting or supine), palpitations, dizziness, chest pain, and sudden shortness of breath should be investigated. Chest pain in particular is a red flag in pregnancy and breathlessness when not moving, particularly when lying supine, is not normal in pregnancy and may indicate cardiac problems (Knight et al., 2019; Resuscitation Council UK, 2021a). Prevention of cardiac arrest also pivots on identification of underlying causes including bleeding and sepsis whilst using a systematic approach to assess and correct reversible causes.

Deterioration and collapse may occur for many reasons, for example:

- Cardiac arrest
- Asthma attack
- Sepsis
- Stroke or neurological event

- Pulmonary embolism
- Caesarean scar rupture
- Placental abruption
- Seizure
- Choking

In all events summoning immediate help for transfer to hospital is vital, alongside a systematic approach to management and continual risk assessment.

MANAGEMENT

It is vital that all clinicians attending the pre-hospital environment are trained in the immediate assessment, recognition, and management of the acutely unwell woman using a systemic ABCDE approach with appropriate corrective actions to ensure that care is administered in a clinical area with appropriate skills, staff, and facilities appropriate to the presentation of the woman recognising the restrictions on providing advanced or anything other than immediate care as a midwife in the community (Resuscitation Council UK, 2021b). Communication must remain clear with an agreed lead for the emergency.

PRINCIPLES OF SYSTEMATIC ASSESSMENT (RESUSCITATION COUNCIL UK, 2021B)

Approach any environment with a view to ensuring your own safety. This includes personal protective equipment as well as environmental factors. Initially a swift 'look, listen and feel' approach will provide information to guide your next steps, acknowledging that some interventions may not be achievable unless paramedic colleagues have arrived or transfer to a hospital setting has occurred. The following general principles of assessment and management may be applied across a variety of situations you may face, adapting for individual situations and clinical presentation, as discussed in this chapter. A full history is vital in providing contextual information.

Airway	• Is the woman talking indicating a patent airway? • Consider an obstruction: is noisy airway?, no breath sounds?, accessory muscles being used?. If choking, follow choking algorithm. • Open airway with appropriate manoeuvres if necessary to open airway (head tilt, chin lift) or insertion of adjunct airway if trained to do so. • Administer high-flow oxygen provided with a mask with oxygen reservoir (15 L/min). • If possible, obtain oxygen saturations aiming for 94–98%.
Breathing	• Look, feel, and listen for signs of respiratory distress including use of accessory muscles, cyanosis (taking into account ethnicity of the woman), abdominal breathing, and perspiration. Also look for airway secretions. • Assess respiratory rate. An increased respiratory rate ($>$20 breaths/min) is a red flag and may indicate imminent collapse or deterioration. • Observe chest for equal chest expansion, depth of breath and pattern of breathing. • Listen for airway sounds such as agonal breathing, stridor, rattling, wheezing indicating obstruction and respiratory distress.
Circulation	• Observe colour of skin, considering presentation in black and brown skin. Are hands, digits, or lips pale, mottled, cyanosed. • Are extremities cold, pallid or warm? • If possible, measure capillary refill. Apply pressure for 5 seconds on a fingertip to cause blanching, release, and count the amount of time for the skin to return to its normal colours. Anything $>$2 seconds may indicate poor peripheral perfusion in the absence of environmental factors such as cold and lighting. • Count the pulse rate by peripheral palpation or auscultating the heart with a stethoscope. Pulse should be assessed for presence, rate, regularity, quality and equality. • Blood pressure. Note that even when presenting with shock, blood pressure may be normotensive due to the compensatory mechanisms present including peripheral resistance. • Consider urine output and reduced consciousness which may indicate poor cardiac output or function. • Consider haemorrhage (see rest of chapter). • Consider 2$\times$ (large-bore) intravenous cannula (14–16 g) in preparation for fluid resuscitation (noting that any collapse or deterioration due to pre-eclampsia and eclampsia will exclude fluids). • If possible, obtain bloods, (acknowledging that this may not be appropriate in a pre-hospital scenario). • If appropriate, administer fluid resuscitation, e.g. Hartmann solution or 0.9% sodium chloride according to local guidelines and policy. • Continually reassess. Do not overload; keep full fluid balance records.

Disability	• Check for reversible causes including opioids.
	• Continually reassess for A–C as the effects such as hypoxia, hypotension, hypertension, and hypovolaemia (list not exhaustive) may be cause of reduced consciousness level.
	• Make rapid assessment of consciousness level. AVPU is a common method (Alert, Voice/ Vocal response, Painful stimuli response, or Unresponsive to stimuli).
	• You may consider a capillary blood glucose reading during ambulance transfer or when in hospital.
	• Neurological assessment may indicate a neurological cause for deterioration and collapse.
Exposure	• Ensure that a full examination of the woman is conducted to exclude causes if not immediately obvious. Ensure dignity and privacy is maintained.
	• Keep the woman warm.
Fetus	• Abdominal palpation to assess uterine tone (if postnatal) and fetal position.
	• Consider fetal auscultation: this will be dependent on the judgement of the midwives in attendance for the individual circumstances and local guidelines. You may consider not doing this for several reasons.
	• If the fetal heart is compromised, will your management change and can you get to the hospital any quicker? May be of little clinical benefit.
	• If compromised, will it increase anxiety of the woman and yourself and compromise the care you are giving?
	• Auscultation in an ambulance may not be safe.
	• There is not always a straightforward answer, and you must use your clinical judgement at the time, as of course listening to the fetal heart may also provide reassurance. Therefore the advice is to consider auscultation based on individual considerations and human factors at the time.
Get Help (Transfer)	• Always recognise when more help is needed and escalate early. Remember that transfer times may vary, so call or help sooner rather than later.
	• All situations should be treated as a time-critical emergency and help summoned as soon as possible
	• Consider how transfer will be facilitated with paramedic colleagues. Consider location of emergency, equipment considerations, pre-alerting the receiving hospital.
	Consider urgency of the transfer and need/ability to stabilise the woman or neonate. Do you want to scoop and go? Communication with the wider multidisciplinary team and paramedics.

Reproduced with the kind permission of Resuscitation Council UK (Resuscitation Council UK, 2021b).

This approach should be revisited and reassessed regularly, correcting any deviations before moving on to the next element of the assessments. Record all observations on a maternal early warning score chart if possible. Communication with colleagues including paramedics, midwives, and those on transfer to hospital requires a systematic communication such as SBAR (NHS Institute for Innovation and Improvement, 2010) and clear agreement on who is leading the emergency should be vocalised, utilising appropriate expertise. In all cases swift transfer is needed for obstetric and/or medical review and possibly a plan to expedite birth if pregnancy. Consider the wider team.

The following describes additional considerations and actions for pregnancy- and birth-related management of specific causes (assuming the ABCDEFG approach is also being undertaken):

Seizure
- Recognise and declare the emergency.
- Summon help as a time-critical emergency. Requires immediate transfer to hospital.
- Take a good history from those in attendance (family/friends) to exclude underlying condition but do not let this process hinder immediate actions.
- Treat as eclampsia in absence of diagnosis of underlying condition, that is, epilepsy, injury, opioids etc.
- If woman is standing or seated, assist in moving her to the floor and make the space safe for them and you.
- Eclamptic seizures are usually self-limiting. Time the seizures and document this.
- If seizure due to underlying condition such as epilepsy, observe for status epilepticus and take all medication to the hospital.
- Once seizure has finished, if possible, place in left lateral and ensure ABCDEF approach is followed.
- Avoid fluid bolus if suspected eclampsia.
- Auscultating the fetal heart during a seizure is likely to add little to clinical picture at this stage. Wait until after the seizure.
- Refer to local guidelines for the management of seizures at home

Cardiac Arrest (Resuscitation Council UK, 2021a, 2021b, 2021c)
- Recognise and declare the emergency.
- Summon help as a time-critical emergency. Requires immediate transfer to hospital.

- If woman is standing or seated, assist in moving her to the floor and make the space safe for them and you.
- Take a good history from those in attendance (family/friends) to exclude underlying condition but do not let this process hinder immediate actions.

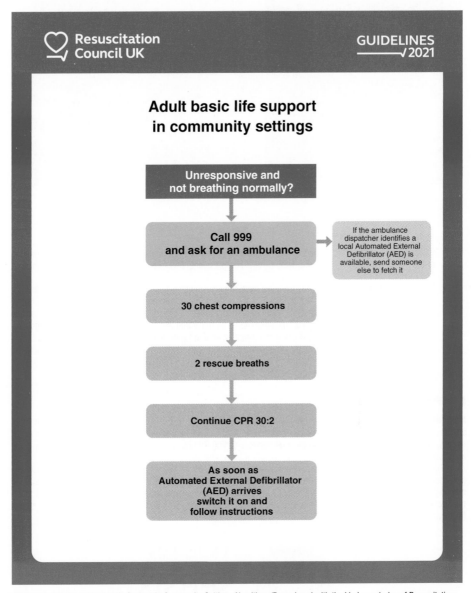

UNFig 11.1 RCUK Adult Basic Life Support in Community Settings Algorithm. (Reproduced with the kind permission of Resuscitation Council UK.)

The resuscitation council special circumstances guidelines (Resuscitation Council UK, 2021a, 2021c) support the following modifications for advanced life support in a pregnant patient:

- Commence basic life support according to the standard guidelines (above) including hand placement or lower half of the sternum if feasible (Resuscitation Council UK, 2021a, 2021c).
- If over 20 weeks pregnant (or uterus palpable above the umbilicus in absence of known gestation), manually displace the uterus to the left to relieve pressure causing aortocaval compression (see Fig. 11.1)

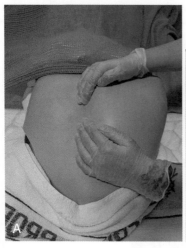
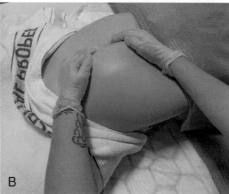

Fig. 11.1 Manual Displacement of the uterus.

- Whilst awaiting paramedic response, the focus of the attending midwives should be on manual displacement of the uterus (as above) and good-quality cardiac compressions. Roles can be swapped during the resuscitation to allow for rest.
- It is possible that an emergency/resuscitative hysterotomy may be required. Critical care attendance in the community will be required for this on site, (acknowledging that this is rare and dependant on local arrangements/ protocols) otherwise potentially undertaken upon arrival to emergency department/ maternity. It should be noted that if >20 weeks pregnant/palpable uterus as described above, emergency hysterotomy is indicated if resuscitation is unsuccessful within 4 minutes, aiming for delivery within 5 minutes of collapse (Resuscitation Council UK, 2021c). It is imperative therefore that no delay occurs in transfer and communication remains effective and resuscitation should continue and not be ceased until in a clinical setting.
- Identify and treat causes (see rest of chapter).

SUSPECTED SEPSIS

Most NHS Trusts now have adopted and are familiar with the 'sepsis six' and an emphasis on instigating recognition and treatment within the first hour (Nutbeam and Daniels, 2021); however, treatment will be limited in the community setting. Emphasis therefore should be on swift recognition, calling for help, and immediate transfer to hospital, where advanced care can be instigated.

Swift recognition and escalation here can improve outcomes. The UK Sepsis Trust publish tools to aid with decision making and instigation of appropriate care pathways and treatments (Fig 11.2). Two tools are available to support screening through the UK Sepsis Trust and may be adopted through local governance processes acknowledging that they need to be supported through training, education, and support, along with audit to ensure compliance and safety (Nutbeam and Daniels, 2021) (Figs 11.3-5).

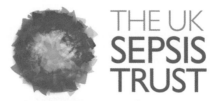

Fig 11.2 UK Sepsis Trust logo. (Reproduced by kind permission of the United Kingdom Sepsis Trust)

SEPSIS SCREENING TOOL COMMUNITY MIDWIVES | **PREGNANT** OR UP TO 6 WEEKS POST-PREGNANCY

01 START THIS CHART IF THE PATIENT LOOKS UNWELL

RISK FACTORS FOR SEPSIS INCLUDE:

☐ Recent trauma / surgery / invasive procedure
☐ Impaired immunity (e.g. diabetes, steroids, chemotherapy)
☐ Indwelling lines / IVDU / broken skin

02 COULD THIS BE DUE TO AN INFECTION?

YES

LIKELY SOURCE:

☐ Respiratory   ☐ Urine
☐ Breast abscess   ☐ Abdominal pain / distension
☐ Infected caesarean / perineal wound
☐ Chorioamnionitis / endometritis

NO ➤ **SEPSIS UNLIKELY, CONSIDER OTHER DIAGNOSIS**

03 ANY RED FLAG PRESENT?

YES

☐ Objective evidence of new or altered mental state
☐ Systolic BP ≤ 90 mmHg (or drop of >40 from normal)
☐ Heart rate ≥ 130 per minute
☐ Respiratory rate ≥ 25 per minute
☐ Needs O₂ to keep SpO₂ ≥ 92% (88% in COPD)
☐ Non-blanching rash / mottled / ashen / cyanotic
☐ Not passed urine in 18 hours (<0.5ml/kg/hr if catheterised)

YES ➤

RED FLAG SEPSIS
START BUNDLE

04 ANY AMBER FLAG PRESENT?

NO

☐ Behavioral / mental status change
☐ Acute deterioration in functional ability
☐ Respiratory rate 21-24
☐ Heart rate 100-129 or new dysrhythmia
☐ Systolic BP 91-100 mmHg
☐ Has had invasive procedure in last 6 weeks (e.g. CS, forceps delivery, ERPC, cerclage, CVs, miscarriage, termination)
☐ Temperature < 36°C
☐ Has diabetes or gestational diabetes
☐ Close contact with GAS
☐ Prolonged rupture of membranes
☐ Bleeding / wound infection
☐ Offensive vaginal discharge
☐ Non-reassuring CTG / fetal tachycardia >160

1 SAME DAY ASSESSMENT BY GP/ TEAM LEADER

2 IS URGENT REFERRAL TO HOSPITAL REQUIRED?

YES

3 AGREE AND DOCUMENT ONGOING MANAGEMENT PLAN (INCLUDING OBSERVATION FREQUENCY AND PLANNED SECOND REVIEW)

NO AMBER FLAGS = ROUTINE CARE / CONSIDER OTHER DIAGNOSIS

COMMUNITY MIDWIFE RED FLAG BUNDLE:

THIS IS TIME-CRITICAL – IMMEDIATE ACTION REQUIRED:

DIAL 999 AND ARRANGE BLUE LIGHT TRANSFER

COMMUNICATION: Ensure communication of 'Red Flag Sepsis' to crew. Advise crew to pre-alert as 'Red Flag Sepsis'. Where possible a written handover is recommended including observations and antibiotic allergies.

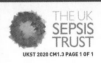

THE UK SEPSIS TRUST

UKST 2020 CM1.3 PAGE 1 OF 1

The UK Sepsis Trust registered charity number (England & Wales) 1158843 (Scotland) SC050277. Company registration number 8644039. Sepsis Enterprises Ltd. company number 9583335. VAT reg. number 293133408.

The controlled copy of this document is maintained by The UK Sepsis Trust. Any copies of this document held outside of that area, in whatever format (e.g. paper, email attachment) are considered to have passed out of control and should be checked for currency and validity.

Fig 11.3 UK Sepsis Trust Community Pregnancy Version 1.3. (Reproduced by kind permission of United Kingdom Sepsis Trust [Nutbeam and Daniels, 2021].)

SEPSIS SCREENING TOOL PREHOSPITAL

PREGNANT
OR UP TO 6 WEEKS POST-PREGNANCY

01 START THIS CHART IF THE PATIENT LOOKS UNWELL

RISK FACTORS FOR SEPSIS INCLUDE:

☐ Recent trauma / surgery / invasive procedure
☐ Impaired immunity (e.g. diabetes, steroids, chemotherapy)
☐ Indwelling lines / IVDU / broken skin

02 COULD THIS BE DUE TO AN INFECTION?

YES

LIKELY SOURCE:

☐ Respiratory
☐ Breast abscess
☐ Urine
☐ Abdominal pain / distension
☐ Infected caesarean / perineal wound
☐ Chorioamnionitis / endometritis

NO → **SEPSIS UNLIKELY, CONSIDER OTHER DIAGNOSIS**

03 ANY RED FLAG PRESENT?

YES

☐ Objective evidence of new or altered mental state
☐ Systolic BP ≤ 90 mmHg (or drop of >40 from normal)
☐ Heart rate ≥ 130 per minute
☐ Respiratory rate ≥ 25 per minute
☐ Needs O₂ to keep SpO₂ ≥ 92% (88% in COPD)
☐ Non-blanching rash / mottled / ashen / cyanotic
☐ Lactate ≥ 2 mmol/l*
☐ Not passed urine in 18 hours (<0.5ml/kg/hr if catheterised)
lactate may be raised in & immediately after normal delivery

YES → **RED FLAG SEPSIS START PH BUNDLE**

04 ANY AMBER FLAG PRESENT?

NO

IF IMMUNITY IMPAIRED TREAT AS RED FLAG SEPSIS

☐ Behavioural / mental status change
☐ Acute deterioration in functional ability
☐ Respiratory rate 21-24
☐ Heart rate 100-129 or new dysrhythmia
☐ Systolic BP 91-100 mmHg
☐ Has had invasive procedure in last 6 weeks (e.g. CS, forceps delivery, ERPC, cerclage, CVs, miscarriage, termination)
☐ Temperature < 36°C
☐ Has diabetes or gestational diabetes
☐ Close contact with GAS
☐ Prolonged rupture of membranes
☐ Bleeding / wound infection
☐ Offensive vaginal discharge
☐ Non-reassuring CTG/ fetal tachycardia >160

YES → **FURTHER INFORMATION AND REVIEW REQUIRED:**

- **TRANSFER TO DESIGNATED DESTINATION**
- **COMMUNICATE POTENTIAL OF SEPSIS AT HANDOVER**

NO AMBER FLAGS OR UNLIKELY SEPSIS: ROUTINE CARE - CONSIDER OTHER DIAGNOSIS - SAFETY-NET & SIGNPOST AS PER LOCAL GUIDANCE

PREHOSPITAL SEPSIS BUNDLE*:

RESUSCITATION:
Oxygen to maintain saturations of >94% (88% in COPD)
Measure lactate if available
250ml boluses of Sodium Chloride: max 250mls if normotensive, max 2000ml if hypotensive. *NICE RECOMMENDS USING LACTATE TO GUIDE FURTHER FLUID THERAPY

COMMUNICATION:
Pre-alert receiving hospital.
Divert to ED (or other agreed destination)
Handover presence of Red Flag Sepsis

*NICE recommends rapid transfer to hospital is the priority rather than a prehospital bundle

THE UK SEPSIS TRUST

UKST 2020 2.2 PAGE 1 OF 1

The controlled copy of this document is maintained by The UK Sepsis Trust. Any copies of this document held outside of that area, in whatever format (e.g. paper, email attachment) are considered to have passed out of control and should be checked for currency and validity. The UK Sepsis Trust registered charity number (England & Wales) 1158843 (Scotland) SC050277. Company registration number 8644039. Sepsis Enterprises Ltd. company number 9583335. VAT reg. number 293133408.

Fig 11.4 UK Sepsis Trust Prehospital Pregnant Version 1.3. (Reproduced by kind permission of United Kingdom Sepsis Trust [Nutbeam and Daniels, 2021].)

SEPSIS SCREENING TOOL PREHOSPITAL — UNDER 5

01 START IF CHILD LOOKS UNWELL, IF THERE'S PARENTAL CONCERN OR PEWS HAS TRIGGERED

RISK FACTORS FOR SEPSIS INCLUDE:

- ☐ Impaired immunity (e.g. diabetes, steroids, chemotherapy)
- ☐ Recent trauma / surgery / invasive procedure
- ☐ Indwelling lines / broken skin

02 COULD THIS BE DUE TO AN INFECTION?

YES

LIKELY SOURCE:

- ☐ Respiratory
- ☐ Brain
- ☐ Urine
- ☐ Surgical
- ☐ Skin / joint / wound
- ☐ Other
- ☐ Indwelling device

NO → **SEPSIS UNLIKELY, CONSIDER OTHER DIAGNOSIS**

03 ANY RED FLAG PRESENT?

YES

- ☐ Doesn't wake when roused / won't stay awake
- ☐ Looks very unwell to healthcare professional
- ☐ Weak, high-pitched or continuous cry
- ☐ Severe tachypnoea (see chart)
- ☐ Severe tachycardia (see chart)
- ☐ Bradycardia (<60 bpm)
- ☐ Non-blanching rash / mottled / ashen / cyanotic
- ☐ Temperature <36°C
- ☐ If under 3 months, temperature 38°C+
- ☐ SpO_2 < 90% on air or increased O_2 requirements

YES → **RED FLAG SEPSIS START PAEDIATRIC PH BUNDLE**

04 ANY AMBER FLAG PRESENT?

NO

IF IMMUNITY IMPAIRED TREAT AS RED FLAG SEPSIS

- ☐ Not responding normally / no smile
- ☐ Reduced activity / very sleepy
- ☐ Moderate tachypnoea (see chart)
- ☐ Moderate tachycardia (see chart)
- ☐ SpO_2 < 92% or increased O_2 requirement
- ☐ Nasal flaring
- ☐ Capillary refill time ≥ 3 seconds
- ☐ Reduced urine output
- ☐ Leg pain or cold extremities

YES → **FURTHER INFORMATION AND REVIEW REQUIRED:**

- **TRANSFER TO DESIGNATED DESTINATION**
- **COMMUNICATE POTENTIAL OF SEPSIS AT HANDOVER**

PREHOSPITAL SEPSIS BUNDLE*:

RESUSCITATION:
Oxygen to maintain saturations of >94%
Measure lactate if available
20ml/kg boluses of Sodium Chloride. Repeat if hypotensive.

COMMUNICATION:
Pre-alert receiving hospital.
Divert to ED (or other agreed destination)
Handover presence of Red Flag Sepsis

*NICE recommends rapid transfer to hospital is the priority rather than a prehospital bundle

Age (years)	Tachypnoea (breaths per minute)		Tachycardia (beats per minute)	
	Severe	Moderate	Severe	Moderate
<1	≥60	50-59	≥160	150-159
1-2	≥50	40-49	≥150	140-149
3-4	≥40	35-39	≥140	130-139

THE UK SEPSIS TRUST

UKST 2020 2.2 PAGE 1 OF 1

Fig 11.5 UK Sepsis under 5 Version 1.3. (Reproduced by kind permission of United Kingdom Sepsis Trust [Nutbeam and Daniels, 2021].)

Additional Management Considerations for Sepsis Alongside Algorithm

- Recognise and declare the emergency.
- Summon help as a time-critical emergency. Requires immediate transfer to hospital.
- Try to obtain a history for possible sources of infection.
- In adults if any red flags present commence pre-hospital sepsis bundle if carrying equipment to enable this/ in communication with paramedic colleagues; however, **rapid transfer to hospital is the priority, NOT the pre-hospital bundle** (Nutbeam and Daniels, 2021):
  - Oxygen measurement to maintain saturation of $>94\%$
  - Measure lactate if available (noting limitations)
  - 250 mL boluses of sodium chloride: max 250 mL if normotensive, max 2000 mL if hypotensive
- If postnatal, ensure then neonate is referred for review in case of neonatal infection.
- If your concern is over a neonate, listen to parents' concerns about behaviours and presentation of neonate including lethargy, poor feeding, not waking for feeds, grunting, and visible signs of respiratory distress (nasal flaring, chest recession, cyanosis taking into account skin colour of neonate). Also refer to chapter *Additional Neonatal Considerations for Homebirth*.
- Prevalent to receiving hospital, emergency department, or other agreed destination.
- CLEARLY hand over your concerns about possible sepsis, making explicit the red flags using an agreed format such as SBAR (NHS Institute for Innovation and Improvement, 2010).
- Refer to local guidelines for the management of suspected adult or neonatal sepsis.

CORD PROLAPSE

Cord prolapse can be defined as the presentation of the umbilical cord through the cervix either below the presenting part (overt) or alongside the presenting part (occult) in the presence of ruptured membranes (RCOG, 2014). Cord presentation is defined as the presence of the cord between the presenting part and the cervix with or without intact membranes (RCOG, 2014). Reasons for cord prolapse might include gestation considerations or prematurity, presentation of the fetus (i.e. breech), a high presentation part, increased liquor volume, for example, polyhydramnios, or multipary. Overall incidence is 1–6 per 1000 births, higher in breech births (1 in 100 births) (RCOG, 2014)

Cord prolapse is a time-critical emergency and requires immediate action and transfer to obstetric unit and timely management is necessary. If the woman or birthing person is in labour, and the cord is prolapsed, this then means that the cord will have pressure applied during contractions and in turn reducing blood flow and oxygen to the fetus.

Recognition is key, then relieving the pressure, and transferring to obstetric unit. Following the next simple steps will ensure that this emergency is managed appropriately.

- **Recognise**: Acknowledge that this is an emergency and call for help. A 999-time critical ambulance is required if not already present. Call ahead to the obstetric unit to prepare for arrival emphasising the time-critical nature of the transfer with a view to transfer straight to labour ward or theatres. Paramedic crew to pre-alert. As soon as recognition has occurred, relieving pressure is the next vital step to minimise cord compression.
- **Relieve**: Consider if the birth is imminent. If yes, then help should still be summoned; however, you may commence pushing, ensuring that neonatal resuscitation is anticipated. If in any doubt that birth is not imminent, commence relief of pressure on the cord through bladder filling (first choice in community setting but never delay the transfer in order to perform this) and apply a dry sanitary pad to keep cord inside the vagina and prevent cold shock and subsequent vasospasm. Avoid excessive handling of the cord.
- **Relieve**: If trained to do so, some midwives may be able to relieve pressure by using the emergency intervention of bladder filling. This will be completed by the midwife that is trained in doing so. A Foley catheter is inserted into the urethra, draining any residual urine and inflating the balloon as normal. Connect a normal intravenous giving set to the drainage port of the Foley catheter and fill the urinary bladder with 500 mL of normal saline. Clamp the set/Foley catheter securely. The intention of this is to lift the presenting part away from the umbilical cord and slow down contractions. This can be used in conjunction with a positional transfer.
- **Relieve**: Ask the woman or birthing person to turn into a knee-to-chest position with buttocks high in the air until transfer is possible.
- **Transfer**: Transfer should be with the woman or birthing person in lateral position, with a cushion/blanket to elevate her lowest hip.
- Consider IV: access and other interventions BUT must only be undertaken if there is time and only then if it does not impede timely and safe transfer.
- Consider fetal auscultation: this will be dependent on the judgement of the midwives in attendance. You may consider not doing this for several reasons.
  1. If the fetal heart is compromised, will your management change, and can you get to the hospital any quicker? May be of little clinical benefit.
  2. If compromised, will it increase anxiety within the woman and yourself and compromise the care you are giving?
  3. Auscultation in an ambulance may not be safe.

There is not always a straightforward answer, and you must use your clinical judgement at the time, as of course listening to the fetal heart may also provide reassurance. Therefore the advice is to consider auscultation based on individual considerations and human factors at the time.

EQUIPMENT

- Gloves
- Dry sanitary pad
- Client's underwear
- Pillow or cushion for transfer
- Bladder filling kit if carried in community (Foley catheter, 500 mL normal saline, IV giving set, clamps)

AFTERCARE

As this is a time-critical emergency, it is absolutely crucial that communication is clear, concise, and compassionate. There will be fear and anxiety, and as healthcare practitioners, we have a responsibility to ensure that we have gained consent for any procedures and that we are calm and concise in our decision making. Ensure that timely debrief has taken place after the event to ensure that questions are answered, and all parties involved are able to reflect and ensure any further needs are actioned.

REMEMBER

- Recognise:
  - Umbilical cord visible or protruding from vagina
  - Cord is palpable on vaginal examination (if this is the case, leave fingers in situ and follow below)
  - Abnormal fetal heart on auscultation
- Call for help: call 999 time-critical ambulance with paramedic.
- Relieve pressure through manual elevation of fetal head if diagnosed on vaginal examination.
- Relieve pressure through bladder filling and apply dry sanitary pad.
- Position woman in knee-to-chest and await transfer to hospital. Consider fetal auscultation.
- Pre-alert hospital en route and keep woman calm and in left lateral position with pillow under hip to elevate.

CASE STUDY 11.1

- Sarah is a 35-year-old G4 P3 who is booked for her 2nd homebirth. She has a previous low-risk obstetric history and has gone into spontaneous labour at 38 weeks and 2 days. The community midwife is in attendance, and Sarah is contracting 3:10 strongly, and her membranes are intact. Sarah has requested a vaginal examination to ascertain cervical dilatation. The vaginal examination is performed in the bedroom upstairs and her husband is present, and mum is downstairs supervising the other children.
- On vaginal examination, the midwife finds that her cervix is 5 cm, fully effaced, and well applied to the presenting part which is cephalic. Membranes are intact, but she feels that part of the cord is in front of the fetal head and can feel it pulsating. The midwife leaves her fingers inside and attempts to relieve pressure by manually elevating the fetal head off the cord. The midwife then calmly explains to the woman and her husband what is happening and asks the husband to call 999 and ask for a time-critical paramedic ambulance.
- Once this task is completed, she asks him to call for another midwife using her phone, instructing him to do so. He then is asked to pass her the bladder filling kit which is in her equipment bag, and she proceeds to fill Sarah's bladder as per guidance, before placing a dry sanitary towel in her underwear and asking her to turn into a knee-to-chest position. The midwife has made the decision to auscultate the fetal heart in view of the fact that the ambulance is en route, the hospital is a 10-minute drive away, membranes are intact, and the cord pulsated at a normal rate. FH was auscultated for 1 minute and was 125–135 bpm.
- In the interim the midwife explains that she will be transferred to the hospital and the obstetric team will be on hand to ascertain the best mode of delivery.
- Paramedics arrive and transfer to hospital with midwife in the ambulance and Sarah in left lateral with a pillow under her hip. On arrival, Sarah is transferred straight to the obstetric theatre, where she was assessed to be 8 cm with cord presenting and membranes intact. A caesarean section was performed under spinal anaesthesia, and a live female infant was born with Apgars of 5/10 at 1 minute, 8/10 at 5 minutes, and 10/10 at 8 minutes.

ANTEPARTUM HAEMORRHAGE

RECOGNITION

Antepartum haemorrhage (APH) is any bleeding from the genital tract after 24 weeks gestation and before the birth of the baby (RCOG, 2011). Causes can sometimes be unknown, but the most important causes are placenta praevia, or placental abruption, but they are not the most common. Similarly to PPH, the amount of blood that is visible is not necessarily the total loss. APH can also be concealed; therefore it is important to consider blood loss that could be accumulating in the abdomen. It is key to remember that mother's life should take priority during the management of an APH.

Symptoms of APH will present in different ways dependent upon the cause. Sometimes women will have visible vaginal blood loss, which needs to be treated and managed immediately. Also, women will present with no visible bleeding but, however, may present with abdominal pain and a tense uterus, indicating potential for concealed bleeding.

Vital signs may be within normal parameters for a short while; however these can deteriorate rapidly in the pregnant woman, and monitoring is vital.

Incidence is around 3–5% of all pregnancies and is a leading cause of perinatal and maternal mortality worldwide (RCOG, 2011). In the majority of homebirth cases APH will be an intrapartum event and as such will require immediate transfer to the nearest obstetric unit. You need to consider the gestation of the woman, the location of the nearest hospital, and the severity of the blood loss.

MANAGEMENT

- On recognition of the APH, call for help immediately via 999 and ask for a time-critical ambulance, stating you have a pregnant woman who is bleeding. You can ask the partner to do this simultaneously with the actions below.
- Simultaneously, reassure woman and assess her colour and her pulse rate and respiration rate using an ABCD approach.
- With consent, place your hand on the abdomen gently to assess if the uterus is soft, contracting, woody etc.
- Assess blood loss, and ensure all garments, pads, and sheets are put into a bag and transferred to hospital for accurate blood loss measurement.
- Ask about fetal movements.
- Consider fetal auscultation.
- If the bleeding continues, insert a wide-bore (16 g preferably) cannula and commence fluid resuscitation with crystalloid as per trust guidance. Have a low threshold for IV fluids.
- Consider Entonox if she is in pain.
- Turn her into left lateral and keep nil by mouth.
- Transfer to hospital as soon as help has arrived and is safe to do so.
- Pre-alert the hospital of transfer and state the severity of the situation.

EQUIPMENT

- Gloves
- Inco sheets
- Sanitary pads
- Crystalloid fluids
- IV cannula (16 g)
- BP cuff/machine, saturation probe

AFTERCARE

Once transferred into hospital care, ensure safe and accurate handover using SBAR tool. Ensure throughout that woman and family are informed of actions, and documentation is contemporaneous and accurate.

Remember

- Upon recognition of APH, call 999 time-critical ambulance.
- Assess if abdomen hard and tender or soft on palpation and observe per-vaginum blood loss.
- Assess vital signs, reassure, and keep woman calm until paramedics arrive.
- Assess fetal movements and consider fetal auscultation on individual basis.
- Gain IV access with wide-bore cannulae and commence crystalloids as per local guidelines.
- Transfer to nearest obstetric unit as soon as possible.

CASE STUDY 11.2

Raveena is a G2, P1 and 37 + 3 weeks pregnant, booked for a homebirth. She has gone into spontaneous labour, and her pregnancy has been uneventful. She has started contracting about an hour ago, but on arrival, the midwife is concerned. During her assessment of Raveena, she finds that in between her contractions, Raveena is experiencing some pain and her abdomen remains tense. She has not felt the baby move for a few hours. The midwife asks her to empty her bladder before she does a full assessment, and Raveena reports some fresh red bleeding. On inspection, the midwife estimates around 100 mL in the toilet and on the tissue.

The midwife explains that she will need to be transferred to the hospital to be assessed and calls 999 for a time-critical ambulance. Raveena's partner is still on his way home from work, and her little boy who is 3 is playing. Raveena is concerned and anxious and calls her parents to come and collect her son whilst the midwife calls the obstetric unit to pre-warn of their arrival.

The midwife considers fetal auscultation as Raveena has just felt the baby move; she auscultates the FH to be 95 bpm, accelerating back to 110 bpm. The paramedics arrive 5 minutes later and transfer Raveena to the hospital 20 minutes away, where the obstetric team are waiting. On arrival, the midwife hands over using the SBAR tool. The fetal heart cannot be auscultated, and an IUD is confirmed by scan 10 minutes later when Raveena's husband arrives. Placental abruption is confirmed.

Q: Would you have auscultated in this situation? In the home environment your management may be different.

Shoulder Dystocia

Recognition

Shoulder dystocia is an acute obstetric emergency which requires immediate skilled intervention to avoid serious fetal morbidity or mortality. Recognition of this emergency swiftly will ensure that the dystocia is resolved as quickly and efficiently as possible.

Risk factors are an unreliable predictor, can make us alert to the possibility of a shoulder dystocia, and should not be relied upon. Shoulder dystocia should therefore be anticipated in all homebirths and planned for accordingly. Many shoulders dystocias are unexpected and thus reinforce the importance of early recognition including early recognition and transfer for labour progress issues in any stage of labour.

Shoulder dystocia should be anticipated if there are any of the following signs:

- Slow progress in any stage of labour.
- Slow delivery of the fetal head by extension.
- Difficulty in delivery of the face and chin.
- When the head is born it remains tightly applied to the vulva.
- The chin retracts and depresses the perineum 'turtleneck' sign.
- Failure of the fetal head to restitute.

Complete recognition is when the anterior shoulder fails to release despite maternal pushing and/or when routine axial traction is applied to assist the birth.

Incidence

- Incidence between 0.58% and 0.7% (RCOG, 2012)
- 1% in infants weighing >4000 grams
- 10% in infants weighing between 4000 grams and 4499 grams
- 23% in infants ≥4500 grams

Management

- Immediately call for help. If alone, call 999 for time-critical ambulance requesting 2 ambulances. Discourage pushing simultaneously.
- Lay woman flat and remove any pillows from bed. See practice point if in the pool.
- Perform McRoberts manoeuvre, thighs to abdomen.
- If another midwife in attendance, perform suprapubic pressure and routine axial traction at the same time. See Fig. 11.6.
- If unresolved, consider episiotomy if this makes internal manoeuvres easier, remembering that this is a bony dystocia and that an episiotomy is unlikely to resolve the dystocia and may be difficult to do. Under no circumstances should performing this slow down any further manoeuvres.

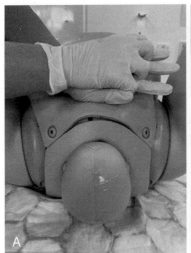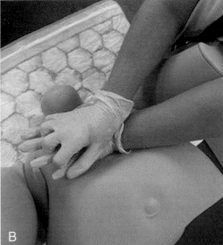

Fig. 11.6 A. Shoulder dystocia 1; B. shoulder dystocia 2.

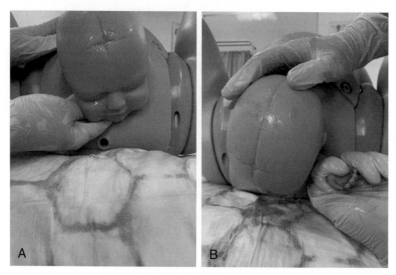

Fig. 11.7 A. Shoulder dystocia 3; B. shoulder dystocia 4.

- Depending on experience and clinical circumstances, attempt delivery of the posterior arm **OR** commence internal rotational manoeuvres. Internal manoeuvres involve inserting the whole hand as if putting on a bracelet into the sacral hollow locating either the anterior aspect of the posterior shoulder or posterior aspect of the posterior shoulder, applying pressure here to internally rotate the shoulders into the oblique diameter. If unsuccessful attempt delivery of the posterior arm by following the upper arm to locate the antecubital fossa, gentle pressure will flex the arm (or indeed the hand may just be sitting there) – gently grasping the hand and wrist, sweep this across the fetal chest and deliver the arm. See Fig. 11.7
- If the above methods fail, turn to all-fours position or repeat from above.
- Immediately transfer to obstetric unit once paramedics arrive.

Practice Point:
- If the woman is in the pool, standing her up and placing one leg on the side of the pool may have the same effect as McRoberts, so sometimes asking her to exit the pool will have the desired effect this should not however, delay egressing the pool.
- Be prepared for neonatal resuscitation at all homebirths, will increase the likelihood of a positive outcome for neonate also.

EQUIPMENT

- Resuscitation equipment as above NLS and area to resuscitate
- Gloves
- Episiotomy scissors
- Perineal repair equipment

AFTERCARE

Anticipate a postpartum haemorrhage.

Depending on the length of time and manoeuvres to resolve the shoulder dystocia, the neonate may need extensive resuscitation. Regardless of degree of neonatal resuscitation, transfer to obstetric unit must be undertaken and a paediatric review undertaken.

Ensure woman and birth partners are fully debriefed on all manoeuvres that have been carried out and also on the condition of the neonate once appropriate. Perineal repair may be required as well as routine postnatal care. Transfer to obstetric unit to allow neonate to be reviewed by paediatricians, despite of what manoeuvres were performed.

Postpartum Haemorrhage

Recognition

Excessive bleeding from the birth canal within 24 hours of the birth of the fetus is known as a postpartum haemorrhage (PPH). One definition can be given based on the amount of blood loss, either minor (500–1000 mL) or major (>1000 mL). Major PPH can be further categorised into moderate (1000–2000 mL) or severe (>2000 mL) (Mavrides et al, 2016). However, care must be taken to only focus on the amount of blood loss and ensure a holistic assessment of the woman is completed, taking into account key observations and your clinical judgement. On this basis, the other definition could be any amount of blood loss that leads to haemodynamic instability, as bleeding could be concealed, in the case of perineal haematoma, for example. This may present in signs of shock or maternal collapse. Bearing in mind that during pregnancy and just after birth, blood pressure can be maintained within the normal range until blood loss has exceeded 1000 mL (Mavrides et al, 2016).

It is important to ascertain the cause of the bleeding in order to decide on the management as quickly as possible. There are 4 commonly recognised causes of postpartum, tone (atony of the uterus, failure of it to contract), tissue (remnants of the placental tissue retained), thrombin (deranged clotting factors failing to allow the blood to clot, which is easily recognised by looking at whether the blood loss is clotting or not), and trauma (any tears sustained to the genital tract during birth). The most likely cause is tone of the uterus, and management depends on whether the placenta has been delivered or not (WHO, 2020).

Incidence

Worldwide, the incidence of PPH is 6%, and a study in Wales (comparative to UK maternity units) found a 4.9% incidence in non-assisted vaginal deliveries and 8.6% in total deliveries (Bell et al, 2020). Incidence of PPH at home is harder to quantify; currently, there is no data to indicate the prevalence of free birthing and being born before arrival (BBA) on top of homebirth data; therefore incidence of PPH is unknown but, however, anecdotally likely to be lower.

> **Practice Point:**
> The availability of oxytocic drugs and other drugs to assist management of bleeding will be dependent on the local guidelines for both paramedics and midwives. These local variations and availability must be taken into consideration when planning births at home, with a full and frank discussion of the limitations of how such situations can and might be managed outside of the hospital.

Management

It is acknowledged that if you are alone, some of this will not be possible, and you will need to wait for further assistance. It is also acknowledged that whilst these are listed actions, some will be done simultaneously and are only designed to aid your thought process as you work through the management. In all cases constant reassessment is necessary revisiting the ABCD approach (see practice point above)

- On recognition of the PPH, call for help immediately via 999 and ask for a time-critical ambulance, stating you have a mother and a baby. You can ask the partner to do this simultaneously with the actions below.
- Lie the woman flat.
- If available, administer high flow oxygen (15 L/min if possible) this via a non-rebreathe mask.
- Place your hands on the top of the fundus in a cupped position to check if the uterus is contracted; if not and it feels soft and spongy, firmly make a circular motion to rub up a contraction, if the **placenta has delivered**. Continue this until help arrives or the bleeding stops. Whilst this is happening, check the blood loss to ensure it is clotting, potentially ruling out any thrombin issues (acknowledging the limitations of this). See Fig. 11.8.
- If the **placenta is not yet delivered**, then if able to, administer an oxytocic, dependent on trust policy if not already administered, to assist separation of the placenta. If unable to administer oxytocin, encourage breastfeeding and skin to skin to aid separation. Perform controlled cord traction to deliver the placenta.
- Simultaneously, reassure and communicate with the woman, and assess her airway, breathing, colour, pulse rate, capillary refill, and respiration rate (list not exhaustive). It is vital to ensure that assessment of colour takes into consideration the presentation with melanated skin. The use of maternity early warning observation charts will assist in tracking deterioration.
- With consent, and if trained to do so, check for any vaginal/perineal tears that may be causing the blood loss. If there are, then apply pressure with a sanitary pad until repair is able to commence.
- When you have help, check the placenta to ensure it is complete.
- When you have assistance, consider catheterisation of the bladder to aid the contraction of the uterus.
- If the bleeding continues, insert 2 wide-bore (16 g preferably) cannulae, and commence fluid resuscitation with crystalloid as per Trust guidance.
- If bleeding is continuing, consider further oxytocic administration. If paramedics are present, consider misoprostol or tranexamic acid (TXA) administration if they carry this. Misoprostol *according to national and*

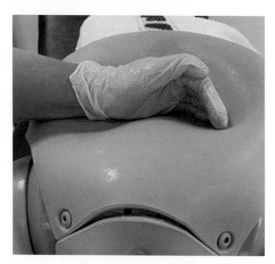

Fig. 11.8 Rubbing up a contraction.

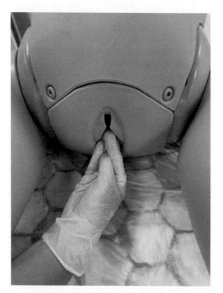

Fig. 11.9 PPH- Bi-manual Compression 1.

local guidelines (Brown et al, 2022) either sublingually or if airway is becoming compromised, give it rectally. TXA can be given 1 g IV over 10 minutes. It is also important here to acknowledge that some midwives will carry some oxytocic drugs, and midwives must adhere to local policy.
- Transfer to obstetric unit must be prepared for, and woman and baby considered. How will they be transferred to the ambulance; are they mobile? Will they need to use stairs? Will the baby come with the woman?
- In the event that bleeding is continuing and deterioration in observations and the woman's condition is occurring, bimanual compression can be considered. Bimanual compression needs to be considered if no other management is effective, as this is an invasive and painful intervention but lifesaving. Bimanual compression may need to be considered an early intervention also.
- When considering bi-manual compression, you need to consider your location. Do you have stairs to get down? How will this be maintained? Will it be easier to commence this in the ambulance when she is on the trolley? Also consider the impact on your safety when transferring.

- Explain the procedure in full and with consent, using sterile gloves, gently insert fingers into the vagina initially (see fig 11.9), then insert whole hand and once inside, carefully form a fist (see Fig. 11.10) to demonstrate position once inside, with the back of your hand facing downwards.
- Place the other hand on top of the fundus and gently fold it forward towards the pelvis, folding over the inserted hand. See Fig 11.11.
- Apply and maintain pressure between your two hands until further assistance has arrived or arrived at hospital.
- Collect ALL blood loss and maintain a running total of this. Weighing pads is important, so ensure this is brought into.
- Aim to stabilise and transfer to obstetric hospital as soon as possible. Midwives should take advice from paramedics in relation to transfer arrangements.

EQUIPMENT

- Gloves
- Oxytocic drugs as per trust guidelines
- Catheterisation pack
- Inco sheets
- Sanitary pads
- Crystalloid fluids
- IV cannula (16 g)
- BP cuff/machine

AFTERCARE

Once the bleeding has subsided, it is important to consider the impact on the woman and also the partner.

Regular observation of vital signs needs to commence to ensure the physical wellbeing of the woman following the PPH, checking particularly for her pulse rate, blood pressure, and respiration rate. Using an Obstetric modified observation chart if available will ensure that any deviations from the normal will be flagged and can be escalated.

Ensure that she is on clean sheets and comfortable and has fresh sanitary pad in situ to ensure visual observation of vaginal bleeding can be observed accurately. Prepare her and neonate for transfer to obstetric unit once help has arrived if not already present.

Ensure clear communication and debrief of situation is communicated to woman and birth partner using an SBAR approach. This will have been a frightening experience, and communication is vital at this point once the initial emergency is stabilised.

Ensure the safe transfer of woman to obstetric unit for review, aiming to keep mother and baby together.

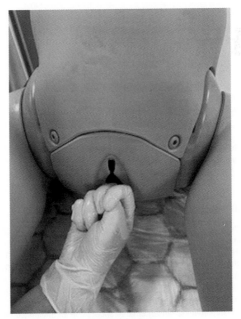

Fig. 11.10 PPH- Bi-manual Compression 1.

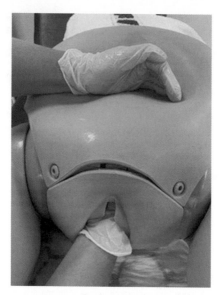

Fig. 11.11 PPH.

CASE STUDY 11.3

Cathy is a 26 years old primigravida who has been booked for a homebirth, with no medical or obstetric history of note, but
her labour progressed rapidly with 2 midwives in attendance at the birth of a live male infant weighing 3.100 kg with Apgars of 9/10 at 1 minute and 10/10 at 5 minutes. The placenta has been delivered with active management, using Syntometrine
1 amp with consent. Shortly after the placenta is delivered there is a constant trickle of blood that appears to be coming from the uterus; blood
loss to this point was estimated at 350 mL, and Cathy is beginning to look a little pale and sweaty.

The midwife places her hand on top of the fundus and ascertains the uterus is soft and boggy, and the blood loss is increasing. The second
midwife calls 999 for a time-critical ambulance and states that she has a PPH and a neonate. Cathy's partner is currently holding the neonate as
Cathy feels too unwell to hold him, and he is keeping the neonate skin to skin to maintain his wellbeing.

The 2nd midwife checks the placenta to check completion, at the same time as ascertaining that there are no thrombin issues as the
blood is clotting on the bed. The 1st midwife continues to rub up a contraction, whilst the 2nd midwife does a visual check of the perineum with
consent. It is concluded that the cause of the PPH is an atonic uterus, and therefore a further oxytocic drug is administered as per their local
guideline.

The 2nd midwife is beginning to prepare for catheterisation and also ensure that they are able to open the door to the paramedics when
they arrive. Once catheterisation has been completed, the blood loss appears to be subsiding slightly; however, Cathy's vital signs indicate she
may be haemodynamically unstable. As the midwife completes a set of observations, the paramedics arrive and a wide bore cannula is inserted
and 1 L of crystalloid is commenced.

Cathy is encouraged to breastfeed her baby to encourage further contraction of the uterus. The blood loss is now under control, and the
midwives are estimating a 1200 mL loss altogether; however, they will collect all sheets and swabs to take to the hospital to weigh and ensure
accurate blood loss estimation.

Cathy and her baby are transferred with midwife present in the ambulance to the nearest obstetric unit for further observation.

Q: What could the midwives have done next had the bleeding not subsided?

Think about this case study in your area, and how may this differ with some of the women you care for and your demographics?

NEWBORN LIFE SUPPORT

Any planned homebirth and those attending should be prepared for the potential of a neonatal resuscitation. Preparation is key and ensuring communication with the woman and partner before labour begins will ensure smooth resuscitation should the need arise. Homebirth will ideally have 2 attendants and staff competent in newborn life support should be available for all births (RCUK, 2021). The woman and her family should be prepared adequately and aware that advanced resuscitation may not be available in the home setting and that any delay in transfer or indeed the process of transfer itself may delay access to advanced resuscitation. Refer to antenatal planning chapter for suggested equipment for planned homebirth and recommendations for safe staffing.

Preparation of the home environment is fundamental to success. In an unplanned homebirth the neonate is at a higher risk of hypothermia and subsequent poorer outcomes (RCUK, 2021).

Ensure that there are no draughts, warm towels are available, and a space is set up for the resuscitation, such as a table or a changing mat on the floor. Ideally this will be next to where the woman births to enable delayed cord clamping and resuscitation to continue without cutting the cord. Make sure that there are plenty of towels and a hat to ensure that the neonate does not get cold.

RECOGNITION

The following guidance is adapted and incorporates the Resuscitation Council UK Newborn life support guidance (2021) (Fig. 11.12).

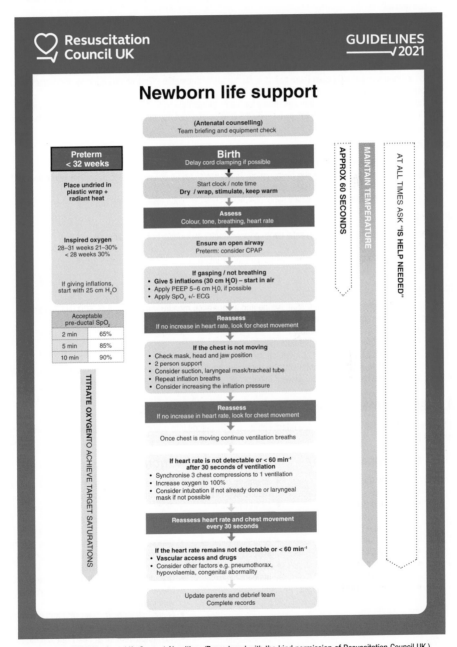

Fig 11.12 RCUK Newborn Life Support Algorithm. (Reproduced with the kind permission of Resuscitation Council UK.)

MANAGEMENT OF THE UMBILICAL CORD

Where possible discuss preferences for cord clamping (also see chapter *Postnatal Care*). RCUK (2021) suggest that in the presence of good thermal care, initial resuscitation can be undertaken with the umbilical cord intact and that clamping and cutting the cord should happen after aeration of the lungs. Clamping after 60 seconds is preferred; however, in neonates >28 weeks gestation, cord milking might be an appropriate alternative.

Once the neonate is born; therefore rapid assessment should occur **before** the cord is clamped and cut:
- Observe tone and colour.
- Dry the neonate vigorously and wrap with dry towels. Apply a hat. Expose only the chest in order to assess rise and fall.
- Assess the adequacy of breathing.
- Count heart rate by apex auscultation with a stethoscope.
- Ensure you keep baby warm during these initial steps.
- Rapid assessment enables the baseline of observations to be set and identifies the need for resuscitation.
- As soon as you recognise the need for further assistance, call 999 and ask for a time-critical ambulance for the woman and baby (in case there needs to be a transfer separately). This can be done by the partner simultaneously with the actions below.
- Rapid assessment also gives the opportunity for tactile stimulation to occur, by drying the infant and gently stimulating them as you dry them, by rubbing the soles of the feet. Try not to rub aggressively, firmly, but gently.

Rapid assessment in more detail:

TONE AND COLOUR

- A very floppy infant is likely to need respiratory support.
- Colour is a poor means of judging oxygenation, as cyanosis can be difficult to recognise. The skin colour of the infant should be taken into consideration.
- Pallor might indicate shock or rarely hypovolaemia – consider blood loss.

BREATHING

Is the infant breathing? – Note the rate, depth and symmetry, work/effort of breathing as:
- adequate
- inadequate/abnormal pattern – such as gasping or grunting
- absent.

HEART RATE

- Determine the heart rate with a stethoscope and a saturation monitor if available +/−ECG (electrocardiogram) for later continuous assessment.
  - Fast ($\geq$100 min^{-1}) – satisfactory
  - Slow (60–100 min^{-1}) – intermediate, possible hypoxia
  - Very slow/absent (<60 min^{-1}) – critical, hypoxia likely

If the infant fails to establish spontaneous and effective breathing following assessment and stimulation, and/or the heart rate does not increase, or decreases if initially fast, respiratory support should be started.

CLASSIFICATION ACCORDING TO INITIAL ASSESSMENT

On the basis of the initial assessment, the infant can usually be placed into one of three groups, as the following examples illustrate.

TRANSITION	ASSESSMENT	ACTIONS
Satisfactory transition: • Good tone • Vigorous breathing or crying • Heart rate – fast ($\geq$100 min^{-1})	• Breathing does not require support • Heart rate is acceptable	• Delay cord clamping for at least 60 seconds • Dry, wrap in warm towel • Keep with mother or carer and ensure maintenance of temperature • Consider early skin-to-skin care if stable
Incomplete transition: • Reduced tone • Breathing inadequately (or apnoeic) • Heart rate – slow (<100 min^{-1})	• Breathing requires support • Slow heart rate may indicate hypoxia	• Delay cord clamping only if you are able to appropriately support the infant; consider cord milking if >28 weeks. • Dry, stimulate, wrap in a warm towel • Maintain the airway, – lung inflation and ventilation • Assess changes in heart rate and breathing • Apply a saturation probe +/− ECG • If no improvement in heart rate, continue with ventilation • Help may be required

TRANSITION	ASSESSMENT	ACTIONS
Poor/failed transition: • Floppy +/− pale • Breathing inadequately or apnoeic • Heart rate – very slow (<60 min⁻¹) or undetectable	• Breathing requires support • Heart rate suggestive of significant hypoxia	• Clamp cord immediately and transfer to the resuscitation platform. Delay cord clamping only if you are able to appropriately support/resuscitate the infant • Dry, stimulate, wrap in warm towel • Maintain the airway – lung inflation and ventilation • Assess changes in heart rate and breathing • Apply a saturation probe +/− ECG. • Continue newborn life support according to response • Help is likely to be required

Reproduced with the kind permission of Resuscitation Council UK (RCUK, 2021).

MANAGEMENT

Management of the newborn needing resuscitation needs to be based on the initial assessment as above and take into consideration your environment, your equipment, your skills, and also whether you have help or not. The NLS algorithm from the Resus Council is included; however, this should be adapted to reflect the situation you are in.

Consider your support and their skills in how you manage the resuscitation and try to communicate throughout with the woman and family if appropriate.

Additional Management Considerations for the Preterm Infant

It is possible that when attending a born before arrival (BBA) or in other circumstances, you may have to adjust your care and resuscitation to accommodate a preterm infant. If help has not yet been summoned, do so as early as possible, as these neonates are likely to require additional support and any delay may contribute to poor outcomes. Immediate transport to an environment with specialist support is necessary. The following are additional considerations for these neonates based on Resuscitation Council UK guidelines (RCUK, 2021):

In general, all preterm neonates should be managed in the same way as term neonates. Consider
- When performing inflation breaths, reduce inflation pressures to between 20 cm and 25 cm H_2O – refer to the RCUK (2021) algorithm for suggested oxygen supplementation guidance.
- Laryngeal masks (LMA) only to be used in neonates >24 weeks (~2000 g); otherwise oropharyngeal airway can be used.
- Consideration of appropriate methods to support thermoregulation, that is, food-grade plastic bag.
- Application of saturation probe as early as possible to inform oxygen supplementation decisions, may use ECG if available.

<28 Weeks Gestation

- Close all windows and doors and exclude draughts; if possible, try to get temperature above 25°C.
- Place into a food-grade plastic bag with head exposed, do not dry, and keep warm by radiant heat source if possible (local maternity and paramedic guidelines may vary on how to achieve this). If radiant heat not available and cord clamping is delayed, ensure thermostability.
- A thermal mat may be appropriate to use (see chapter *Paramedic Transfer and Multidisciplinary Working with Ambulance Services*).
- Consider a hat.

Skin to skin is possible; however, in extreme premature neonates and those who are compromised through growth restriction, this may be difficult. Avoid hypothermia in all cases.

≤32 Weeks Gestation.

- Completely cover the neonate with a polyethylene wrapping such as food grade plastic bag, keeping the face clear. Do not dry the neonate. Place neonate on/under a radiant warmer if available. Place a hat on the neonate.
- If no resuscitation required, and the neonate is well, consider drying and placing the neonate skin to skin and cover both with a towel or covering, ensuring you monitor both temperature and respiratory effort. Skin to skin is possible; however, in extreme premature neonates and those who are compromised through growth restriction, this may be difficult. Avoid hypothermia in all cases.

Suggested Equipment (RCUK, 2021):

- Self-inflating bag – 500 mL with 40 cm blow-off valve
- Round soft silicone masks for the preterm and term baby – (× 2 of each size)
- Stethoscope
- Laryngoscope handle – with long and short blade (0,00)

- Oropharyngeal airways – sizes 0 (6 cm), 00 (5 cm), and 000 (4 cm) or laryngeal mask for infants >34 weeks gestation (2000 g).
- Paediatric Yankauer suckers – ($\times$ 2)
- Soft suction catheters sizes 12 or 14 FG
- Syringes (5 mL $\times$ 2)
- Elastoplast/hypofix/cotton tape
- Spare bulbs, batteries, and disposable blades for laryngoscope if necessary
- Gloves
- Small gauze squares – ($\times$ 2 packets)

Additional:
- Changing mat/heated mattress
- Hats ($\times$ 2)
- Towels ($\times$ 4)
- Good portable light, for example, torch
- Sterile packs of cord scissors and umbilical clamp ($\times$ 3)
- Scissors
- Sharps disposal container
- Clock/stopwatch
- Record keeping charts
- Identification bracelets

POST RESUSCITATION CARE

It is vital to recognise that any neonate that has had any degree of resuscitation may later deteriorate; therefore transfer to a clinical environment that may support close monitoring should be expedited. All care during and post-resuscitation must be clearly and contemporaneously documented. Thermoregulation is crucial following resuscitation; therefore ensure that neonate is able to have skin-to-skin contact and encourage early feeding. Resuscitation can be traumatic for all involved especially parents, so thorough debriefing is an essential element of the process, ensuring time for questions and time to process events. Review in hospital is essential to ensure that any adverse outcomes are identified and managed appropriately. Early feeding to avoid hypoglycaemia is vital.

Practice point:

Remaining calm during this situation is challenging; remember that you are trained for this and have the skills to adequately resuscitate the newborn and that up to 85% of infants will breathe spontaneously without intervention, and a further 10% respond after simulation, drying, and airway manoeuvres. Around 5% require positive pressure, and less than 2% require intubation (Resuscitation Council UK, 2021). However, preparation is key, and more than likely will lead to successful resuscitation.

Call for help early.

CONCLUSION

This chapter is aimed to support other chapters throughout this book in providing a guide and a clear management of some of the obstetric emergencies that you may encounter in the home environment.

Human factors play a key role in healthcare and ensuring that consideration of this during training will help to minimise errors in patient safety and maternity care. As homebirth midwives, it is crucial that MDT training is prioritised to ensure all staff have the knowledge and up-to-date skills to deal with emergencies as they arise. In the vast majority of cases women who plan for a homebirth will have no additional needs, therefore reducing some risks of additional needs; however, as midwives we know that often emergencies cannot be predicted.

Being prepared for any eventuality, being that one step or even two steps ahead, will ensure that should your skills in managing emergencies be needed, you are up to date with evidence-based skills to deal with it.

Having supported many women to birth in their own home throughout her career, the author concludes this chapter by reminding midwives that there is nothing more rewarding than supporting a family within their own environment, and remember, you are a guest in their space, it is sacred, and as such with respect for the process of birth, respect for the importance of the environment around you, trust in the process and empower the women, and emergencies will be few and far between.

REFERENCES

Bell, S. et al., 2020. Incidence of postpartum haemorrhage defined by quantitative blood loss measurement: a national cohort. BMC Pregnancy Childbirth 20, 271. Available at: Incidence of postpartum haemorrhage defined by quantitative blood loss measurement: a national cohort – PMC (nih.gov)

Brown, S.N., Kumar, D.S., James, C. and Mark, J. (eds.) (2019) JRCALC clinical guidelines 2019. Bridgwater: Class Professional Publishing.

Clinical Human Factors Group (CHFG), 2021. *What are clinical human factors*. Available at: What are clinical human factors? | CHFG – Clinical Human Factors Group

Knight, M., Bunch, K., Tuffnell, D., Patel, R., Shakespeare, J., 2021. Saving Lives, Improving Mothers Care – Lessons Learned to Inform Maternity Care From the UK and Ireland Confidential Enquiries Into Maternal Deaths and Morbidity 2017–19. National Perinatal Epidemiology Unit, University of Oxford, Oxford.

Knight, M., Bunch, K., Tuffnell, D., Shakespeare, J., Kotnis, R., Kenyon, S., Kurinczuk, J., 2019. Saving Lives, Improving Mothers Care – Lessons Learned to Inform Maternity Care from the UK and Ireland Confidential Enquiries Into Maternal Death and Morbidity 2015–2017. National Perinatal Epidemiology Unit, University of Oxford, Oxford.

Mavrides, E., Allard, S., Chandraharan, E., Collins, P., Green, L., Hunt, B.J., Riris, S., Thomson AJ on behalf of the Royal College of Obstetricians and Gynaecologists, 2016. Prevention and management of postpartum haemorrhage. BJOG 124, e106–e149. Available at: Prevention and Management of Postpartum Haemorrhage – 2017 – BJOG: An International Journal of Obstetrics & Gynaecology – Wiley Online Library

NHS Institute for Innovation and Improvement, 2010. Safer Care. SBAR Situation • Background • Assessment • Recommendation Implementation and Training Guide.

Nutbeam and Daniels (2021) on behalf of the UK Sepsis Trust. Clinical Tools. Available at sepsistrust.org/professional-resources/clinical/, date last accessed 13th April 2023.

Ockenden, D., 2021. Findings, Conclusions and Essential Actions From the Independent Review of Maternity Services at the Shrewsbury and Telford Hospital NHS Trust. House of Commons, London.

RCUK, 2021. Newborn Resuscitation and Support of the Transition of Infants at Birth Guidelines.

Resuscitation Council UK, 2021a. Adult Advance Life Support Guidelines.

Resuscitation Council UK, 2021b. The ABCDE Approach.

Resuscitation Council UK, 2021c. Special Circumstances Guidelines.

Rowe, R., Draper, E., Kenyon, S., Bevan, C., Dickens, J., Forrester, M., Scanlan, R., Tuffnell, D., Kurinczuk, J., 2020. Intrapartum-related perinatal deaths in births planned in midwifery-led settings in Great Britain: findings and recommendations from the ESMiE confidential enquiry. BJOG Int. J. Obstet. Gynaecol. 127, 1665–1675. https://doi.org/10.1111/1471-0528.16327

Royal College of Obstetrics and Gynaecology (RCOG), 2011. *Antepartum Haemorrhage Green-top guideline no. 63*. Available at: Antepartum Haemorrhage (Green-top Guideline No. 63) | RCOG

Royal College of Obstetrics and Gynaecology (RCOG), 2012. *Green-top guideline 42: Shoulder dystocia*. Available at: https://www.rcog.org.uk/guidance/browse-all-guidance/green-top-guidelines/shoulder-dystocia-green-top-guideline-no-42/

Royal College of Obstetrics and Gynaecology (RCOG), 2014. *Umbilical cord prolapse: Green-top Guideline No.50*. Available at: Layout Proof (rcog.org.uk)

Timmons, S. et al., 2015. Implementing human factors in clinical practice. Emerg. Med. J. 32, 368–372.

World Health Organization (WHO), 2020. WHO Recommendations for the Prevention and Treatment of Postpartum Haemorrhage. WHO, Geneva. Available at: WHO recommendation on routes of oxytocin administration for the prevention of postpartum haemorrhage after vaginal birth

CHAPTER 12

PARAMEDIC TRANSFER AND MULTIDISCIPLINARY WORKING WITH AMBULANCE SERVICES

Aimee Yarrington and Lydia Miller

INTRODUCTION

In this chapter we hope to explain more about how the ambulance service works in the UK and what you could expect from your colleagues in Green when dealing with emergency or other transfers from home. The chapter will discuss technical issues and national policy as well as provide helpful practical tips to ensure smooth multi-disciplinary working; after all, patient care is at the centre of both professions, and the better we work together, the better the patient outcome will be. Maternity calls make up a very small proportion of the overall call volume, so prehospital clinicians have minimal exposure to pregnancy, labour, and birth, so team working is essential to ensure the care for mother and baby.

UNITED KINGDOM AMBULANCE SERVICE

These are all run with individual management and leadership structures. There may also be private ambulance services working within some individual trusts, for example, St John ambulance service, who may have been commissioned to assist with pressures or short staffing. If these are employed, they must all comply with the same governance structure and are CQC regulated, as are the ambulance trusts. In the remote areas of Scotland the RAF are often called upon for transfer, and within ambulance services, there are often charity-run Helicopter Emergency Medical Services (HEMS) who are staffed by paramedics with enhanced skills, which will be explained below.

The Association of Ambulance Service Chief Executives (AACE) is the overarching strategic organisation that ensures the national objectives are adhered to and implements national policy frameworks. AACE also oversee the Joint Royal Colleges Ambulance Liaison Committee (JRCALC).

JRCALC are responsible for the development and updating of national clinical guidelines (Association of Ambulance Service Chief Executives [AACE] JRCALC Clinical Guidelines 2022 [2022]) that all paramedics and pre-hospital clinicians adhere to. They assist in the uniformity of service delivery and high-quality patient care. They are developed by experts in the clinical arena and cover an extensive range of topics from resuscitation, medical emergencies, trauma, and medicines to major incidents and staff wellbeing. As you can imagine, ambulance clinicians are required to know a little bit about a lot of areas of healthcare and whilst there are specialist roles, ambulance crews cannot be selective about which emergencies they attend. Therefore the JRCALC guidelines are extensive in order to support the clinicians as best as possible when dealing with less common conditions and situations. JRCALC have developed an electronic app containing all of the guidelines and each individual Ambulance Trust can add their own specialist policies to it. This app will be held on either the clinicians' personal electronic device or accessible via a tablet on the vehicle. The maternity management section is guided by the national maternity leads group. This group has representation from each ambulance service, many of whom have midwives in post, or a senior paramedic who has maternity within their portfolio. Currently, there are two consultant midwives within two ambulance services in the UK, a valuable resource and one which is likely to be expanded in the future to strengthen the safety of mothers and babies who birth unexpectedly in the pre-hospital arena.

WORKING WITH THE EMERGENCY SERVICES – WHO IS WHO?

Working within the services, there are differing levels and grades of clinicians, from a volunteer driver only to a consultant paramedic. Unfortunately, there is no uniformity, and these are often given different names depending on the service.

There are several levels of unregistered clinicians who have been through a certified training course and will wear rank slides appropriate to their level of training.

Here is a brief description of some of the levels of clinicians that you may encounter. This list may not be definitive as there may be variation in some areas; however, if you are ever in doubt, then please ask the individual about their scope of practice. You may wish to record this as part of your contemporaneous record keeping.

COMMUNITY FIRST RESPONDERS (CFRs)

These are volunteers who assist mainly in rural areas with life-threatening calls where there may be a delay in the ambulance arrival. They are trained to FPOS (first person on scene) level and carry a basic life support kit as well as an AED (automated external defibrillator). CFRs often respond in their own cars but should always carry identification from the trust they work for.

EMERGENCY CARE ASSISTANT (ECA)/EMERGENCY CARE SUPPORT WORKER (ECSW)/AMBULANCE CARE ASSISTANT (ACA)

These clinicians are trained in emergency driving and assisting the clinician with illness and injury. Their primary role is to support. They are not autonomous clinicians and are not registered but do receive approx. 9–12 weeks of basic training. Some will have additional technician drugs and some will be able to place an advanced airway. This varies around the UK.

ASSOCIATE AMBULANCE PRACTITIONER (AAP)

A person who has followed a completed 18-week educational course will work supervised by a qualified member of staff until the end point assessment and portfolio sign-off. Once this process is complete, the employee is a qualified AAP and may wear technician rank slides.

TECHNICIAN

A clinician who either has completed an approved IHCD (Institute of Healthcare and Development) technician course and qualified via this route or is a qualified AAP awaiting a university course.

STUDENT PARAMEDIC (STP)

A clinician may wear student paramedic rank slides who is in the apprenticeship technician role stage of their employment. The Student Paramedic title will also be worn by external university students who are completing placement hours within their allocated ambulance service. They will be identifiable by wearing a university uniform.
- Level 1 – AAP (trainee)
- Level 2 – Qualified AAP or technician
- Level 3 – Qualified AAP or technician enrolled on DipHE or BSc Paramedic course. L3s will practice their Paramedic skills under direct supervision of a qualified paramedic only. This does not include the administration of PGDs (patient group directions) or CDs (controlled drugs).

There are 3 levels within the STP program, which are as follows:

PARAMEDIC

A clinician who is registered and maintains the standards of the HCPC (Health and Care Professions Council) register. They must adhere to the HCPC code of standards, performance, and ethics (2018). The term paramedic, like midwife, is a protected title and only those who have passed a university degree-level program are entitled to use the term paramedic. Some of the key practical differences between a paramedic and a non-registrant are skills such as cannulation and advanced airway as well as training and knowledge base. If in doubt, it is okay to ask the Clinician in attendance. Every Paramedic starts as a Newly Qualified Paramedic for the first 2 years of their career and progresses to Band 6 after demonstrating a range of competencies.

ADVANCED PARAMEDIC

In certain trusts the term advanced paramedic may be used for clinicians who have undergone further training and enhanced skills in diagnostics, treatment, and management. These are commonly solo paramedics who will respond in a rapid response vehicle (RRV) who have advanced patient treatment skills but do not have the ability to convey patients to hospital. For example, in some Trusts these Paramedics will carry magnesium sulphate for the management of eclampsia, where this would be outside of a normal paramedic's scope of practice.

CRITICAL CARE PARAMEDIC (CCP)

A clinician who is a qualified paramedic and has completed an approved master's level 7 qualification and is employed in a critical care role, for example, within the Helicopter Emergency Medicine Service (HEMS).

CONSULTANT PARAMEDIC

Not usually patient facing, often works within the medical directorate to update policy and provide expert opinion on various projects. Many will act as a strategic on-call provider to assist in the provision of complex cases. There is always a senior paramedic on call for this, with many services now having multiple consultants to provide this experience and expertise.

DUAL QUALIFIED PRACTITIONERS

There are some clinicians who have qualified and are registered in dual roles. It will depend upon the individual's contract of employment as to what skills they are permitted to practice within their roles with the ambulance service. For example, there are operating department practitioners (ODPSs) registered with the HCPC who are also paramedics and they will generally only be employed as paramedics. There are also a few dual qualified midwives and paramedics. Many are employed in specialist maternity roles and not working clinically as a pre-hospital midwife at this moment in time but there is always development for the future!

Who Might Attend Your Call

	Dispatched to Maternity Cases	Managing Normal Birth	Managing Maternity Complications	NLS	Ability to Cannulate	Ability to Administer Drugs	Enhanced Skills
Community first responder (CFR)	Not commonly will depend on area			✓			
Emergency care assistant (ECA)	✓	✓		✓			
Technician	✓	✓	✓	✓			
Student Paramedic	✓	✓	✓	✓	*		
Associate ambulance practitioner	✓	✓	✓	✓			
Paramedic	✓	✓	✓	✓	✓	✓	
Advanced paramedic	✓	✓	✓	✓	✓	✓	✓**
Critical care paramedic	✓	✓	✓	✓	✓	✓	✓

*Some student paramedics will have the ability to cannulate and provide appropriate treatment under the direct supervision of a qualified paramedic depending on their level of training/duration.
**May not be in maternity-related skills.

Ambulance Trusts aim to send the most appropriate resource to each patient based on the information gained during the emergency call. For many obstetric emergencies, this will mean an advanced paramedic or CCP will be listening to the call as it comes in and may choose to dispatch that additional resource immediately.

COMMON EQUIPMENT ON VEHICLES

Due to the differences in the commissioning for each ambulance service, each trust will choose which equipment it wishes to purchase for its fleet of vehicles. There will be similarities, of course, but it is up to the individual service which equipment it chooses. NHS England (2021) has a specification document that must be adhered to for double-crewed ambulance (DCA) vehicle construction to ensure the safety of clinicians and patients carried within it. In general, the equipment carried is largely similar but the layout may be strikingly different between services. Even within the same service, as the Trust transition from one model of ambulance to a newer fleet, differences might be noted. At the time of writing, London Ambulance Service have just introduced their first electric fleet of ambulances. This is an area which is likely to constantly be changing as technology develops and the NHS fulfils its commitment to becoming more sustainable.

MATERNITY EQUIPMENT

This will vary dependant on area; however, there is a standard list of equipment that is recommended by Association of Ambulance Service Chief Executives (AACE). This includes a pack containing (Fig 12.1):

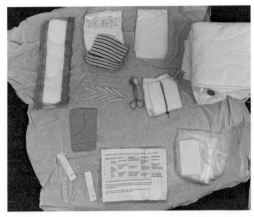

Fig. 12.1 2× hooded towels; nappy; hat; 4× cord clamps; umbilical scissors; placenta bag and label; yellow clinical waste bag and tie; 10× x-ray detectable swabs; 1× maternity pad; 1× plastic apron; 2× identity bracelets; 1× Apgar score chart; 1× sterile field/package wrap. (Picture credit: Aimee Yarrington.)

Some Ambulance Trusts will carry smaller hats and nappies for premature babies as well as food-grade plastic bags for use for extremely premature infants. All ambulances should have a stock of 2 maternity packs at all times, but practically speaking, this may not always be the case if restocking has not been possible for availability reasons.

MATERNITY EMERGENCY DRUGS

Within the JRCALC guidance paramedics are permitted to administer:

Syntometrine – 1 dose only; however, very few services carry it now due to expiration and storage issues.
Misoprostol – 800 mcg single dose. This is the most commonly carried and can be administered in cases sublingual or rectal without storage issues.
Tranexamic Acid (TXA) – carried by all paramedics widely used in the ambulance service in major trauma and now indicated for PPH too.
Carbetocin – not a standard JRCALC drug but is used by some ambulance services under a patient group directive (PGD).

NEWBORN RESUSCITATION EQUIPMENT (Fig 12.2)

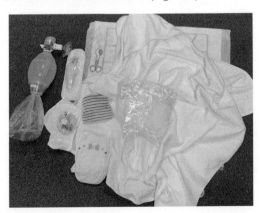

Fig 12.2 Towels, hat, and nappy from maternity pack; 250 mL bag valve mask (BVM); size 0 mask; size 1 iGel; newborn oxygen saturation probe; plastic bag for preterm baby under 32 weeks; heated exothermic mattress (Picture credit: Aimee Yarrington.)

DIAGNOSTIC EQUIPMENT

All frontline emergency vehicles will carry a monitoring device capable of performing defibrillation, ECG monitoring, non-invasive blood pressure (NIBP), SPO$_2$ monitoring (all ages), capnography monitoring, and heart rate monitoring. Often called by their branded name such as Lifepack or Zoll, they may also be referred to as 'the monitor'. They are a mandatory piece of equipment to respond to any emergency call.

As well as the monitor, the clinician will carry a blood glucose monitoring kit, tympanic thermometer, pen torch, and a stethoscope

MANUAL HANDLING EQUIPMENT

For moving patients, there will be at least one type of carrying chair to enable recumbent extrication, as well as a carrying sheet/extrication device for patients who need to be kept flat or where resuscitation is in progress. Most services will carry a range of equipment to assist with lifts where possible such as slide sheets, handling belts, and lifting cushions to assist patients from the floor who have fallen. For bariatric patients, many trusts will have specially commissioned vehicles with equipment capable of lifting patients over 30 stones. Most trusts have given the extra responsivity to their hazardous area response team (HART) as they have the capabilities within their remit for training and deployment.

PERSONAL PROTECTIVE EQUIPMENT

Since the start of the COVID-19 pandemic, the minimum PPE that was expected to be worn by pre-hospital clinicians was level 2 (mask, apron, gloves, and eye protection) as standard, with many Trusts utilising air filtration hoods as well for confirmed COVID-19 cases and aerosol-generating procedures (AGPs). This should also be joined with sleeve protectors for birth as a minimum standard. The guidance on this is constantly changing; however, even pre-pandemic most ambulance crews will wear some form of PPE when attending a birth.

UNDERSTANDING 999 AND 111 CALL PROCESSES

When a 999 call is made you will first be asked by the operator which service you require; once you state ambulance service you will be put through to your local ambulance service according to your location at the time.

> **Practice Point:**
> If you are phoning from an area of poor signal, try to use the landline. This will not only be a more reliable line but also help to quickly locate you. It is worth considering if a woman is choosing to homebirth against advice as part of your risk mitigation.

An emergency call handler will answer. They are specially trained in using the telephone triage system which is a clinical decision support system (CDSS). It takes the call through a series of questions to establish the correct level of assistance. Call handlers are not clinicians and so may not understand the complex clinical nature of certain requests. There are 2 different CDSSs in use within the UK ambulance services; these are NHS Pathways and AMPDS (Advanced Medical Priority Dispatch System). Although the two have different elements the basics are the same in that they aim to establish the most appropriate response to make as well as send the appropriate help. Not all 999 calls will result in an ambulance dispatch, so establishing early on that you are a healthcare professional requesting the transport is essential, but at the correct point. When you are passed over to the ambulance service, there are 4 key questions that must be answered first, in order to arrange the ambulance; these will not delay the ambulance but help to establish the essential details needed for dispatch. These are:

1. Is the patient breathing? *(This is a Yes/No Question)*
2. What address are you calling from? *(You will be asked to confirm this twice)*
3. What number are you calling from? *(In case you get cut off and need to be called back)*
4. What is the reason for the call? *(Give the specific reason, for example, 'I am a community midwife requesting an emergency transfer for a postpartum haemorrhage')*

The CDSS will take the call handler through a set sequence of questions based upon the information that you give to them. They need to understand the nature of the request in order to ensure you get the correct response and at the correct level of urgency. There are four categories of calls that the ambulances are assigned to in order of priority. These are a national standard set out by NHS England in 2017 and are adhered to by all ambulance services, known as Ambulance Response Programme (ARP) (NHS England 2018). All ambulance services are monitored and ranked according to their performance in the ARP (see Fig. 12.3)

Due to the nature of the different time frames attached to the calls, it is imperative that the questions asked as part of the triage system are answered fully, as an incorrect response may result in a delay in the priority of ambulance dispatched.

Category 1
Defined as life threatening which requires a targeted time critical response of 7 minutes with an average of 15 minutes to attend. Types of call within this category might include a birth in progress or a cardiac arrest.

Category 2
Defined as an emergency call which has the potential to be serious necessitating a rapid assessment, treatment, intervention, and transport. Types of call within this category might include stroke or chest pain. The target for response is 18 minutes.

Category 3
Defined as an urgent call with no average response target time. These types of calls usually represent a problem that is not automatically life threatening but requires an assessment and management strategy that may include a telephone triage or a face to face assessment and transport to an appropriate care centre. Conditions such as a fall with no apparent injuries.

Category 4
Defined as a less urgent call that present as less or non-urgent that require assessment and potential transport to a clinically appropriate destination. This may be handled by a non-paramedic response and have no average response target time.

Fig. 12.3 Categories of call (NHS England, 2018).

You as the caller cannot demand a certain category of call; the triage system will do this for you. Clinicians within the control room may up- or downgrade a call after speaking to the caller during a call back.

Whilst it is unlikely you will need to access the 111 system during a homebirth situation, it is useful to understand the process for reference. Within the 111 system, there exists the same CDSS used to support the call taker in making the correct choice of care for the caller. This non-emergency system has many outcomes or dispositions to offer the caller. They may advise the caller to make their own way to a hospital or an out-of-hours (OOH) centre or a GP visit may be arranged. There is also the disposition for self-care advice and instructions on how to manage conditions at home without the need to speak to a clinician. In some complex cases the offer of a clinician call back is advised to ascertain more information on the patient in order to provide the best outcome. If it becomes apparent that an ambulance is required, this can also be dispatched from the 111 CDSS as an emergency response.

Many call handlers now are becoming dual trained in both 111 and 999 call taking. All calls received by the Emergency Operations Centre (EOC) are recorded for training and audit purposes. Call handlers are regularly audited and must adhere to a strict script to ensure safety and consistency. If a call handler fails an audit as they did not adhere to the script, then they may face disciplinary proceedings and even have to retrain.

Whilst this process can be frustrating, it is important to remember that triage systems are in place for a reason. Whilst the emergency you are dealing with may be critical, you must remember a dispatcher is looking at a screen full of people who feel the same as you. Under current pressures, there are only so many resources for the amount of ambulances required. Although it may be tempting to claim the patient is more unwell than they are to try and get an ambulance quicker, that may cause an ambulance to divert from someone significantly injured or dying. It may be your colleague down the road dealing with another more serious obstetric emergency that is then denied an ambulance. The system has been designed to get the right outcome and all of the lines are recorded for transparency and learning. That being said, patients do deteriorate, so if something has changed, please ring 999 back and get re-triaged. If you do not update the ambulance service when something serious changes, it may delay getting help to you.

Occasionally the triage system does not work as intended, so it is important in these circumstances to report it through appropriate channels such as DATIX and work with your local service to debrief and learn from these incidences.

INDICATIONS FOR TRANSFER

When attending a homebirth, or a birth in a stand-alone MLU, there are several reasons why you may need ambulance transfer. They may not all require a blue light response and women who book for care in this type of birth must be counselled appropriately on the length of time it may take to summon help, and this should always form part of the individual dynamic risk assessment.

Non-emergency transfer:

These can face up to a 2-hour wait for an appropriate vehicle. Indicators for these transfers include but are not limited to:

- Maternal request transfers
- Post birth suturing where woman is haemodynamically stable
- Retained placenta where woman is haemodynamically stable

Emergency transfer:

Conditions may include but are not limited to:

- Cord prolapse
- Severe pre-eclampsia with risk of eclampsia
- Eclampsia
- Antepartum/intrapartum haemorrhage
- Fetal heart rate abnormalities
- Significant meconium
- Unplanned? Breech presentation in active labour
- Transverse or unstable lie
- Shoulder dystocia
- Postpartum haemorrhage
- Maternal collapse/arrest
- Newborn collapse/arrest

It is important to note that ambulances cannot be 'on standby' for your emergency. Whilst it may form part of risk assessment to inform the ambulance service about a woman with particular complexities that may affect her birth due to occur in the community, an emergency ambulance cannot be pre-booked to arrive and stay until after the birth has happened.

MAKING THE CALL

When a maternity emergency arises, the decision to make the call must be clearly tasked to one of the clinicians in attendance. This should be practiced, and regular training should take place so that when the emergency arises, it is 'muscle memory' and not forgotten. The clear instruction 'call for an ambulance' should be given, and then the delegated clinician should feed back once the call has been placed. This is called closed-loop communication and will ensure tasks get completed (Salik et al. 2021).

If there is only a single clinician at a birth there should be consideration of utilising the speaker function. If you have to utilise the birthing partner, be conscious of the fact that they may not convey the appropriate message and this could cause a delay in achieving the correct response. Be clear in your instruction to them and if possible ask them to repeat the information back to you.

As previously discussed, once the operator has put the call through to the ambulance service, the call handler will ask 4 specific questions to ascertain the nature of the call.

1. Is the patient breathing? *(This is a Yes/No Question)*
2. What address are you calling from? *(You will be asked to confirm this twice)*
3. What number are you calling from? *(In case you get cut off and need to be called back)*
4. What is the reason for the call? *(Give the specific reason, for example, 'I am a community midwife requesting an emergency transfer for a postpartum haemorrhage')*

Having the patients' details written down to hand will assist with this process. Having a note or proforma similar to the one below will help with the details required in this situation:

Name	
Address (inc. postcode)	
Telephone number	
Gestation	Parity
Antenatal history	
Labour history	

The responding resources will be the nearest and most appropriate resources that the ambulance dispatcher can find. This may be a solo clinician on a car, followed by an ambulance, or this could be 2 ambulances straight away. If a solo clinician turns up on a car do not be disheartened; they are a very useful extra pair of hands and have direct communication with the control room.

MANAGING A TRANSFER (TRANSFER OR EMERGENCY)

Once the ambulance arrives, you will be expected to give a full SBAR handover to the attending crew. Utilising SBAR will prevent key information from being missed and ensure everyone caring for that patient has some shared situational awareness (Brennan et al. 2020). Whilst most ambulance personnel will understand terms such as eclampsia you may need to explain what this means if you are speaking to a non-Paramedic. Most services should aim to send you a paramedic response; however, regardless of the clinician grade, as the midwife, you remain the lead clinician. The exception to this may be a maternal resuscitation scenario where the ambulance clinicians will have more experience, but in every other situation the midwife will remain the lead. The Ambulance clinicians will be able to be led by you and, as long as it is within their PGDs, fully utilise all of their equipment and drugs for you. The exception to this may be the rare situation where you have 2 patients and are not able to oversee the entire event. If you have an unwell baby and an unwell woman, you will need to consider who is best for you to travel with. If there are 2 midwives, this decision is easy and you would likely split up to manage each patient. If there is only 1 midwife on scene, it will be on a case-by-case basis, but there is *unlikely* that you will be needed to continue clinical care to a neonate. Communication with ambulance colleagues is paramount in this case. As a midwife, you have an extended scope of practice for a compromised woman, compared to an ambulance crew, so it would likely be more likely that you travel with the woman.

Maintaining the 'helicopter view' on the event is critical to ensure that no one becomes task focused to prevent a delay in moving the patient to hospital. The ambulance service is well trained in this concept and may send an officer to scene to help manage the situation. Becoming task focused on a complicated or emergent scene is one of the most common reasons why mistakes are made in healthcare (Brennan et al. 2020). Spending time with your local ambulance service to practice and drill these scenarios together can be extremely useful in preparing you for this situation. Ensuring leadership is established early could be the difference in whether the woman or neonate has a good outcome (Hunziker et al. 2011).

There are generally 2 different types of transfer:

- The emergency
- The non-emergency.

The ambulance clinician may ask you as the midwife what sort of transfer you require. An emergency transfer will be for situations where you want to move quickly to an obstetric unit. This will be under emergency conditions with the use of blue lights and sirens. This is the quicker way to get the woman to the obstetric unit; however, there is obviously an added risk to driving with blue lights, so it needs to be justified and 'just to not sit in traffic' is not a valid justification if the patient is not unwell.

Not all transfers require emergency conditions, and it is up to you as the lead clinician to decide how you wish to transfer.

Once you are in the ambulance with your woman, you must take your seat and put your seatbelt on. As you are not an employee of the responding ambulance service, you are not covered by the service insurance the same as the pre-hospital clinician. The responding clinician has an exemption in the law to be out of their restraint ONLY when actively providing treatment; other than that, they should be restrained with their seatbelt also. If you are injured as a result of an accident sustained within the ambulance and you were not restrained, you are not covered by insurance and are not entitled to be compensated, etc., as road traffic law is still required to be followed.

If you do not already know what your local ambulance service vehicles look like, it would be useful to approach them for training. Have a look in the back of the ambulance at the layout and where the equipment is so that you can think through your positioning if you were dealing with an emergency. These can be highly stressful situations to deal with and often we wish to be as prepared as possible, so it's worth understanding as much as you can about the ambulance that will be coming to help you (Fig 12.4).

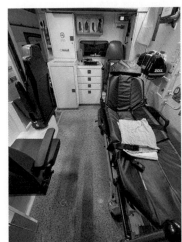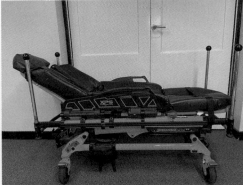

Fig 12.4 Photo of the back of an Ambulance (Left) and Ambulance Trolley bed (Right) (Images by kind permission of South Western Ambulance Service NHS Trust)

The other thing to consider is what equipment you actually need to take with you on the transfer. As you will have seen above, there is a vast amount of equipment carried on the ambulance, stored with easy access if required. If you do need to take some of your own equipment with you, then this must be safely stowed on the vehicle, and not loose on the floor, so this does not become a missile in the unfortunate event of a road traffic collision. Ambulance personnel are good at storing equipment safely; for example, often patients wish to bring a suitcase with them. If you are not sure where your bag should go, just ask one of the crew members.

COMMUNICATION

The SBAR handover tool is widely utilised within the NHS to ensure safe and effective handovers as well as to highlight any clinical situation that requires immediate attention (NHS Institute for Innovation and Improvement 2010).

This tool is known and taught to ambulance clinicians. Each aspect of the handover creates a key building block for communication and cuts out the unnecessary information which may prevent the critical message from coming across (Shahid et al, 2018).

How it is used (Fig 12.5):

S – Situation
Identify yourself and skill grade
Identify the patient by name and the main reason for the communication/what the concern is
B – Background
Any specific antenatal history, medical history, risk factors
Type of birth if relevant and the time this took place
A – Assessment
Vital signs
Contraction pattern
Clinical impressions
R – Recommendations
Explain what you need specifically and give time frames
Make suggestions
Any treatment given or required
Ask if there are any suggestions or ideas if relevant

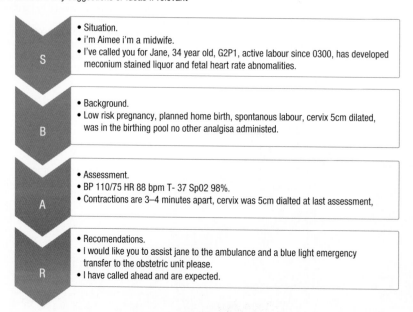

Fig. 12.5 Example of an SBAR handover

In addition to an SBAR, it can be useful to 'Headline' your handover.

Headlining is identifying the problem as your opener before starting your handover. Although this is done as part of the 'Situation', if you have a time-critical patient, it is good practice to headline as it ensures the person you are handing over to is listening and they can already start wheels in motion for any immediate action required.

For example:

Midwife: 'Hello, I'm dealing with a PPH here. Are you happy for a quick handover?'

Paramedic: 'Yes and I'm just going to ask my crewmate to start getting some necessary equipment to help you; go ahead.'

Midwife: 'Okay, my name is....'

This just expedites any immediate action and instantaneously gets all clinicians on the same page. The full SBAR should still happen and is very important, but this can be simultaneous to any necessary actions.

You may also receive a handover from an ambulance crew in an ATMIST format. This is similar to SBAR but often utilised in either trauma patients or pre-alerted medical patients (patients who are extremely unwell). This stands for: Age, Time of injury, Mechanism of injury, Injuries sustained, Signs and Symptoms, and Treatment/needs (JRCALC, 2022). If this happens, try not to interrupt and ask for an SBAR instead. The information is largely similar and if you need something clarifying you can always ask a question at the end.

MEDICAL ACRONYMS

Medical professionals all love an acronym, and this is no exception for paramedics and midwives. Occasionally some of these acronyms are exactly the same; however, they may mean a completely different thing to a Paramedic than they do to a midwife. Here are some of the more common ones that can get misinterpreted.

Acronym	To a Midwife Means...	To an Ambulance Person Means...
MI	Male Infant	Myocardial Infarction
ARM	Artificial rupture of membranes	An arm, attached to your body
LSCS	Lower segment Caesarean section	Lumber spine, cervical spine
Liquor	Amniotic fluid	Alcohol?
AF	Artificial feeding	Atrial fibrillation
OA	Occipito-anterior	On arrival
OP	Occipito-posterior	Oropharyngeal airway
OT	Occipito-transverse	Overtime!

Generally speaking, it is all about context. If a midwife said to a Paramedic, 'This woman has had an MI' it may be misunderstood as a completely different emergency. Whereas if a midwife said, 'This woman has given birth to a MI', the Paramedic is likely to work out very quickly what that means.

When we are handing over to a multi-disciplinary team in an emergency it can be easy to use acronyms that only you understand. Be cautious and try to avoid this if possible.

If you hear something that doesn't quite make sense it's probably because it means something entirely different; just ask.

BORN BEFORE ARRIVAL

When a baby is born before the arrival of the midwife the ambulance service will often request the presence of a midwife to discharge the woman on scene if she does not require hospitalisation. Paramedics and ambulance clinicians are told very clearly that they must not leave a newly birthed woman and baby on scene without handing over in person to a midwife. In many areas due to staffing pressures this often does not happen, and women and babies are transferred to the maternity unit for assessment.

If, however, a midwife is able to travel to scene, the Ambulance practitioner will deliver an SBAR handover and wait for the midwife to perform her assessment.

Indications to transfer postnatally include:

- No extensive suturing required
- Placenta intact
- Baby warm/no neonatal issues
- Mother haemodynamically stable
- No safeguarding issues

Once the midwife is confident that there is no indication to transfer the crew can then be discharged from the scene, giving the name of the midwife taking charge to their emergency control room (EOC).

BED vs CHAIR

As discussed above each Ambulance has at least one form of wheelchair and a stretcher. If the woman is unable to walk, one of the two may be required. For certain emergencies such as cord prolapse the woman should be encouraged to walk and if unable must be placed on a stretcher rather than a chair, to minimise pressure on the cord.

This may be suitable if the house or flat is on the ground floor. When the woman is upstairs. However. a chair may be required as the stretcher cannot be taken upstairs unless there is a lift that fits the length of the stretcher. If a woman must be carried out flat, it is likely the ambulance crew may request additional resources to help them, and a scoop stretcher will be used to extricate the patient (Fig 12.6).

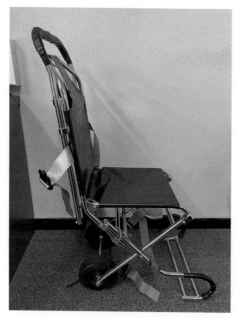

Fig. 12.6 Ambulance Carry Chair (Images by kind permission of South Western Ambulance Service NHS Trust)

Practice Point:
If requesting an ambulance when your patient is relatively stable, try to get to the ground floor whilst walking is an option. If there is any chance of deterioration, being on the ground floor will expedite the transfer.

Transferring the newly birthed mother and baby postnatally is often a challenge. There is not currently a nationally agreed safe way of transferring a mother and baby together in an ambulance. Some services utilise an extra small child restraint, but this device requires the separation of mother and baby in 2 different ambulances, which is not ideal for the newly birthed mother or baby. They may choose to use the mother's own car seat/infant carrier if they have one, but these can only be placed on a forward-facing chair and this often means that the baby's face is out of the direct line of vision.

Each Ambulance service will have its own policy on this and it's worth enquiring with your local one about what this is. If Mother and baby are well it may be possible for them to travel in the same Ambulance. Check with your local ambulance service on what their policy is.

BABY BORN WITH THE AMBULANCE CREW

As discussed Paramedics are required to know a little bit about a lot of things, so how much do we know about the various obstetric emergencies that may occur in the community and how often do we get training in these? The following briefly outlines the more common emergencies and what you might expect from your ambulance colleagues.

MECHANISMS OF NORMAL BIRTH

Sometimes despite it being a 999 call when the ambulance service arrives on scene everything happens smoothly and the only emergency is the fact that it was unexpected and perhaps a midwife wasn't on scene. A 'normal birth' should be able to be managed by most pre-hospital clinicians, although they may find this incredibly daunting. If everything has run smoothly the ambulance crew may request a midwife to scene, but as discussed this may not always be possible and transfer to hospital may be the only option.

Undergraduate and then postgraduate training in normal birth is variable across the UK and can range from an afternoon of lectures to an entire week placement on a maternity ward depending on the level of qualification and area.

As far as experience goes, some ambulance crew members are lucky enough to have seen and been involved in many births. Others can have a 30-year career and not support the birth of a single baby. Experiences therefore will vary and exposure can be very low and confidence in managing obstetric emergencies will therefore vary as exposure to these patients can be very low. Simulation training with mannequins may be the only experience that ambulance staff have had. Some ambulance clinicians enjoy attending maternity jobs and others would rather avoid them but mostly because it feels scary as it is something we have very little exposure to.

PRETERM BIRTH

Preterm birth is something ambulance clinicians may be exposed to due to the nature of it often being unexpected. Depending on the gestation, JRCALC will guide the paramedics with how to proceed, falling in line with national guidance around premature birth and viability.

There is very little in terms of management that the ambulance service will do for a baby born at 32 weeks compared to a term baby and the focus remains on thermoregulation. Some trusts will carry a food-grade plastic bag to place the baby in if the skin is very delicate and requires protection. It is clear in the guidance that this should be accompanied by a radiant heat source. Many Trusts have a warming mattress available which will provide a radiant source if the mother is unable to do this. Training in this may be sparse and theory is likely to be covered more commonly than practice, as lifelike mannequins are expensive for the Trusts to purchase.

NEONATAL RESUSCITATION

Although rare, these do happen in the community and it can be devastating when they do. Ambulance clinicians will likely have very little exposure to these but should have a fairly reasonable level of competence. As most of the emphasis is on airway and breathing all levels of ambulance clinicians will have had training in this and should be proficient in the algorithm. Update training should happen approximately annually and many Ambulance Trusts will have online training and continuous professional development to take part in should an individual wish to update. Occasionally an ambulance crew may be called to assist a midwife because a baby has collapsed post birth, even up to many days old. We recognise that midwives are trained in newborn life support and not always paediatric life support. The Resus Council (2021) advise that a newborn is considered to be the period just after birth and an infant is under the age of one. Given how stressful these scenarios are it may be best to adhere to the algorithm you remember and support each other to do your best for the patient.

POSTPARTUM HAEMORRHAGE (PPH)

As discussed above ambulance crews (if a paramedic crew) may carry a few drugs for the treatment of PPH. Clinicians are able to perform fundal massage if the placenta has been born and should be aware of the main causes of bleeding. No ambulance clinician will conduct a VE, but a paramedic should be able to identify a poorly contracted uterus from palpation and may be able to identify whether the bleeding is caused by a tear from a visual inspection or the history. Suturing a tear is not within the scope of practice for a paramedic and will always be referred to a midwife to perform. Severe haemorrhage generally is something most ambulance clinicians will have seen and dealt with, but exposure to a postpartum haemorrhage will be very low. Ambulance clinicians will likely have similar difficulties estimating blood loss (EBL) as midwives do (Wiklund et al., 2022) and are taught to convey all incontinence sheets etc. to hospital to assist with EBL. Drugs will only be given by a Paramedic; they will not be able to give extra doses under your registration. JRCALC advises ambulance clinicians to wait 20 minutes for the placenta (AACE, 2022); after this the guidance prompts a swift extrication to hospital. Uterotonic drugs are not able to be given by Paramedics to expedite the arrival of the placenta and can only be given for PPH.

Paramedics will not generally be trained in bimanual uterine compression; however, in JRCALC there is a section which allows for Paramedics who have completed appropriate additional training to undertake the lifesaving manoeuvre (AACE birth imminent guideline section 5.4 (4)).

SHOULDER DYSTOCIA

Ambulance clinicians in general are quite terrified of shoulder dystocia and as a large number are unpredictable, it is an emergency they will want to be prepared for. Ambulance clinicians are taught the McRoberts position as their first option, suprapubic pressure as their second option, rocking suprapubic pressure as their third option, and finally, all-fours-position if all of that doesn't work. Training may come up annually or be completed by Paramedics as part of their CPD. JRCALC (AACE, 2022) have diagrams and there are various prompt cards that may be in the maternity pack to assist them with how to manage a shoulder dystocia step by step.

BREECH BIRTH

Breech birth is possibly less likely than shoulder dystocia to occur in the prehospital environment because it is more predictable, and therefore women may already be in hospital; however, they do happen. Training in breech is largely inconsistent across the UK, with some ambulance clinicians completing additional CPD in this to boost confidence and others having only watched a PowerPoint. If the Ambulance crew arrive before the midwife and recognise this is happening they may phone into the unit to ask for advice. Try to be patient with them as it's likely they've never seen it before and it may have been years since their last training. An ambulance crew may phone into labour ward to be talked through how to manage a breech birth.

MATERNAL COLLAPSE

Fortunately this is rare; however, maternal out-of-hospital cardiac arrests are very challenging to attend to, for both clinical reasons and because these can be highly emotive patients to deal with.

Ambulance clinicians should have had training in manual displacement of the uterus. This has been in JRCALC (AACE, 2022) for some years now, and you shouldn't come across wedges of any kind. Whilst training in Resuscitation is frequent, there are some key differences with a pregnant woman and specific maternal cardiac arrest training is less common. Some specialist resources within the ambulance service will carry mechanical CPR devices which have been approved for use with pregnant women according to local protocol (LUCAS, 2021). Mechanical CPR brings the benefit of improved compressions during motion. Obtaining effective compressions in the back of a moving ambulance is very difficult to achieve; given that CPR will never be terminated on a pregnant woman in the community, there should be early consideration for a mechanical CPR device (AACE, 2022).

This can be very brutal to watch and ambulance crews will have a low threshold for requesting HEMS teams to scene. If they are available and attend, they may perform a resuscitative hysterotomy in order to improve resuscitation efforts of the mother (AACE, 2022). If a healthy baby is delivered as part of this then that's excellent, but this procedure is recommended in order to optimise the mother's chances of survival (Resuscitation Council UK, 2021).

Although considered 'scary' to most ambulance clinicians, obstetric emergencies are rare, and the majority of the time the ambulance service attends to babies that just couldn't wait for either the hospital or for the midwife. Although often happy occasions one of the biggest challenges with babies born prehospitally is ensuring thermoregulation. In the hospital/MLU (midwife-led unit) or birth centre the temperature is often carefully regulated. In the woman's own home in an emergency, it is often a challenge. Some babies are also born outside of hospital or home, such as in the back of a car or taxi... One of the largest complaints received by the ambulance services is that of the newborn being cold on arrival at the maternity unit. The JRCALC (AACE, 2022) guidelines give the following advice to the prehospital clinician:

- Always dry the baby thoroughly, paying particular attention to head.
- Remove the wet towel used for initial drying
- Place the baby skin to skin with a warm mother or relative – cover with at least 2 layers
- An exothermic warming mattress, is recommended; however, it is up to the individual service to purchase these.
- Babies born under 32 weeks' gestation are placed into a suitable food-grade plastic bag wrapped and a warming mattress used (AACE, 2022).

SPECIAL CIRCUMSTANCES

Occasionally the ambulance service may deal with a particularly challenging case. These could range from an un-booked woman to an abandoned baby.

Un-booked woman may choose to present to the ambulance service if something happens that she is not expecting. Free-birthing is on the rise and this presents similar challenges to the ambulance service as it does to midwifery services. If a woman hasn't had any antenatal care little is known about the condition of the baby or the health of the mother. Ambulance clinicians will in this case have a lower threshold for travelling to hospital earlier in case of a twin pregnancy or complication. If a woman presents to the ambulance service as un-booked it will be the responsibility of the nearest obstetric unit to accept her. Local policies exist to support this and each patient is dealt with on a case-by-case basis.

Similarly if a woman is travelling away from home and requires emergency treatment it will be the responsibility of the nearest unit to accept her rather than the ambulance travelling miles further to her booked unit.

Abandoned babies are rare but often dealt with first by the ambulance or police service. If the police are not on scene they will be requested by the ambulance service to become guardians of the baby until social services arrive. These will almost always be pre-alerted into hospital by the ambulance crew, as little is known about the health of the baby or the mother.

SUPPORTING WOMAN OUTSIDE OF GUIDELINE DECISIONS

Occasionally a woman may make a decision that a healthcare professional deems outside of guideline decisions about her care. This may be in the antenatal period, for example birthing outside of guidelines or choosing a homebirth when she is deemed high risk. Or this may be during labour or postpartum, for example, wishing to have a physiological third stage despite beginning to seriously bleed.

As this book is being written many maternity services across the UK are transitioning to electronic notes. This has many benefits for both the patient and the maternity care provider; however, it poses a risk to ambulance clinicians. Solutions are being explored and as technology develops I'm sure ambulance clinicians will be able to access the information they need. Whilst in this transition period it may cause an increase in phone calls to the hospital to obtain the information they need on scene as the notes are unavailable. It's worth remembering that even if the notes are available when dealing with an emergency our hands can be full and taking time to read the notes isn't always possible, so the ambulance service may ring for information or they may ring for advice. Remember, we have very little exposure to these emergencies and may have had very little training, so try to be patient and supportive in these circumstances; teamwork is key to a positive outcome for the mother and baby.

DEBRIEF FOLLOWING EMERGENCY

Where possible it's best practice for the whole team to have a hot debrief and if necessary a cold debrief once the patient's journey has come to a conclusion Kolbe et al. (2021). A framework for this is TAKE STOCK (Sugarman et al., 2021). However, many other proformas exist and can be utilised. Hot debriefs allow for all staff involved to process what happened and why it happened and identify any learning for next time. The benefit of ensuring this is that a multi-disciplinary debrief allows the team to address any gaps in knowledge or flaws in policy or procedure across profession boundaries. This could identify a need for a change in practice or for new procedures to be put in place. Without this debrief it can be challenging for each member of the team to fully evaluate their own performance and how they could improve (Gilmartin et al., 2020).

Practice Point:
Depending on the nature of the case this may have included the call handler and they should be considered when organising a cold debrief.

SUMMARY

Working within a multi-disciplinary team can be challenging, especially when dealing with an emergency. I would encourage you to work with your local ambulance service to establish regular training both within the hospital and in the community. Communicate when things have gone wrong and learn from each other. Transferring a woman into hospital can be a difficult task made easier by crossing the organisational boundaries to facilitate regular multi-disciplinary training.

REFERENCES

AACE, 2023. Structure of the UK Ambulance Services [WWW Document]. Assoc. Ambulance Chief Exec. URL https://aace.org.uk/uk-ambulance-service/ (accessed 4.16.23).

Association of Ambulance Service Chief Executives (AACE) (2022) *JRCALC Clinical Guidelines 2022*. Bridgwater: Class professional publishing.

Brennan, P.A. Holden, C. Shaw, G. Morris, S. Oeppen, R.S. (2020) What can we do to improve individual and team situational awareness to benefit patient safety*? British Journal of Oral and Maxillofacial Surgery*. Vol. 58 (4) P404–408. (Online) available at: Leading article: What can we do to improve individual and team situational awareness to benefit patient safety? – ScienceDirect

Gilmartin, S. Martin, L. Kenny, S. Callanan, I. Slater, N. (2020) Promoting hot debriefing in an emergency department. *British Medical Journal*. Vol. 9 (3) (Online) available at: Promoting hot debriefing in an emergency department I BMJ Open Quality

HCPC (Health and Care Professions Council) (2018) Standards of conduct performance and ethics (online) available at: https://www.hcpc-uk.org/standards/standards-of-conduct-performance-and-ethics/ [accessed on 23/08/22].

Hunziker, S. Johansson, A.C. Tschan, F. Semmer, N.K. Rock, L. Howell, M.D. Marsch, S. (2011) Teamwork and leadership in cardiopulmonary resuscitation. *Journal of the American College of Cardiology*. Vol. 57 (24) (Online) available at: Teamwork and Leadership in Cardiopulmonary Resuscitation I Journal of the American College of Cardiology (jacc.org)

Instructions for Use (2021) LUCAS 3 chest compression system (Online) available at: 1757365_101034-00 Rev G LUCAS 3 IFU US_lowres.pdf (lucas-cpr.com)

Kolbe, M. Seelandt, J.C. Schmutz, J. (2021) Team debriefings in healthcare: aligning intention and impact. *BMJ* (Online) available at: Team debriefings in healthcare: aligning intention and impact I The BMJ

NHS England (2021) Double-crewed ambulance specification. (online) available at: https://www.england.nhs.uk/wp-content/uploads/2018/09/B0356_National-specification-base-vehicle-and-conversion_October-2021.pdf [accessed on 14/4/22].

NHS England (2018) Ambulance response programme review. (online) available at: https://www.england.nhs.uk/wp-content/uploads/2018/10/ambulance-response-programme-review.pdf [accessed on 20/04/22].

NHS Institute for Innovation and Improvement (2010) Safer care: SBAR situation background assessment recommendations; Implementation and training guide. (online) available at: https://www.england.nhs.uk/improvement-hub/wp-content/uploads/sites/44/2017/11/SBAR-Implementation-and-Training-Guide.pdf [accessed on 24/8/22].

Resuscitation Council UK (2021) Paediatric basic life support. (Online) available at: Paediatric basic life support Guidelines I Resuscitation Council UK

Resuscitation Council UK (2021) Special circumstances. (Online) available at: Special circumstances Guidelines I Resuscitation Council UK

Salik, I. Ashurst, J. (2021) Closed loop communication training in medical simulation. *In: StatPearls* (Online) available at: Closed Loop Communication Training in Medical Simulation – PubMed (nih.gov)

Shahid, S. Thomas, S. (2018) Situation, background, assessment, recommendation (SBAR) communication tool for handoff in health care-a narrative review. *Saf Health.* Vol. 4 (7) (Online) available at: Situation, Background, Assessment, Recommendation (SBAR) Communication Tool for Handoff in Health Care – A Narrative Review | SpringerLink

Sugarman, M. Graham, B. Langston, S. Nelmes, P. Matthews, J. (2021) Implementation of the 'TAKE STOCK' hot debrief tool in the ED: A quality improvement project. *Emergency Medicine Journal.* Vol 38 (8) (Online) available at: Implementation of the 'TAKE STOCK' Hot Debrief Tool in the ED: a quality improvement project | Emergency Medicine Journal (bmj.com)

Wiklund, I. Fernandez, S.A. Jonsson, M. (2022) Midwifes' ability during third stage childbirth to estimate postpartum haemorrhage. *European Journal of Obstetrics & Gynaecology and Reproductive Biology.* Vol. 15 (Online) available at: Midwives' ability during third stage of childbirth to estimate postpartum haemorrhage – ScienceDirect

CHAPTER 13

HOMEBIRTH IN THE PRESENCE OF COMPLEX NEEDS

Anna Madeley and Dr Claire Feeley

INTRODUCTION

So far within these chapters, we have discussed planning and support for homebirth in a cohort of women who are generally healthy, with a lower risk of complications, and who would be offered homebirth as an option aligned with national and local guidance. However, for some who sit outside of these parameters, homebirth might still be requested. This chapter will explore who might be considered 'complex' in planning homebirth, either by virtue of prior medical and obstetric history, social and economic factors, geographical location, or birthing and pregnancy preferences and choices. This chapter will also discuss the legislation in support of maternal autonomy and the considerations required of health professionals to support these birth choices. This chapter does not include those who freebirth (see chapter *Home Alone – Choosing Freebirth*); however, the authors note that similarities may exist.

WHAT DO WE MEAN BY COMPLEX NEEDS?

The term 'out of guideline homebirth' care has come to encompass women who might be deemed 'high risk' and choose to birth at home. This, however, can oversimplify the nature of women with complex needs who, for whatever reason, may choose to labour and birth outside of institutional and national guidelines at home, attended by midwives. These complex needs might be:

- Medical and obstetric/physiological complexity
- Psychological complexity (including previous trauma, phobia etc)
- Social and economic complexity
- Rural and remote, highlands and islands (see chapter *Antenatal Planning*)
- Housing locations/travelling communities

For the purposes of this chapter, we are focussed on those individuals who might fall outside the recommendations for birth at home illustrated by NICE (2017), that is, women healthy, at lower risk of complications. It is important to note that complexities are often simplified into a binary categorisation of 'low' or 'high' risk, with care pathways designed around this binary. However, such a simplistic approach may mask important nuances and contextual factors pertaining to women's health and subsequent chance for complications during pregnancy and birth. For example, there is a difference between someone presenting with significant cardiac disease and someone with a previous third-degree tear following a forceps birth – however, both are typically deemed 'high risk'. The former will clearly benefit from obstetric care, yet the latter opting to birth at home might may reduce the chance of repeated perineal trauma (Reitsma *et al.*, 2020). Conversely, those deemed 'healthy' or at 'low risk' of complications may have emerging pathologies that require action but may be missed due to an assumption made about their health status. Complexities therefore need to be seen as a spectrum, with any woman potentially requiring additional support, yet equally, it is vital that assumptions are not made and care is tailored to the individual. For the maternity professional, we need to be simultaneously alert to deterioration in any birthing woman or person *and* to avoiding over-medicalised approaches when not warranted. Therefore NICE recommendations (NICE, 2017. p12) are not static 'rules but an opportunity for maternity professionals to factor in specific considerations when discussing birthplace options'. "Women may therefore with informed consent, still decide to birth at home in the presence of biopsychosocial factors and complicating factors."

> **Practice Point:**
> Reflect on your guidelines and policies. What groups of women or birthing people are excluded locally from a recommendation for homebirth and is this evidence based? Does it reflect NICE guidelines?

> **Practice Point:**
> Does your local Trust routinely collect data about who requests outside guideline care at home? If so, who collects this data and what is it used for? Is this something that could be implemented to guide future strategic service planning?

LEGALITIES IN THE UNITED KINGDOM

One of the more complex and challenging issues that healthcare providers face when a request for homebirth outside of guidance or against recommendations are the perceived issues around the legal responsibilities of the individual health-care professional (midwife, obstetrician etc) in relation to discharging duties of care. The Human Rights Act (1998) ensures that public bodies such as the NHS and those who work within them fulfil their legal obligation to ensure human rights are respected, protected, and fulfilled. Fundamental in this process is a firm and working understanding of the rights of the woman or birthing person, where maternal bodily autonomy is enshrined in UK legislation, even if health professionals deem a decision to be one that might jeopardise the wellbeing and safety of either the woman/birthing person or the fetus (*St George's Health Care NHS Trust v SR v Collins and others ex parte S*, 1998) The right to choose the location of birth is firmly situated within a human rights framework, underpinned by both international and national laws and the principles of choice, autonomy, equality, dignity, and respectful care (Birthrights, 2017). The Universal Declaration of Human Rights, undoubtedly the historical cornerstone of protected rights, was agreed upon and adopted internationally in 1948 (United Nations, 1948). The UK was a founding signatory of the UDHR, which set out 30 rights and freedoms which formed the basis of firstly the European Convention on Human Rights (Council of Europe, 1950), which was then incorporated into law in the United Kingdom by the Human Rights Act (HMSO, 1998).

EUROPEAN CONVENTION ON HUMAN RIGHTS

The Council of Europe consists of 46 member states, including the UK (who were founding members in 1949), all of whom have signed and therefore are committed to upholding the European Convention on Human Rights (ECHR). The convention forms the basis of protection for human rights, guaranteeing specific rights and freedoms for those residing in member countries whilst also prohibiting treatment that might be harmful, prejudicial, or discriminatory. The convention is arranged into articles:

- Article 2   The right to life
- Article 3   Freedom from torture
- Article 4   Freedom from slavery
- Article 5   The right to liberty
- Article 6   The right to a fair trial
- Article 7   The right not to be punished for something that wasn't against the law at the time
- Article 8   The right to respect for family and private life
- Article 9   Freedom of thought, conscience, and religion
- Article 11   Freedom of assembly
- Article 12   The right to marry and start a family
- Article 14   The right not to be discriminated against in respect of these rights
- Protocol 1, Article 1   The right to protection of property
- Protocol 1, Article 2   The right to education
- Protocol 1, Article 3   The right to participate in free elections
- Protocol 13   The abolition of the death penalty
-

The convention is interpreted through applications made to the European Court of Human Rights (ECHR).

(Council of Europe, 1950)

Any choices made in pregnancy and childbirth are protected by both Article 2 (the right to life, in the case of the UK the pregnant woman and not the fetus) and Article 8 (the right to respect for private and family life) of the ECHR. Article 8 involves protection of both physical and psychological safety and wellbeing (Council of Europe, 1950). Article 9 is a qualified right and under some circumstances it might be appropriate to restrict a right. However, these decisions must meet the 3 legal tests of:
- Is the restriction lawful?
- Is there a legitimate aim for the restriction?
- Is it necessary?

Such tests have been tried in the European Court of Human Rights (see table *Ternovszky v Hungary* [2010]), which have gone on to establish the right to respect for a private life which includes choice of where to birth your baby.

TERNOVSZKY v HUNGARY (2010)

Ms Ternovszky was a pregnant woman in Hungary who had chosen to birth at home. She had previously been supported by a midwife, Agnes Gereb, at her first homebirth and was now seeking confirmation that the midwife would not be prosecuted for attending Ms Ternovszky's second birth at home. At that time in Hungary, the laws meant that midwives would be unavailable to attend her birth at home as there was a risk of liability for practising outside the law. The European Court of Human Rights ruled in this case that Hungary's laws and professional rules governing birth outside of a hospital prevented Ms Ternovszky's choice of homebirth and consequently violated her autonomy to choose birth at home and that this violated Article 8 of the European Convention on Human Rights. The court asserted that homebirth should be a matter of personal choice and that licensed medical services must be provided within the country to support women to birth at home; thus independent midwives were permitted to apply for licenses.

Ternovszky v. Hungary (2010).

Practice Point:

Much anxiety and confusion exist around how far registrants are protected when supporting women/birthing people making choices outside of guidelines. The NMC Code (2018) supports registrants to uphold women's choices such as these in the following sections (non-exhaustive):

1.3 avoid making assumptions and recognise diversity and individual choice

1.5 respect and uphold people's human rights

2.5 respect, support and document a person's right to accept or refuse care and treatment

4.1 balance the need to act in the best interests of people at all times with the requirement to respect a person's right to accept or refuse treatment

4.2 make sure that you get properly informed consent and document it before carrying out any action

8.1 respect the skills, expertise and contributions of your colleagues, referring matters to them when appropriate

8.2 maintain effective communication with colleagues

8.5 work with colleagues to preserve the safety of those receiving care

8.6 share information to identify and reduce risk

9.3 deal with differences of professional opinion with colleagues by discussion and informed debate, respecting their views and opinions and behaving in a professional way at all times

13.1 accurately identify, observe and assess signs of normal or worsening physical and mental health in the person receiving care

13.2 make a timely referral to another practitioner when any action, care or treatment is required

13.3 ask for help from a suitably qualified and experienced professional to carry out any action or procedure that is beyond the limits of your competence

---

Reproduced with kind permission of the author of the Code, The Nursing and Midwifery Council (2018).

INFORMED CONSENT

Informed consent is an ongoing, dynamic process that, once given, can be withdrawn at any time. Informed consent is an integral foundation for protecting bodily autonomy, agency, and human rights–centred care and without informed consent, no intervention, recommendation, or examination can be lawfully undertaken. Moreover, women should remain the final decision makers in each and all the choices offered during pregnancy. Published guidance exists to provide support in facilitating informed consent (GMC, 2020) alongside key UK court rulings, which have helped shape how we approach discussion with women (UKSC, 2015). Fundamentally, all women have the right to not only be involved in decisions about their care but should remain central in that process, free from coercion. The process of decision making should revolve around a meaningful conversation with the aim of exchanging relevant information, including the material risks involved in recommendations (and reasonable alternatives) (UKSC, 2015). In order to do this, an exploration of what matters to that woman must form the basis of an unbiased exchange of evidence-based information and the risks and benefits of all recommended options and alternatives, including importantly, the option to do nothing (GMC, 2020). The key test of materiality was defined in the key UK case *Montgomery v Lanarkshire Health Board*, UK Supreme Court (2015) (see Vignette). The test of 'Materiality' means understanding what is important or significant to the woman and providing information, including alternatives, led by women's needs. This can only be achieved by individualised and tailored discussions with health professionals being guided by what matters to the woman by asking them and sharing relevant information in a way that can be understood (GMC, 2020).

Practice Point:

How is informed consent practiced where you work? Reflect on your own guidelines and policies for women who choose to birth outside of guidelines at home. What pathways and support networks are there for you and for the woman/birthing person? What challenges have you faced or observed that relate to providing appropriate, nonbiased information and thereby support informed consent

MONTGOMERY v LANARKSHIRE HEALTH BOARD (2015)

In 1999, Mrs Montgomery became pregnant with her 1st child. Mrs Montgomery was short in stature and an insulin-dependent diabetic. Evidence at the time suggested that those with diabetes were at risk of having a larger-than-average baby and more likely (9–10% risk) to have a shoulder dystocia with the inherent fetal and maternal risks such as brachial plexus injury, hypoxic brain injury, and severe genital trauma. Mrs Montgomery was noted to therefore have a high-risk pregnancy and was informed that her baby was above average size, and she subsequently voiced her concerns about vaginally birthing her baby. She was encouraged to agree to an induction of labour and not told of the risk of shoulder dystocia in labour. Her consultant said that whilst the risk of shoulder dystocia was high, she considered that the risk occurring was small and so failed to discuss it with Mrs Montgomery, noting that in the consultant's opinion if they discussed shoulder dystocia with every diabetic woman, they would opt for a caesarean section which they believed wasn't in their best interest. Mrs Montgomery was therefore encouraged to birth vaginally, during which time a shoulder dystocia occurred. This resulted in her son sustaining a brachial plexus injury, paralysis of his arm, and later a diagnosis of cerebral palsy. The court found that as the risk of shoulder dystocia was substantial, Mrs Montgomery should have been advised of the risk and that had this been the case, Mrs Montgomery would have probably opted for a caesarean section.

GUIDELINES

Clinical guidelines should provide evidence-based recommendations and/or care pathways to facilitate informed discussions. Used well, they can be an invaluable source of information and a tool to guide consultations and personalised care planning with women (Frohlich and Schram, 2015). However, used inappropriately, as 'rules to follow' wherein women are coerced into staying 'within' guidelines and/or used interchangeably with policies, protocols, or procedures, they become problematic (Kotastaka 2011; RCM, 2022). Women have the right to make choices, assert agency and protect their bodily autonomy; guidelines cannot and should not replace or override these rights. Supporting autonomy therefore sometimes requires moving outside of recommendations made by guidelines, either because the guideline does not support the individual's circumstances or because the woman's perception and acceptability of risk versus benefit differs from the recommendation even when the quality of evidence supporting the recommendations is strong (Kotaska, 2011). Therefore women's perceptions of safety must be viewed with a biopsychosocial-cultural-spiritual model (Feeley, 2022) and 'materiality' of what constitutes safety to the individual must guide the care planning.

This may cause anxiety and discomfort in clinicians who do not have mechanisms to support complex care planning, particularly when women decline recommended care (Feeley, Downe and Thomson, 2021). Research has shown clinicians may behave coercively to gain compliance and to protect themselves (Jenkinson, Kruske and Kildea, 2017). Recent cases within the United Kingdom (*Sanderson v Guys and St Thomas' NHS Foundation Trust*, 2020) have tested the extent to which guidelines should be evaluated, interpreted, and contextualised in light of the clinician's decision making process.

SANDERSON v GUYS AND St THOMAS' NHS FOUNDATION TRUST (2020)

The claimant was born in 2002 and during her birth suffered a moderate cerebral palsy after an acute episode of hypoxia in the time immediately before her birth. The 2 allegations during the case were that a breach of duty occurred in 2 instances, firstly the decision to perform fetal blood sampling rather than performing an immediate delivery and secondly that there was a delay in proceeding to instrumental birth after a period in which a bradycardia occurred. The judgement in the case highlighted important considerations around not only the length of time between the incident occurring and the litigation being brought being such that it was difficult to reconstruct a timeline of events, but importantly in how guidelines are applied within a clinical context. The judgement found that contradictions in guidelines for the action to take following a 3-minute bradycardia challenging and stated that interpretation of guidelines must be done alongside and considering clinical judgement, not being used as a substitute for such, rejecting a 'formulaic application'. The Court emphasised a necessity to consider how a reasonably competent clinician would act, which is not the same as rejecting or defying the guidance. The obstetrician was therefore found to have acted reasonably in both the fetal blood sampling and not expediting the birth of the Claimant. The issues of delay around performing an instrumental birth due to retrieving the necessary equipment to perform a safe procedure were rejected, with the Judge ruling that the obstetrician should not be criticised as she had acted as quickly as she could have in the context of the 'real world'.

(Sanderson v Guys and St Thomas' NHS Foundation Trust (2020)).

MENTAL CAPACITY

Maternal autonomous decision-making is contingent on 'mental capacity'. Mental capacity refers to an individual's ability to be able to make decisions about and for themselves, including choices to consent to recommendations for intervention and treatment, but importantly also withholding consent or declining care. The Mental Capacity Act (2005) provides a legal framework to support those lacking mental capacity. Crucially, the Act assumes capacity, and a person should not be treated as lacking capacity simply due to a decision that healthcare professionals did not agree with. It is relatively rare in the context of maternity care for someone to lack mental capacity. An individual is deemed to have capacity where they:

- Can understand the information that is relevant to the choice or decision they are making
- Can retain that information
- Use the information to inform that decision
- Can communicate that decision

It would be wrong to assume that someone lacked capacity merely because of having decided that health-care professionals disagree with their decision, a diagnosed mental ill health or learning disability, being a young person or socially vulnerable/under local authority care, being a drug or alcohol user. If doubts exist around an individual's capacity to decide, then advice should be sought, and formal pathways of assessment carried out as per local Trust pathways. However, using this assessment as a means of trying to change someone's mind or influence a particular decision is coercive and inappropriate. Sometimes capacity can be lost temporarily, for example, the influence of opiates, alcohol, psychotic episode, or injury – however, in these cases, and where appropriate, healthcare professionals might wait until capacity is regained to then support decision making (Office of the Public Guardian, 2007).

Practice Point:
How might you assess the mental capacity of anyone in maternity care? What support networks and pathways are there in your local area to support you in this process?

Practice Point:
Referral to social services for women making informed choices to birth outside of guidelines is highly inappropriate in the absence of safeguarding concerns. The legal issues highlighted in this chapter serve to illustrate that whilst a clinician may not agree with a decision a woman or birthing person is making, it is not their role to make them change their mind through coercive and bullying practices such as vexatious social services referrals or threats to do so. Anecdotal evidence suggests this is on the rise. Before making a referral, think. Why is this appropriate? Consider reviewing local guidelines for automatic referral in the event of an outside-of-guideline request.

COURT OF APPEAL, S v St GEORGE'S HEALTHCARE TRUST (1998)

A woman, S, had a previous diagnosis of moderate depression and was offered an induction of labour to prevent harm to her unborn baby, having also been diagnosed with severe pre-eclampsia. S expressed the wish to have a 'natural' delivery and therefore declined induction of labour. S was then sectioned under the Mental Health Act of 1983 to undertake a mental health assessment. She was transferred immediately after being sectioned, against her will to the hospital (who had at that point applied for a dispensation to requiring consent for a caesarean section, having advised incorrectly that S had been in labour for the previous 24 hours.) The dispensation was granted, and a caesarean section performed to deliver the baby. S was returned post caesarean to the mental health facility, from which she discharged herself 48 hours later. S appealed the decision to enforce a caesarean section and the court held that S indeed that the right to decline treatment even if it meant the life of S or her baby was put in danger and the initial ruling was overturned. The application by the Trust failed to make distinct the need for urgent treatment and S depression diagnosis necessitating the section under the Mental Health Act and subsequent detention, with her condition being a medical one, not a mental one. The court held that pregnancy does not reduce the entitlement for a woman to decide to consent or not to undergo treatment and that the unborn child's rights do not prevail over hers. The unborn is not a distinct and separate person from the woman and she is entitled to not be forced into anything including treatment. Importantly this underlines the principle of the Mental Capacity Act of 2005 in that everyone has an immediate presumption of capacity.

(St George's Health Care NHS Trust v SR v Collins and others ex parte S (1998)).

COURT OF APPEAL, Re MB (1997)

MB was 40 weeks pregnant when she was admitted to hospital. During her pregnancy she had attended antenatal appointments where she declined bloods due to being needle phobic and had not attended other appointments that were made for her. The day before her admission she had attended a clinic where the ultrasound scan had confirmed her fetus was in the breech position and she was offered and advised to have a caesarean section, to which she agreed. During MB's admission she signed consent forms for the caesarean section but declined venepuncture for blood samples due to her needle phobia. MB continued request that the caesarean section go ahead and the following day she signed consent forms again for the operation; however when the anaesthetist attended insert a cannula, MB declined, and the caesarean section was subsequently cancelled as she declined both a cannula and any anaesthesia administered by needle. MB agreed to administration of anaesthesia via a mask and the caesarean was again rebooked. Two days later during a conversation with the consultant anaesthetist, the risks of aspiration with anaesthesia with a mask were discussed, which subsequently resulted in MB declining consent for the caesarean section. MB then started to labour but was not talking to the midwife or obstetrician, so her GP talked to her and discovered she was indeed happy to have the caesarean provided she did not feel or see any needles, which included IV lines and catheters. A consultant psychiatrist was then involved, after which MB agreed again to the caesarean. During preparation on the theatre table, MB then refused consent for anaesthesia and the caesarean was cancelled. The hospital at this stage had already consulted with their legal team, who sought a court order to proceed with the caesarean section. MB appealed this through her own appointed legal team. The court of appeal held that every person with the capacity to consent to or decline medical treatment has the right to do so regardless of potential consequences, but that temporary factors may contribute to a lack of capacity to make decisions and in this case that MB did not have capacity due to her needle phobia. The court held therefore that it would be lawful in this case to undertake an emergency caesarean section if it were in the patient's best interests and that she lacked capacity, and MB's appeal was dismissed. MB did in fact consent to the operation in the end. The ruling established that a pregnant woman who is deemed competent and therefore with capacity can decide for any reason or 'no reason at all' even if the consequences may lead to the death or serious injury of her or her fetus/newborn.

(Re MB (Medical Treatment) (1997) EWCA Civ 3093 (1997)).

MOTIVATIONS FOR OUTSIDE-OF-GUIDELINE PREGNANCY AND BIRTH AT HOME

Understanding birthing women and people's motivations for 'out-of-guideline' pregnancy and births or withholding consent to interventions is an evolving field of enquiry. Within the UK emphasis has been on exploring specific phenomena such as freebirth (Feeley and Thomson, 2016; Plested and Kirkham, 2016), decision making, risk perception, information use, and interactions with health professionals when planning 'high-risk' homebirth (Lee, Ayers and Holden, 2016, 2016c, 2016b, 2016a), water vaginal birth after caesarean (McKenna and Symon, 2014), or how health professionals facilitate alternative care choices (Madeley et al, 2019; Feeley, Thomson and Downe, 2020; Westbury and Enion, 2021). Internationally, an evidence base has also emerged over the last decade. For example, in Australia, where homebirth is not as established nor adopted within most traditional maternity systems, research has explored those who might be considered 'high risk' or with complicated pregnancies reject in whole or in part conventional pathways and locations for pregnancy and birth, preferring to birth at home either with no healthcare provider present or with unregulated birth workers (Rigg *et al.*, 2017, 2020). Jackson, Schmied, and Dahlen (2020) found that hospitals births were rejected by some women due to previous experiences such as limited autonomy, a lack of emotional safety within the institutional environment (likening it to being a 'cattle yard'), and fear of institutional birth which they felt influenced an overuse of interventions in birth (Jackson, Schmied and Dahlen, 2020).

Similar findings were identified in the Netherlands, whose maternity system is vastly different from that of Australia, in that homebirth is an integrated part of primary care provision. Hollander *et al.* (2017) explored why 21 women opted for homebirth outside of medical advice and found that birth without intervention and freebirth were common choices, fear being overarching motivator (see chapter *Freebirth*). Vaginal birth after caesarean/homebirth after caesarean (HBAC) was also a common option inferring previous birth experience was a factor in decision-making, evident in a London hospital 'outwith guidelines' clinic (Hattan, Flohlich, and Sandall, 2016) who confirmed HBAC as their most common 'complex' choice. Keedle *et al.* (2015) explored the experiences of women planning and birthing at home after a previous caesarean section. The authors highlighted an overarching theme of 'it's never happening again', revealing that for some women and birthing people, homebirth was protective, a way to avert another negative experience in hospital, to one experienced as profoundly empowering. Moreover, women reported that the homebirth experience was a way to reclaim control over their previous experience. Across all studies it is clear however that a significant influence and common motivator for choosing complex homebirth is the desire to avoid further trauma experienced in previous maternity care, which the authors refer to as a *pathway of traumatic experience* (Holten, Hollander and de Miranda, 2018; Hollander, 2020).

It is important to note that in much of the qualitative data, women express that they are willing to take responsibility for the potential consequences of their choices regardless of the degree of risk and potential poor outcome (Symon *et al.*, 2009). Additionally in cohorts of women rejecting medical recommendations to birth in hospital, studies have demonstrated that women will access care if they feel it is necessary, or if needed (Jackson, Dahlen and Schmied, 2012; Jackson, Schmied and Dahlen, 2020). In this way women are making their own risk assessment (Feeley and Thomson, 2016); while this may be counter to a clinical risk assessment, we as clinicians must accept their decisions. These decisions are situated within the context of women's wider lives, For which which 'safety' encompasses more than clinical outcomes with psychological, social, spiritual, and cultural elements that we may or may not be privy to (Feeley, 2019).[1]

In the UK a secondary analysis of the UK Birthplace study (Brocklehurst *et al.*, 2011; Hollowell *et al.*, 2015) explored the socio-demographic and clinical characteristics of women with complicated pregnancies planning to birth outside of an obstetric-led setting (alongside or freestanding midwifery-led unit or homebirth). The researchers found that compared to those planning to birth in an obstetric-led unit, they were more likely to be of white ethnic background, older, domiciled in less deprived areas, married, or living with a partner, multiparous having had more than one previous birth. Common complexities present in those planning to birth outside obstetric-led settings were:

- Previous caesarean section
- Post term pregnancy
- BMI > 35 kg/m^2
- known group B streptococcus carriage

Broadly supporting the range of complexities seen in the 'outwith' guidelines clinic discussed previously (Hattan, Flohlich and Sandall, 2016). Interestingly for those women who planned complex birth in a non-obstetric-led setting, fewer pregnancy-related 'complicating conditions' (prolonged rupture of membranes, meconium liquor, abnormal fetal heart rate, hypertension, vaginal bleeding, non-cephalic presentation, proteinuria) were noted at the beginning of labour compared to their counterpart planned OU births. In terms of likelihood of transfer from non-obstetric-led unit (OU) to OU, there was broad congruence across all settings, with nulliparous women reflecting a higher rate (45–56%) and multiparous women 18–23%; however interestingly, in relation to homebirth, there was no difference in transfer rates between healthy and those with complex pregnancies for nulliparous women. However, for multiparous women with complex needs, they were more likely to be transferred than those with healthy pregnancies. It should be noted that many women will not remain static in their presentation of risk – it may increase or decrease. Safe care involves recognising these changes, adapting to every individual situation, and responding in a timely manner. More research is needed to understand the experiences of women and birthing people who choose homebirth in the presence of social and psychological complexities, as these seem to be missing from the data.

OUTCOMES AND SAFETY DATA

Li *et al.* (2015) in their secondary analysis of the Birthplace Cohort Study suggested that in women with complexities:

> '...compared with planned OU [obstetric unit] birth, planned homebirth was associated with a significantly reduced risk of "intrapartum related mortality and morbidity" or neonatal admission within 48 hours for more than 48 hours. The difference reflected a higher neonatal admission rate in planned OU births'
>
> (Ibid, p. 747)

Moreover:

> 'Compared with planned OU birth, planned homebirth was associated with a significantly lower risk of intrapartum interventions and adverse maternal outcomes requiring obstetric care in both nulliparous and parous "higher risk" women and a significantly higher probability of straightforward vaginal birth in both nulliparous and parous "higher risk" women'
>
> (Ibid, p. 746)

As noted in the chapter *Homebirth – The Evidence*, no evidence demonstrates that intrapartum perinatal deaths are more likely in a midwife-led setting compared to an obstetric unit for low-risk women (Scarf *et al.*, 2018; Hutton

---

[1]Highlighting the gravity and impact poor experiences of institutional maternity can have on maternal decisions and neonatal outcomes, an early piece of work exploring homebirth in the context of provision and autonomy was carried out by Symon et al. (2009). They compared, in an anonymised matched cohort analysis, 1462 women cared for by UK-based independent midwives (IM) (and therefore the majority birthed at home) and matched them to women who birthed within the NHS (n = 7214). Their findings demonstrated that those under IM care experienced an increased likelihood of spontaneous labour and vaginal birth and with less need for analgesia, but unexpectedly also an increased rate of stillbirth and neonatal death (Symon et al., 2009). However, the authors acknowledge that if women with risk factors and pre-existing medical conditions and previous obstetric conditions within the IM cohort were excluded, the difference between NHS and IM perinatal mortality disappeared. Moreover, contextual factors to these deaths were identified in a follow-up qualitative study (Symon et al., 2010). The researchers interviewed 15 IMs and analysed their case notes pertaining to the perinatal deaths the IMs were involved with. While 8 of the deaths were likely avoidable, in all cases, the IMs had appropriately identified fetal compromise. However, the mothers declined the suggested interventions such as transfer to hospital, due to a strong fear of NHS care. Having suffered previous significant trauma within the NHS, these women opted to remain home, with devastating consequences. Therefore it is imperative that we deliver trauma-informed, respectful, and dignified care if we are to improve outcomes.

et al., 2019); indeed existing evidence is supportive of the safety of homebirth overall (Brocklehurst *et al.*, 2011; Hutton *et al.*, 2019; Reitsma *et al.*, 2020), while favourable findings from Li et al.'s (2015) study acknowledged that a much larger study would be required to rule out clinically important differences between those planning birth at home and obstetrics units with complexities. Other data suggests that care could be improved to prevent poor perinatal outcome and for women opting for homebirth with complex needs. The 2020 ESMiE confidential enquiry of the quality of pregnancy, intrapartum, birth and postnatal care investigated perinatal deaths in births planned in midwifery-led settings. Data were examined using MBRRACE methods (Draper *et al.*, 2017), focussing on outcomes between 2015 and 2016 in alongside midwifery units and between 2013 and 2016 for freestanding midwifery units and homebirths. Of the 64 deaths included within the enquiry, 15 women planned to have their baby at home. Of these 15, 10 planned a homebirth while having complexities, and 5 of the 10 against explicit medical recommendations. For 4 perinatal deaths, homebirth against recommendations was considered a contributory factor and the panel reported '*health professionals could have done more to engage with the mother*' (Rowe *et al.*, 2020, p. 1669). Common contributing factors to the 10 perinatal deaths were found to include: a lack and/or delay in appropriate antenatal and intrapartum escalation for complexities, women not engaging with recommended antenatal care or not disclosing health concerns and/or women declining interventions including transfer when they were offered and delays in the decision to transfer, arrival if the paramedic/ambulance response, and delayed obstetric review once arrived in hospital. Interventions declined included scans, induction of labour, vaginal examinations, fetal monitoring, and transfer to an obstetric unit. However, the report does not account for the decision-making process and motivations behind and why women and birthing people chose outside guideline care, decline interventions and pathways, and choose to birth at home with a complicated pregnancy. Clear recommendations arising out of ESMiE aimed at providers of all midwifery-led services, including homebirth, were made. As such the following should be considered as part of all homebirth service planning, and especially for those where women with complexities choose to birth at home:

- Fully and accurately documented discussions between the woman/birthing person, the midwife, and/or obstetrician including risks and benefits of all birth settings, considering existing complexities or those which might arise. Discussions should be evidence based, unbiased, considering the woman's needs, values, and preferences, demonstrated effective planning for managing complexities that might arise, intervention, and transfer rates (specific to that Trust [see chapter *Antenatal planning – Organisational considerations*]). There should also be an opportunity to revisit the care plan at period intervals during the pregnancy and at the start of intrapartum care.
- Audit of the use of monitoring in labour, including the frequency and timing, benchmarked against national and local guidance.
- The development of a standardised risk assessment too that can be commenced at the beginning of the intrapartum period and continued through the duration of labour, to support swift and appropriate identification and escalation of deviations from normal physiological processes.
- Development and maintenance of guidelines for the management of the compromised neonate in any community setting (see also chapter *Homebirth in undergraduate, postgraduate and clinical education*). This should be revisited annually in mandatory training and include in situ skills and drills and the multidisciplinary team (including ambulance colleagues).
- Adoption of a standardised means of communication to relay urgency of transfer with emergency services and the receiving obstetric and neonatal unit.
- Transfer guidelines, pathways, and protocols developed alongside local ambulance trusts to facilitate safe, effective, and prompt transfer. This should include discussions such as attendance and transfer times as well as ensuring urgent transfer prompts urgent obstetric and neonatal assessment.

Overall outcome and safety data related to individual complexities is beginning to emerge but however remains limited in range and scope. Emphasis on personalised approach to both risk assessment and complex care planning with the woman/birthing person and their caregivers should underpin every conversation with woman or birthing people making these choices (NHS England, 2016, 2021), especially in the presence of co-complexities which require careful consideration considering a constantly evolving evidence base. More information on keeping up to date with evidence can be found in the section '*useful contacts, organisations, and resources*' at the end of this book.

PRACTICAL SUPPORT FOR COMPLEX HOMEBIRTHS

Having established birthing women and people opting for homebirth have the legal right to do so, with decisions spanning a spectrum of complexity and motivations, this section will explore the role of maternity professionals in delivering complex homebirth care. Research recognises that for maternity professionals 'out of guidelines' care can be challenging and a site for tension or conflict (Jenkinson, Kruske and Kildea, 2017; Madeley et al, 2019; Feeley, Thomson and Downe, 2019). For some maternity professionals, their values and beliefs may not align with maternal autonomous decision-making, viewing complex birthing decisions in conflict with fetal wellbeing (Kruske *et al.*, 2013; Thompson, 2013). For others, a lack of institutional and leadership support cultivates fear of blame and repercussions should an adverse outcome occur, thus creating a 'reluctance' to support complex physiological births (Cobell, 2015; Westbury and Enion, 2021). Conversely, other maternity professionals report competence and confidence and, even where there is a lack of institutional support, are (mostly) managing to successfully support these birth choices

(Madeley et al, 2019; Feeley, 2019; Westbury and Enion, 2021). Regardless of personal opinions or feelings, our moral, legal, and professional obligations require maternity professionals to uphold respectful and dignified care including in circumstances we may not choose for ourselves. Therefore learning from those maternity professionals who have facilitated complex homebirths can provide insights to support other professionals in their clinical practice.

> **Practice Point:**
> Take some time to reflect on how you feel when someone requests care outside of guidelines. What is it about the request that makes you feel a certain way? Only by recognising and addressing our own unconscious biases and knowledge/skills gaps can we then begin to address how we might respectfully approach challenging conversations with both women/birthing people and the multidisciplinary team.

PRINCIPLES OF CARE

Based on previous research (Feeley, Thomson, and Downe, 2020) there are several principles of care to guide approaching supporting complex homebirths:

- *Supported and/or informed decision-making* is the recognition that birthing women and people's autonomy and agency is paramount. Here, the role of maternity professionals is to provide unbiased information regarding the benefits and risks of all the available options, including doing nothing, to which the decision resides with woman.
- *Relationship building and connection* is the recognition that safe care is actualised through meaningful relationships. Taking the time to understand and get to know the birthing woman or person, to actively listen to their perspectives and how they arrive at their decisions, will build connection and offer insights to appropriate information-giving. For example, enquiring about the woman's 'non-negotiable' components of care can form the foundation of an acceptable plan of care (see Fig. 13.1).
- *Relationship building and support* is the recognition that proactively convey support and demonstrate a commitment to facilitating a complex birth decision is a building block of trust. While conveying support is trickier in fragmented care models, it can be achieved through verbal support, reading and respecting birth plans, and conveying agreement and understanding in a non-judgemental way.
- *Relationship building and trust* is the recognition that where these earlier principles are applied mutual trust (hopefully) occurs. Trust is pivotal in all care encounters but especially important within complex physiological

> *"Trish, a senior midwife, was caring for a woman with multiple medical complexities who wanted a twin home waterbirth. While the community midwives were alarmed at such a decision, Trish found through careful listening, the woman revealed the extent and impact of her previous traumatic hospital birth experience; to reclaim control was through homebirth. Taking the time to understand the woman's position Trish asked what her birthing 'non-negotiables' were:*
>
> *'…The things that were non-negotiable though were not to do with clinical care. She wanted everyone who came in her room to introduce themselves, no one to touch her without asking permission and all changes to the plan to be explained to her first…'*
>
> *This finding was extremely important, Trish got to the heart of what constituted safety for this woman, less about birthplace and even midwifery-led care, but an issue of dignity and respect in the birth room (Morton & Simkin, 2019) - emotional safety. As it turned out, over time and in their ongoing relationship the woman did decide to have a hospital birth (with a very successful outcome). Where a hospital birth may have been the safer physical option, had this woman's emotional safety needs not been met first, it may have deterred engagement with maternity professionals. Where women do not feel supported, and/or lack trust in their caregivers, they are increasingly opting out of maternity care altogether (Greenfield et al., 2021; McKenzie & Montgomery, 2021). For midwives who may be nervous in this situation, Trish's actions (and others in the study) highlight that through understanding the woman, what appears to be a seemingly radical (and perhaps alarming) complex birth decision becomes simplified and less alarming - such is the power of relationships."*

Fig. 13.1 Understanding non-negotiables, extract from Feeley (Forthcoming 2023).

birth planning; without trust, women may opt out of the service altogether or, in situations of a deteriorating clinical picture, disbelieve the caregiver (Plested and Kirkham, 2016). Therefore, behaving and *being* trustworthy is an acute responsibility of maternity professionals. Trust can be viewed as an essential component of safe care (Feeley, Thomson, and Downe, 2020).

CARE PLANNING

Ideally trusting relationships are built within the antenatal period creating the opportunity for birthing women and people to share and discuss their birth preferences. For those seeking complex homebirths, the antenatal period offers time and space to consider all options; develop care plans; discuss with the multidisciplinary team as appropriate, plan any preparation as required; and consider contingencies (Feeley, Thomson, and Downe, 2020). For example, someone who has suffered a previous traumatic postdate induction of labour resulting in a caesarean section and is now seeking a homebirth may consider two care plans – a primary care plan and a contingency. In this example assuming the woman will not accept any form of induction should postdates reoccur, the primary care plan will focus on the homebirth in the event labour begins spontaneously.[2] The complex (HVBAC) homebirth care discussions and plans would consider the usual suggestions regarding a homebirth while ensuring information is provided around the signs and symptoms of scar dehiscence (urgent action required) and uterine rupture (emergency action required) and with transfer times a key discussion point. A contingency conversation and plan might include the possibility of labour not starting spontaneously, and therefore a planned caesarean section, should that be preferred.

Key components of care planning must include offering women up-to-date information with a range of options tailored to their decision and personal circumstances. This requires maternity professionals to have sound knowledge of evidence-based information underpinned by the latest research and beyond that of their local guidelines.[3] Wider sources include NICE, RCOG, RCM, latest research, professional networks, and accessing other Trust guidelines that may differ. Furthermore, the ability to read, assess, and apply research findings is a core skill, along with, where evidence is lacking, the ability to apply sound anatomy and physiology knowledge to unique circumstances (Feeley, Thomson, and Downe, 2020). An advantage of antenatal planning is the time it affords for maternity professionals who may need to seek out further information to inform the conversations. It is fair that maternity professionals may have gaps in their knowledge base regarding certain conditions, particularly those that are rare. However, it is the professional's responsibility to take time to source appropriate information as required – which is also a trust-enhancing activity.

While many birthing women and people will have good knowledge of their options, it is important not to make assumptions and be ready with a 'tool bag of ideas' (Feeley, Thomson, and Downe, 2020) to explore a range of possible options or modifications to usual care pathways. These discussions should be captured and documented as a care plan which are typically written by maternity professionals but should be based on the woman's decisions. Care plans should reflect the discussion of risk/benefit for each option, alternatives, and an individualised risk assessment (while appreciating for multiple complex needs, an accurate, individualised risk assessment may not always be possible). When used well, care plans are tools to support birthing women and people's decisions, reflecting a commitment to support and a way to reduce repetitive risk conversations from other health professionals and to communicate with and/or support professionals delivering the intrapartum care (Feeley, Thomson, and Downe, 2020). Additionally, women should have a copy of their care plan to maintain a sense of ownership that it is theirs and as a tool of communication with other professionals if/when needed.

Moreover, care planning conversations should ideally include contingency plans should the events of labour and birth unfold differently from expectations. Contingency planning is an ideal opportunity to support individualised care for any possibility, facilitating women to consider what is important to them (their non-negotiables) in different scenarios, thus remaining the decision-maker and in control. Crucially, these conversations and care plans must not be reduced to a tick box exercise or information overload regarding 'risk' or infer a disclaimer.[4] They must be led by the woman's initial preferences, needs, and desires for her birth and ideally held over a period, so space is created for women to consider the information, ask further questions, and consider all options available. This also gives maternity professionals the time to consider and plan or implement any preparation required (if necessary).

Within the care planning, and where necessary, additional safety measures may need to be considered and planned for. Such measures will vary depending on the complexity of the homebirth choice and the level of experience and competence the local community midwives' levels have (Feeley, Thomson, and Downe, 2020). Therefore additional safety measures are not hard-and-fast rules but locally determined and contingent on these factors. However, these may include 'skills and drills' practice for community midwives, refresher days, training sessions, or setting up specific on-call teams with the appropriate skill sets (see chapter *Homebirth in Undergraduate, Postgraduate and Clinical Education*). One aspect required for all complex homebirths is robust lines of communication amongst the staff for disseminating the care plans to the appropriate care settings, including consideration of informing the ambulance service and other professionals as necessary. Additionally, community midwives must have a mechanism of support during the intrapartum care episode, with transparent documented escalation plans should they be needed.

---

[2]Note that this is not exhaustive but an example of a complex birth decision.

[3]While NICE provides national guidance each hospital Trust is not obligated to follow them and develop their own local guidelines. Therefore there are variations of what is deemed 'complex' or 'out of guidelines' depending on the organisation.

[4]Within the legal context it is essential that maternity professionals understand they are not responsible for women's decisions and that any perceived risk is theirs to take. However, maternity professionals still maintain responsibility for the clinical care provided; therefore disclaimers do not protect practitioners or Trusts if poor or negligent care is found during an adverse event.

> **Practice Point:**
> In your local area how is multidisciplinary team working with local Ambulance services facilitated? Is there a way of identifying to them any potentially complex cases that need to be flagged in the event of an emergency? Many Ambulances Trusts now have consultant midwives who will be delighted to discuss cross-professional work and arrangements for discussion.

In some Trusts complex care plans including those for homebirth are carried out by consultant midwives or obstetricians. This is typically an offer for referral to the senior professional and is not compulsory, for all maternity professionals should be equipped to have informed decision-making discussions. Therefore care must be taken that offers of referrals are not used in a coercive or threatening manner. However, senior input may be advantageous and often is a supportive mechanism to ensure the woman's decision is respected and upheld (Feeley, Thomson, and Downe, 2020). Consultant midwives typically have responsibility of ensuring the wider community midwifery teams are equipped to provide adequate intrapartum care, such as implementing the safety measures outlined above (Rogers and Cunningham, 2007; Robinson, 2012). For women with medical and obstetric conditions, where possible, it is helpful to have a link obstetrician. Where community midwives have a primary obstetric contact, it facilitates better communication and positive interprofessional relationships (Madeley et al, 2019; Feeley, Thomson, and Downe, 2020), thus likely to improve safe care (Kings Fund, 2008). Additionally, complex homebirth planning may require multidisciplinary input to ensure the care plan is based on appropriate and best available evidence. In some complex situations, for example, if someone has medical and obstetric co-morbidities, several specialists may need to be involved (see Fig. 13.2). Some organisations have robust pathways where MDT meetings are embedded as part of everyday care and practice, and in others it may require the lead midwife to orchestrate.

> **Practice Point:**
> Who in your workplace is responsible for care planning when a request for outside-of-guideline care is received? Some NHS Trusts will have dedicated birth choices clinics, or a consultant midwife clinic – for some midwives may be empowered and supported to have these conversations with women and birthing people. Is there a dedicated Obstetrician responsible for engagement with women who make similar choices?

INTRAPARTUM CARE DELIVERY

Complex homebirths are typically attended to by community midwives but occasionally paramedics may be the first to arrive (e.g. in the event of rapid labour or an emergency). Depending on the level of complexity, it may be arranged to have two on-call midwives from the start of the care episode or occasionally a consultant midwife or other senior midwife may also provide care. If newly qualified midwives or those new to the community setting are part of the on-call rota, it is helpful to have an experienced midwife to attend together. This is an ideal opportunity to provide proactive help, support, and guidance while maintaining appropriately safe care (Feeley, 2019). Consideration also needs to be made for those birthing women and people who do not disclose their birthing intentions nor have an antenatal care plan in place, as women are not obliged to disclose (Feeley, Thomson, and Downe, 2020). For example, arriving at a homebirth where a woman is postdate and has declined induction of labour without a complex care plan requires midwives

> Kerry highlighted an extensive collaboration between herself, obstetricians, neonatologists, and specialist doctors to support a woman with a blood born virus requesting a homebirth. Kerry emphasised the value of working alongside the MDT, crucially recognising the limits to her scope of practice while also contributing to the MDT discussions as expert in homebirth (her team had 35% homebirth rate). Thus, demonstrating valuable interprofessional collaboration and good communication to meet the needs of the woman:
>
> *'I think it is always the same thing, just the communication being really honest and listening to them as well and making sure, cos I'm not an expert in the follow-up care but reassuring them that I am an expert in normal birth, our homebirth rate was 35% so I was very confident that if things weren't going to happen we would transfer in and definitely listening to them, and knowing I wasn't that expert because although we were happy to support her but there may have been specialist genuine reasons why we'd have to think of alternatives and stuff.'*

Fig. 13.2 MDT specialist care planning (extract from Feeley, 2019).

to be flexible and attend to her needs, retaining a human rights approach. Or in other situations where the clinical picture changes for someone with an antenatal complex care plan, this too requires skilled care and a preparedness to adapt to changing needs, all while maintaining woman-centred care and respecting decisions that are made.

For complex homebirths, intrapartum care is delivered in line with midwives' usual scope of practice; it is not 'bringing the hospital to home' and thus requires usual care as outlined within the rest of this book. Any additional measures that have been agreed upon with attending clinicians and the woman should be undertaken with the express recognition that any care provided will be limited and this may result in a delay in obtaining medical and emergency assistance should this be required. Transfer times from home to hospital for obstetric or neonatal emergency care can be an issue, either due to the local ambulance Trust response times or due to the limited nature of interventions that can be accommodated at home. Midwives are usually adept at managing the unexpected; however, they should always work within the scope of their own competence and code of conduct. For those situations where the clinical picture changes during the intrapartum period and discussions/consent are required. Immediate and appropriate escalation should be ensured.

Practice Point:
Care planning for complex homebirth should include a clear understanding from all parties that the care provided at home, either standard midwifery care or emergency care, will be limited by the resources on the ground – both equipment and staffing. This might include increased transfer times to an obstetric or neonatal unit or access to medications and drugs. This should feature in any care planning and considerations for how early to transfer. Also refer to chapter on *Antenatal Planning*, *Paramedic Transfer*, and *Emergency Care*.

CONCLUSIONS

This chapter has highlighted some of the evidence and practicalities around care planning for complex homebirth including legalities and protections for midwives supporting choice. Key to respectful care is a framework of trusting relationships between women and their givers. It would be easy to provide a list of 'to dos' when someone presents with choices for complex homebirth; however, in doing so this would do a disservice to the need for personalised care planning necessary for safe and individualised care. This chapter therefore has provided some points for consideration, including understanding why women and birthing people make choices. Motivations for choosing a complex homebirth are multifaceted, which negates a standard tick box approach to planning care. More evidence is needed to evaluate outcomes both for specific and individual medical complexities and for women or birthing persons with psychological, social, and economic needs.

REFERENCES

Birthrights (2017) *Human rights in maternity care, Birthrights.* Available at: http://www.birthrights.org.uk/library/factsheets/Human-Rights-in-Maternity-Care.pdf (Accessed: 29 January 2021).

Brocklehurst, P. *et al.* (2011) 'Perinatal and maternal outcomes by planned place of birth for healthy women with low risk pregnancies: The birthplace in England national prospective cohort study', *BMJ (Clinical Research Ed.)*, 343, pp. d7400–d7400. Available at: https://doi.org/10.1136/bmj.d7400.

Cobell, A. (2015) *What are midwives' experiences of looking after women in labour outside of Trust guidelines.* Masters. Kings College, London.

Council of Europe. (1950) "Convention for the Protection of Human Rights and Fundamental Freedoms." Council of Europe Treaty Series 005, Council of Europe

Draper, E. *et al.* (2020) 'MBRRACE-UK Perinatal Mortality Surveillance Report, UK Perinatal Deaths for Births from January to December 2018'. The Infant Mortality and Morbidity Studies, University of Leicester.

Feeley, C. (2019) *'Practising outside of the box, whilst within the system': A narrative inquiry of NHS midwives supporting and facilitating women's alternative physiological birthing choices.* Doctoral. University of Central Lancashire.

Feeley, C., Downe, S. and Thomson, G. (2021) '"Stories of distress versus fulfilment": A narrative inquiry of midwives' experiences supporting alternative birth choices in the UK National Health Service', *Women and Birth* [Preprint]. Available at: https://doi.org/10.1016/j.wombi.2021.11.003.

Feeley, C. and Thomson, G. (2016) 'Why do some women choose to freebirth in the UK? An interpretative phenomenological study', *BMC Pregnancy and Childbirth*, 16(1), p. 59. Available at: https://doi.org/10.1186/s12884-016-0847-6.

Feeley, C., Thomson, G. and Downe, S. (2019) 'Caring for women making unconventional birth choices: A meta-ethnography exploring the views, attitudes, and experiences of midwives', *Midwifery*, 72, pp. 50–59. Available at: https://doi.org/10.1016/j.midw.2019.02.009.

Feeley, C., Thomson, G. and Downe, S. (2020) 'Understanding how midwives employed by the National Health Service facilitate women's alternative birthing choices: Findings from a feminist pragmatist study', *PLOS ONE*, 15(11), p. e0242508. Available at: https://doi.org/10.1371/journal.pone.0242508.

Feeley, C. (2022) The Asset Model: What midwives need to support alternative Physiological Births (Outwith Guidelines), *Practising Midwife*, 25, pp. 28–30.

Frohlich, J. and Schram, R. (2015) 'Clinical guidelines: Hindrance or help for respectful compassionate care?', in S. Byrom and S. Downe (eds) *The roar behind the silence*. London: Pinter and Martin, pp. 119–126.

GMC (2020) 'Decision making and consent'. General Medical Council. Available at: https://www.gmc-uk.org/-/media/documents/gmc-guidance-for-doctors—decision-making-and-consent-english_pdf-84191055.pdf.

Greenfield, M., Payne-Gifford, S. and McKenzie, G. (2021) Between a rock and a hard place: Considering "Freebirth" during Covid-19, *Frontiers in Global Women's Health*, 2, pp. 603744. doi:10.3389/fgwh.2021.603744

RCM and RCOG. (2020) Guidance for provision of midwife-led settings and homebirth in the evolving coronavirus (COVID-19) pandemic.

Hattan, J., Flohlich, J. and Sandall, J. (2016) '"Outwith guidelines" care planning and care delivery outside and obstetric unit: Outcomes and experience.' London: Kings Health Partners. Available at: https://view.officeapps.live.com/op/view.aspx?src=https%3A%2F%2Fwww.npeu.ox.ac.uk%2Fassets%2Fdownloads%2Fukmidss%2Fstudy-day-2016-presentations%2F06%2520Study%2520Day%25202016%2520-%2520Julie%2520Frohlich%2520-%2520utwith%2520guidelines%2520care%2520planning.pptx&wdOrigin=BROWSELINK (Accessed: 26 May 2022).

HMSO (1998) *Human Rights Act.*

Hollander, M. (2020) 'Birthing in the Netherlands', in H. Dahlen, B. Kumar-Hazard, and V. Schmied (eds) *Birthing outside the system: Canary in the coal mine.* 1st edn. Oxford: Routledge.

Hollander, M. *et al.* (2017) 'Women's motivations for choosing a high risk birth setting against medical advice in the Netherlands: A qualitative analysis', *BMC Pregnancy and Childbirth*, 17, pp. 1–13. Available at: https://doi.org/10.1186/s12884-017-1621-0.

Hollowell, J. *et al.* (2015) The Birthplace in England national prospective cohort study: Further analyses to enhance policy and service delivery decision-making for planned place of birth. *Southampton: Health Services and Delivery Research*, 3. Available at: https://www.ncbi.nlm.nih.gov/books/NBK311289/pdf/Bookshelf_NBK311289.pdf.

Holten, L., Hollander, M. and de Miranda, E. (2018) 'When the hospital is no longer an option: A multiple case study of defining moments for women choosing homebirth in high-risk pregnancies in The Netherlands', *Qualitative Health Research*, 28(12), pp. 1883–1896. Available at: https://doi.org/10.1177/1049732318791535.

Hutton, E. *et al.* (2019) 'Perinatal or neonatal mortality among women who intend at the onset of labour to give birth at home compared to women of low obstetrical risk who intend to give birth in hospital: A systematic review and meta-analyses', *The Lancet*, 14, pp. 59–70.

Jackson, M., Dahlen, H. and Schmied, V. (2012) 'Birthing outside the system: Perceptions of risk amongst Australian women who have freebirths and high risk homebirths', *Midwifery*, 28(5), pp. 561–567. Available at: https://doi.org/10.1016/j.midw.2011.11.002.

Jackson, M.K., Schmied, V. and Dahlen, H.G. (2020) 'Birthing outside the system: The motivation behind the choice to freebirth or have a homebirth with risk factors in Australia', *BMC Pregnancy and Childbirth*, 20(1), p. 254. Available at: https://doi.org/10.1186/s12884-020-02944-6.

Jenkinson, B., Kruske, S. and Kildea, S. (2017) 'The experiences of women, midwives and obstetricians when women decline recommended maternity care: A feminist thematic analysis', *Midwifery*, 52, pp. 1–10.

Keedle, H. *et al.* (2015) 'Women's reasons for, and experiences of, choosing a homebirth following a caesarean section', *BMC Pregnancy and Childbirth*, 15(1), pp. 206–206. Available at: https://doi.org/10.1186/s12884-015-0639-4.

Kings Fund (2008) 'Safe birth: Everybody's business'. Kinds fund. Available at: http://www.kingsfund.org.uk/sites/files/kf/field/field_publication_file/safe-births-everybodys-business-onora-oneill-february-2008.pdf (Accessed: 29 January 2021).

Kruske, S. *et al.* (2013) 'Maternity care providers' perceptions of women's autonomy and the law', *BMC Pregnancy and Childbirth*, 13(1), p. 84. Available at: https://doi.org/10.1186/1471-2393-13-84.

Kotaska, A. (2011) Guideline-centered care: A two-edged sword, *Birth*, 38, pp. 97–98.

Lee, S., Ayers, S. and Holden, D. (2016a) 'Decision-making regarding place of birth in high-risk pregnancy: a qualitative study', *Journal of Psychosomatic Obstetrics & Gynecology*, 37(2), pp. 44–50. Available at: https://doi.org/10.3109/0167482X.2016.1151413.

Lee, S., Ayers, S. and Holden, D. (2016b) 'How women with high risk pregnancies perceive interactions with healthcare professionals when discussing place of birth: A qualitative study', *Midwifery*, 38, pp. 42–48. Available at: https://doi.org/10.1016/j.midw.2016.03.009.

Lee, S., Ayers, S. and Holden, D. (2016c) 'Risk perception and choice of place of birth in women with high risk pregnancies: A qualitative study', *Reconceptualising Risk in Childbirth*, 38, pp. 49–54. Available at: https://doi.org/10.1016/j.midw.2016.03.008.

Lee, S., Holden, D. and Ayers, S. (2016) 'How women with high risk pregnancies use lay information when considering place of birth: A qualitative study', *Women Birth*, 29(1), pp. e13–e17. Available at: https://doi.org/10.1016/j.wombi.2015.07.010.

Li, Y. *et al.* (2015) 'Perinatal and maternal outcomes in planned home and obstetric unit births in women at "higher risk" of complications: Secondary analysis of the Birthplace national prospective cohort study', *BJOG*, 122, pp. 741–753.

Madeley, A.-M., Williams, V. and McNiven, A., 2019. An interpretative phenomenological study of midwives supporting homebirth for women with complex needs. British Journal of Midwifery 27, pp. 625–632. Available at: https://doi.org/10.12968/bjom.2019.27.10.625.

McKenna, J.A. and Symon, A.G. (2014) 'Water VBAC: Exploring a new frontier in women's autonomy', *Midwifery*, 30(1), pp. e20–e25. Available at: https://doi.org/10.1016/j.midw.2013.10.004.

McKenzie, G. and Montgomery, E. (2021) Undisturbed physiological birth: Insights from Women Who Freebirth in the United Kingdom. *Midwifery*, 101, pp. 103042. doi:10.1016/j.midw.2021.103042

Montgomery v Lanarkshire Health Board [2015] SC 11 [2015] 1 AC 1430

Morton, C. and Simkin, P. (2019) Can respectful maternity care save and improve lives? *Birth*, 46(3), pp. 391–395. doi:10.1111/birt.12444

NHS England (2016) 'National maternity review. Better Births'. NHS England.

NHS England (2021) *Maternity Transformation Programme, england.nhs.uk.* Available at: https://www.england.nhs.uk/mat-transformation/ (Accessed: 5 May 2021).

NICE (2017) 'Intrapartum care for healthy women and babies.' National Institute for Health and Care Excellence. Available at: https://www.nice.org.uk/guidance/cg190/chapter/recommendations#pain-relief-in-labour-nonregional (Accessed: 29 January 2021).

Nursing and Midwifery Council. (2018) *The code: professional standards of practice and behaviour for nurses, midwives and nursing associates.* Available at: http://www.nmc.org.uk/globalassets/sitedocuments/nmc-publications/revised-new-nmc-code.pdf

Office of the Public Guardian (2007) 'Mental Capacity Act Code of Practice: Code of practice giving guidance for decisions made under the Mental Capacity Act 2005.' The Stationery Office.

Plested, M. and Kirkham, M. (2016) 'Risk and fear in the lived experience of birth without a midwife', *Midwifery*, 38, pp. 29–34. Available at: https://doi.org/10.1016/j.midw.2016.02.009.

RCM (2022) 'Care outside guidance. Caring for those women seeking choices that fall outside guidance'. Royal College of Midwives. Available at: https://www.rcm.org.uk/media/5941/care_outside_guidance.pdf.

Reitsma, A. *et al.* (2020) 'Maternal outcomes and birth interventions among women who begin labour intending to give birth at home compared to women of low obstetrical risk who intend to give birth in hospital: A systematic review and meta-analyses', *EClinicalMedicine*, 21, pp. 100319–100319. Available at: https://doi.org/10.1016/j.eclinm.2020.100319.

Re MB (Medical Treatment) (1997) EWCA Civ 3093 (1997).

Rigg, E.C. *et al.* (2017) 'Why do women choose an unregulated birth worker to birth at home in Australia: A qualitative study', *BMC Pregnancy and Childbirth*, 17(1), p. 99. Available at: https://doi.org/10.1186/s12884-017-1281-0.

Rigg, E.C. *et al.* (2020) 'A survey of women in Australia who choose the care of unregulated birthworkers for a birth at home', *Women Birth*, 33(1), pp. 86–96. Available at: https://doi.org/10.1016/j.wombi.2018.11.007.

Robinson, A. (2012) *The role of consultant midwife: An exploration of the expectations, experiences and intricacies.* University of Southampton. Available at: https://eprints.soton.ac.uk/349088/.

Rogers, J. and Cunningham, S. (2007) 'Pregnancy. A consultant midwives' clinic: A catalyst for cultural change?', *MIDIRS Midwifery Digest*, 17(2), pp. 201–206.

Rowe, R. *et al.* (2020) 'Intrapartum-related perinatal deaths in births planned in midwifery-led settings in Great Britain: Findings and recommendations from the ESMiE confidential enquiry', *BJOG: An International Journal of Obstetrics & Gynaecology*, 127(13), pp. 1665–1675. Available at: https://doi.org/10.1111/1471-0528.16327.

Sanderson v Guys and St Thomas' NHS Foundation Trust (2020).

Scarf, V.L. *et al.* (2018) 'Maternal and perinatal outcomes by planned place of birth among women with low-risk pregnancies in high-income countries: A systematic review and meta-analysis', *Midwifery*, 62, pp. 240–255. Available at: https://doi.org/10.1016/j.midw.2018.03.024.

St George's Health Care NHS Trust v SR v Collins and others ex parte S (1998).

Symon, A. *et al.* (2009) 'Outcomes for births booked under an independent midwife and births in NHS maternity units: Matched comparison study', *BMJ*, 338, p. b2060.

Symon, A. *et al.* (2010) 'Examining autonomy's boundaries: A follow-up review of perinatal mortality cases in UK Independent Midwifery', *Birth*, 37(4), pp. 280–287. Available at: https://doi.org/10.1111/j.1523-536X.2010.00422.x.

Thomson, A. (2013) 'Midwives' experiences of caring for women whose requests are not within clinical policies and guidelines.', *British Journal of Midwifery*, 21(8), pp. 564–570.

Ternovszky v. Hungary (2010). European Court of Human Rights judgement

UKSC (2015) *Montgomery v Lanarkshire Health Board.*

United Nations (1948) 'Universal Declaration of Human Rights'. United Nations. Available at: https://www.un.org/en/about-us/universal-declaration-of-human-rights.

Westbury, B. and Enion, A. (2021) 'Matricentric or medically responsible: An exploration of midwives' attitudes towards caring for women and birthing people who choose to birth outside of guidelines', *The Practising Midwife* [Preprint].

REFLECTIVE VIGNETTE

CAROLYN ROOTH

My interest in homebirth almost certainly began as a small child. I recall saying goodbye to my mother, who was in strong, active labour prior to leaving for my day at primary school, and I clearly remember the excitement of seeing her cradling my newborn sister on my return home. I remember the calm cheerfulness of the midwife in her blue community uniform and hat. It all seemed like a very normal life experience. Little did I know that midwifery was a career pathway I would eventually follow and in some small way my mother's experience was influential in my choice of career. I also remember my mother's wish for a homebirth some years later when she was expecting my brother, a choice supported by her family doctor but not by the midwife attached to the surgery, who had an obvious dislike of homebirth. The beliefs and attitudes of healthcare professionals undoubtedly impact both positively and negatively on the choices made by those who use our maternity services. In this case I have no idea of the catalyst for the midwife's homebirth aversion, but it was highly influential on my mother giving birth in the local maternity unit.

As a student midwife in the late 1980s the influence that healthcare professionals have on the options given to women and the choices they subsequently make was also apparent. My community placement was in a small semi-rural market town and my midwife mentor was a keen advocate of homebirth as a choice for women considered low risk. I recall some interesting discussions on the topic as we travelled in her car between clients, and it seemed to me at the time that such women comprised a significant proportion of her caseload. Whilst time has inevitably impacted my recall and I doubt that women opting for homebirth really were in the majority, choice of place of birth appeared to be routinely discussed at booking appointments and homebirth was seemingly presented both as a positive and real option. Continuity of care and where possible carer was considered the norm and I learnt to trust the ability of women's bodies to birth their babies whilst being encouraged to maintain a healthy respect for labour and birth as an unpredictable phenomenon where things do not always go to plan. I also learnt the importance of keeping women at the centre of midwifery care and offering real options for birthplace way before the concept of informed choice became the accepted norm. On reflection, I now recognise that whilst some demand for homebirth came from women themselves the impact of a woman's named midwife was an important influencing factor in their decision making. The beliefs and values of midwife supervisors and mentors also impact the impressions and experiences of students. As a clinical midwife, manager, and educator over the years I have witnessed how these shape beliefs and values of others. I have witnessed how those students in placement with a midwife who holds a positive attitude towards promoting homebirth choice are more likely to reflect this ethos and in turn promote homebirth as a viable choice themselves.

As a student midwife, I felt that the family doctors I had contact with were fairly ambivalent towards homebirth but were seemingly willing to support a woman's choice in the absence of known risk factors. There appeared to be an unwritten understanding that there was no requirement for a GP to be involved in the labour or birth itself which supported a feeling of status quo. Although very unlikely to be universal, it was clear that the GPs knew and respected the skills of the community midwife attached to their surgery which in turn appeared to promote confidence amongst women and their families that homebirth was a real choice.

By the time I became a community midwife myself some 6 years after qualification I had met and cared for a woman, who I will call Jenny. She had recently moved with her husband into the geographical area of the surgery where I was based and had no relevant medical or obstetric history. Jenny was in the mid-trimester of her first pregnancy and wanted to labour and give birth at home. She had attempted to register at the GP surgeries locally, requests which were declined because of her desire to have a homebirth and although not acknowledged perhaps her expressed interest in complementary therapies. I got to know Jenny and her husband well during pregnancy and the usual care offered throughout pregnancy was accepted by the couple. Jenny laboured at 39 weeks gestation, with her immediate family present and using only homeopathic medicines and practising meditation (perhaps what we would now recognise as hypnobirthing). She gave birth to her baby boy standing after an uneventful first stage of labour, had a physiological management of the third stage, minimal blood loss, and an intact perineum. I supported her to bath her baby as she requested before the cord was cut. It was a calm, almost magical experience where instinctively I knew that Jenny had been enabled to birth as she wanted and that her choices had been respected. Jenny will never know how much my experience of looking after her has influenced my practice or how it reinforced my belief in women having choice. I will always be grateful to her.

It is little wonder that doctors and, in particular, obstetricians are wary of birth at home. After all it is to those practitioners to whom we turn for assistance when faced with situations that fall outside the expected normal physiology.

Faced with assisting with emergency situations or the requirement to manage complicated childbirth on a daily basis, this inevitably becomes the practitioner's norm and leads to beliefs that childbirth is uncomplicated only in retrospect. Overall, I have found most medics supportive of the midwives caring for women at home, although a dissection of midwifery practice appears commonplace when transfer to hospital becomes necessary. Many midwives too have become increasingly medicalised in their approach to childbirth and, additionally, are required to care for women in times when staffing issues and financial constraints have become commonplace. Reports of adverse outcomes may also contribute to anxieties in clinical practice and as a result, some are fearful of physiological labour and birth. This may result in a reduction in the number of women who are offered the option to birth at home and see increasing numbers of women who now feel that it is necessary to exert their human rights to request to labour and birth in the place of their choosing.

In recent years I have seen an increase in the numbers of requests for homebirth from women with known risk factors who wish to exercise a right to choose homebirth. These may be in the minority but also inevitably create anxiety for the midwives required to provide care for women at home in the presence of complications. I understand these anxieties, having cared for women at home who have had previous caesarean sections, a previous shoulder dystocia, third-degree tear, or haemorrhage. The women for whom I have personally cared for in these circumstances have laboured and given birth uneventfully. In this respect I have been fortunate but as a former consultant midwife, I believe that provision of accurate information, detailed care planning, and discussion were key to women making informed choices both about their place of birth and care preferences. I recognise that women have a right to make choices which as professionals we would advise against or to choose options for care when we would prefer selection of an alternative option. I appreciate that not all midwives I have encountered feel the same way and for whom the provision of individualised support and the involvement of a senior midwife is essential. Although rare, on occasion we may need to seek legal advice. For example, the case of the woman who still wishes to birth at home at 46 weeks gestation or the woman who lacks decision making capacity. When the need has arisen, I have found this helpful when exploring the need to provide in complex and difficult situations.

My time as a midwife has undoubtedly seen changes in how choices for women are promoted, and how maternity care is delivered. In many cases a woman's maternity care has become fragmented, with many women seeing several different midwives during pregnancy and childbirth. Birth in hospital is often promoted as the safest option for place of birth despite available evidence which supports home as a safe place of birth for women without complications. As a midwifery manager, I was once sent the old birth registers by a relative of a midwife who had recently died for safekeeping. These illustrated how in the late 1950s and early 1960s the majority of women birthed at home with GPs often in attendance. However, our local population demographics have now changed, the average age of maternity service users has risen, and our caseloads comprise a greater number of women with medical and obstetric risk factors. Attitudes to childbirth have changed and as midwives we now practise in quite a different world. Labour and birth in hospital maternity units have become the norm reflecting a greater risk-averse society. As a midwife, for me this emphasises the importance of ensuring that women are given options which provide real choice about place of birth and that respect for individual birth preference remains more important than ever.

CLARAK HAKEN

When I was tasked with writing this reflection, I was asked to explore how I support homebirth as a consultant midwife and what the associated challenges and rewards are. I decided to approach this by undertaking a 6-minute splurge. When I considered homebirth, I thought of a delicate balancing act, like that of a tightrope walker.

Imagine there is someone on a tightrope, journeying from one side of the big top to the other, carefully putting one foot in front of the other, working to safely undertake their endeavour. They may have a harness. Or not. They may have a safety net below them, or perhaps just part of one. They may have excellent self-knowledge and self-belief. This may or may not be justified. They may be well rehearsed, experienced, and skilled, with the benefit of reliable equipment and an expert support team. Or they may not have these things ... or at least not things well suited to the situation.

When the clinical situation is relatively straightforward the tightrope feels like it's low to the ground. Undoubtedly there can still be a fall from height, but perhaps you'd be unlucky if that caused lasting harm. Sometimes the tightrope is at vertiginous height, under the glare of spotlights, and far removed from those looking on. The absolute risk of falling may still be low but the consequences are more significant, particularly where the safety measures requiring effective communication, training, equipment, and shared understanding are lacking. How scary to be on the tightrope knowing that those things are missing.

The tightrope walk is not a stunt or a hedonistic spectacle. Some parties feel that this is something they do not want to be associated with. They are often fearful of both harm to those involved and being called upon to explain or manage the situation if a complication occurs. They are likely to voice their disquiet and, if their warnings are not heeded, want to leave the tent altogether.

When I support homebirth as a consultant midwife, I am more likely to be formulating individualised plans of care with women planning birth outside of guidance rather than contributing to the day-to-day functions of homebirth. This has shaped the nature of my reflection.

I have no doubt of the joys and merits of birthing at home. I came later to homebirth than some, qualified 10 years before I attended a birth at home despite longing to do so. In part this was due to my working in maternity services, where homebirth was on the fringes and where it was largely unusual, unseen, and unimportant. This meant no exposure to homebirth as a student midwife or when working in the obstetric unit in terms of both practical experience and acknowledgment of home as a reasonable option for birth. For me being on the 'fringe' is an important context for homebirth. It was seen as peripheral, an added embellishment, a 'nice to have' but not core business in addition to the robust fabric of maternity service designed to envelop the majority of those receiving care, but not something woven into the body of it. Whist the 'fringe' itself may be seen as alternative, unnecessary, or even decadent by some, it also provides a dynamic, comforting, and tailored contrast to the uniformity.

Things have changed since my early career. Publication of the Birthplace evidence in 2011 gave new legitimacy to the practice and the policy direction of Better Births helped to bring homebirth in England into focus as a service priority. However, the challenges of maintaining a safe and effective homebirth service in the context of contemporary staffing crises, increasing clinical complexity, and diminishing confidence in midwives and midwifery care have exacerbated historic problems. We are not at a stage where birth at home is an everyday occurrence in the majority of maternity services. It may be closer to core business for women who are at low risk of complications, but it remains vulnerable to these challenges. Birth at home for women who are not at low risk but have social, medical, psychiatric, or obstetric complexities is fraught with additional perils.

The perils I refer to are not those associated with the clinical complexities themselves, the risks of thromboembolism, psychosis, shoulder dystocia, or uterine rupture. These are obviously important and often subject to repeated discussion. The perils for me are associated with birthing on the peripheries of a service when the implicit, and often explicit, expectation is that birth will occur in an obstetric setting, with the concomitant recommended interventions. This means the realities of managing the clinical complication or the absence of our usual safety measures at home are not anticipated, so there can be no mitigation.

The expectation that women will birth in what we deem to be the best possible place is something many professionals cannot see beyond. It may not be an unwillingness to do so but without understanding the unique context of homebirth the default is that women will, logically, reduce any potential risk and come in. The perspective is one borne from the notion that birth at home inherently increases risk rather than recognising that the poor transferability of our safety culture is part of the issue. In antenatal clinic consultations intended place of birth is not directly considered and opportunities to create shared understanding are lost. Women may be hesitant to engage with specialties they don't feel share their values or priorities for birth and so trust and open communication may be diminished. The potential for weaving a safety net is not explored.

One example of this is seen in our local and national guidance. Guidelines and their recommendations are ascribed value by setting standards for safe care and offering quality assurance in that standardisation. Local guidelines often omit place of birth, assuming the default of the obstetric unit with multidisciplinary care. Thresholds for obstetric review and consideration of intervention do not reflect the possibility of a woman being off the labour ward and how that should influence decision making, time thresholds, or clinical management. This phenomenon places women and midwives in a perilous situation when it's not acknowledged, and no mitigation is made.

National guidance offers steer on where birth should occur but limited if any clinical direction for birth at home when national steer does not align with the woman's preference. Whilst not every circumstance or combination of risk factors can be considered within guidance, care out with guidance may not have organisational or clinician's confidence. It may feel risky. Of course, risk and complexity are not absolute. Just as low risk of obstetric complication does not mean without risk, those at high(er) risk do not have a certainty of poor outcome if they do not follow the recommended advice. Of course, risk is not always about the woman and her characteristics; it's also about the characteristics of those caring for her. Are they experienced, up to date, competent? Are they supported by right systems and processes?

How, then, can care be given safety? Is it up to the individual midwife to apply their knowledge and expertise and hope for the best? Should they just follow the guideline as if care were being given in hospital and save the CTG monitoring/cannula/obstetric review? Is there realistic opportunity for constructive multidisciplinary team working and agreement on a bespoke plan of care? Can a plan of care be shared effectively and be deliverable? All may depend upon the organisational culture and the willingness to have responsive systems. There is also a fundamental question about forging relationships with women and families.

When I was considering homebirth and my role, I thought about advocacy for women and for midwives, organisational requirements and professional standards and I thought about balance. That led me to the tightrope. Why walk the tightrope? For me, I am propelled by a desire to support and meet the needs of others. Women are, after all, walking that same tightrope. I am acutely aware that for many homebirth is not just 'an' option; it is 'the' option, the only tenable choice in a situation far from ideal. Women choose home not only for all its inherent benefits but as an active avoidance of that associated with the hospital birth alternative: loss of agency and control and expected compliance with guidelines. Fragmented care, obstetric (or midwifery) interference, technology, and intervention are available at the push of a button. Fear and experience combine for women to make homebirth the better choice. That's not always a choice to celebrate if it comes from failing to meet women's needs, but it is one that needs an effective response.

We know that the lack of trust families understandably carry as a result of past trauma is not easily overcome. I have encountered women who engage with care but on guarded terms, offering apparent compromise or collaboration in order to access what they need but without confidence or conviction. They may opt to change their plans publicly and inform us that we cannot meet their needs but this often a private decision. This may lead to disengagement from care, birthing unattended or having hard lines where they will no longer follow professional advice despite careful planning and previous agreement. This becomes about survival for some women, and it can throw the midwife off balance. Negotiated plans that provided assurance to midwives and to services are no longer reliable and the mental model of care needs fast and flexible reworking.

As registrants we have clear duties and as employees well-drawn responsibilities. The tightrope walker's task is to respect these whilst prioritising being present with the woman and listening and offering sensitive and responsive care. The consultant midwife is ideally placed to help keep this balance. To aid the organisation, the midwife and the woman find shared understanding and agree on safety measures for their journey. As a consultant midwife my role is to contribute to this, but it can never be effective in isolation. There must be a sense that BIRTH is core business—not hospital birth, or spontaneous vaginal birth, but birth in all its guises. That means that safety measures need to work in all those guises too.

KAT HASSELL

Understanding why I love homebirth so much involves explaining my own personal experiences. I had 2 wonderful birth experiences at home after a very traumatic first birth after an induction of labour for preeclampsia.

Whilst I needed the medical input, the issues and trauma that I experienced could have been prevented by the power of the language used, things not explained, and choices not having been given. I felt unsafe, unsupported, and alone. I went on to find some healing birth experiences, and although I needed some medical support from the midwives as I didn't have straightforward births, I will say the benefits from being at home were huge. I had midwives attend to me because, if needed, they can act in the best interests of the woman and the baby and support healthy births.

I'm currently a Doula and well, I love it! I work with families no matter what their choice of birth environment is but I am definitely a huge homebirth advocate and have been for many years.

My tales of homebirth span the last 11 years, from my own homebirth leading into setting up a free homebirth support group with my very close friend (also a midwife and homebirth mummy), working alongside some amazing and inspiring midwives as a support worker prior to my doula journey.

Reflecting on all the homebirths I've been to, whether they were long, short, fast, loud, peaceful, transfers into hospital, water births, land births, supported by midwives, or birthed fully without any hands on, they all have some similar things in common in retrospect.

All the homebirth families made informed choices to birth at home. They read up, they questioned, and they got education and support. These may have been 'high-risk' women who declined to follow that pathway. They all have similar stories of how people have met them with the quote 'you're brave' and 'is it safe though?' when sharing the homebirth plan. These families are not reckless and don't plan to be unsafe.

I have also found that they all went into labour and birth much more relaxed; the hormones allowed them to do their job while the mothers rested, ate, danced, walked, cleaned, watched funny films, chatted, or even at a recent birth watched the Queen's funeral! Pets and other children could be in the home or sent off to family or friends. Partners and dads seem so much more in control of the environment, feeling free to make food and drinks, walk around, and support the mother in the birth process. They are more confident and take a place next to the birthing woman; they shelter and care for them without feeling a little in the way.

I have been able to learn from some just amazing midwives along my own journey, being able to watch a woman and see the body and her change through the journey. When you sit back and just become very in tune and see these changes it never fails to amaze me how truly powerful and strong women are when they birth. Birth is incredible and very instinctive. Being in your own home really allows for you to go within and find these powers. The emotions of when the baby is born, the pride and sheer elation of what they have just done is just breath-taking and a lot of the time a very emotional moment in time. Time almost stands still during the last throes of labour and early birth/postnatal time.

Watching and waiting was something I really did get taught by midwives. They would show me all the signs that things were moving and changing. They would advocate and support the families' choices, giving them time to process and make evidence-based choices. I will never forget one such birth where things I thought were going quite well and baby would be born soon, but things then changed, slowed, and stopped. The midwife explained to me that we will feed her and give her a drink, pop her in bed with the lights low, and her partner could snuggle up with her keeping some oxytocin flowing and allow her to rest. This rest and be thankful stage would give her the energy she needed to birth. We went home and the midwife said that she will call me in a few hours and that she will birth fast, and she did. I woke up to the call you're coming baby catching these calls were always in whispers the excitement would fill and I'd be up dressed and driving through the night to support the midwives and families. This lady had a beautiful, fast water birth, and the midwife knew, not from examinations but from watching with many years of experience of homebirths and truly being with women.

I can safely say several births have made me cry. I'm a person who is emotional but the hardest thing I ever see is siblings meeting their new brother or sister. They make my eyes leak! The excitement, especially when the other kids have stayed fast asleep, not knowing the story unfolding below, with the mother who roars her baby into the world, then slowly moves into the living room to be checked after birth, has some food and a hot drink to let that adrenaline slow, and gets ready to welcome her other children who now seem so big and grown.

I have been at a number of births and none have been the same; the home environment allows much more space for families to move and use the pool, bath, shower, bed, sofa, and stairs (I have definitely supported many mums to use the upstairs loo over the downstairs one, these steps are your friend!). Lots of mothers will go to the bathroom and stay put; the dark, small safe space and opening of the pelvis can all support the birth of a baby.

Water birth provides this space as well. Mothers feel almost covered and move quite a lot in a pool; it brings warmth and relaxation. Several times I've seen this power of relaxation that water has when the woman sinks away between her surges and fully follows her body.

When you're welcomed into someone's home and are able to watch and support a new family member being birthed however that birth goes, it feels like such an honour to be part of something very natural and special of our human nature. As a doula I support the family however they need; my last role was much more clinical and under midwife instruction, and now my focus is much more family based, which I love. Just holding space sounds so simple but can really change a birth.

I have many funny stories from my homebirths, from dads being sick at my making a placenta smoothie to rushing to fill a birth pool with pans of hot water to rushing to a birth to be stood on the doorstep in the rain hearing the birth unfold on the other side (door locked). I've spent time unplugging pumps cloaked with membranes. One wonderful mama stopped birthing to ask if I wanted a brew! I have had babies born to Nirvana and piano music. Large and small ones, babies who needed more support to birth, and ones who just came fast or slow. Every woman is different, and birth is unique.

MEG HILL

When I fell pregnant the first time I fell into the trap of believing homebirths are for hippies, that people 'like me' didn't have them and I made *that face* when anybody suggested it – you know the one, slightly between a wince and a grimace with a side order of horror.

Then I had a traumatic hospital birth. Physical recovery was difficult, and my mental health was poor. I knew I couldn't endure anything like that again, so when we started discussing the idea of expanding our family, I tried to get support for tokophobia. Unfortunately, at the time it was something nobody understood; after receiving a shrug of the shoulders from the GP I took matter into my own hands by hiring a doula and planning a homebirth.

At 1:30 am on Christmas Eve morning, I woke up in labour. I dozed for a couple of hours before waking again, this time with stronger contractions. My husband and I crept downstairs so we didn't wake our elder child, where we pottered about making tea and contemplating what time we ought to call reinforcements. As my first birth took 00:46 am we didn't envisage anything exciting happening anytime soon.

Well, that was wrong! At about 4:10 am my contractions jumped from being roughly 9 minutes apart to 3–4 minutes apart. Hurried phone calls were made to my parents to collect our son, to our doula Abbie, and also to the local midwife team. Far from the serene homebirth I'd envisaged, the house was chaos at that point, with my parents and my son getting ready to go, my husband trying to clear the room where the birthing pool was going to be, and my doula and my midwife doing their thing! I decided to get in the bath as the pain was getting a bit much; to be honest I also wanted a bit of peace and tranquillity. Only a few minutes later was the birth pool ready, so I took a heave on the gas and staggered downstairs.

I'd tried a waterbirth with my first and it wasn't a pleasant experience: the water felt far too cold in such a big room in hospital, so I had initially been wary of being in water again, but this was heaven! Toasty and warm and like a cocoon. The gas and air combined with oxytocin and endorphins did their thing and zoned me out from my surroundings.

After about an hour I started to feel the need to push. Or at least I thought I did! I doubted myself because I had never felt it with my first. I also didn't know if I was supposed to tell anyone or just push! As I was so zoned out it took several contractions to work up to being able to speak and tell everyone that things were hotting up. Abbie came into her own here and persuaded me to move from my sitting position to a kneeling position, which was much easier to give birth in.

At 8:46 am, in a couple of pushes, our baby was born with membranes still intact. Coated in vernix and puffy from the delivery, she was the most beautiful thing I'd seen. She healed me in ways I can't even describe, mending many of the scars from my firstborn.

After that experience it was a no-brainer that I'd plan a homebirth for my third child.

I was due on 14 December, coincidentally the same due date as my second child's, and although I'd been having contractions on and off from around 33 weeks the pregnancy was dragging. By New Year's Eve I'd decided enough was enough and requested a caesarean section during a monitoring appointment, which was booked in for the following Monday. I was offered an immediate induction but due to the trauma from an intervention-heavy first birth I declined everything but a sweep.

I had mild cramping when I got home at tea time but they died off quickly. And then, at five to midnight they started up again. I knew instinctively that this was 'it' and that it was going to be quick.

To give the midwife an opportunity to say Happy New Year to her nearest and dearest, I held off phoning her until after midnight – then promptly told her she needed to come very quickly! She arrived swiftly, not long after our photographer. I was already upstairs pacing at this point, in my room where we'd had a birthing pool set up for weeks. They set up while I climbed in the pool ... and it felt like only minutes later I needed to bear down.

I felt it all so much. I felt the change between the types of contractions, feeling the downward ripples as I moved into stage two. I felt myself going into transition – adrenaline rising, heart pumping, recognising that my body needed to work. I was about to meet her, and it was amazing. And I was so happy this was happening before my booked C-section.

It was incredible. At 1:15 am my daughter was born and it couldn't have gone better. It was the perfect birth. The placenta took an hour to come and we spent that hour in the pool together while her siblings came to have a peek at their new sister. There wasn't a single second of this birth where I didn't feel completely and utterly in control of what was happening – a far cry from my first birth.

If there was one thing I could go back and change it would be planning a homebirth for my first baby too. I truly believe that a lot of trauma and long-term physical and mental harm could have been avoided if I'd done so. Maternity services need to get better at making sure all families know and understand their birthplace choices. And while I owned my power during my second and third births, some of the treatment I received during the pregnancies tried to take that away from me and that simply isn't ok. My body, my baby, my choice.

SAMANTHA PHILLIS

As I looked up through the glass ceiling of the conservatory, the black clouds parted, the late spring rain stopped, and the sunlight streamed down. The phrase which sprang to mind was 'other worldly'. I could not believe my good fortune to be present, at this moment, about to bear witness to a warrior mama birth her third baby in the safety and protection of her home surrounded by her family. I am not a religious person but that moment felt heaven sent.

At this point in my career I had been a qualified midwife for 6 months and had slowly been building my confidence and competence at homebirths with the organisation I worked for (One to One Midwives). The general rule was: witness 3 homebirths, be a 2nd midwife at 3 homebirths, then step up as a 1st midwife leading on care.

By this point, I had already been the first midwife at a few homebirths but this one was different; this was a woman on my caseload. I knew her. I knew her family, I knew her children, I knew her husband and heard his anxieties … I even knew the dog!

As a student midwife I had not had the privilege of being present at a homebirth. When qualifying I was offered 2 preceptorship jobs, one within a traditional preceptorship model, working my way around the wards and ticking off skills, and one within a continuity, caseloading model completing my preceptorship caring for women and families from conception to 6 weeks postnatal.

I knew from starting my training that I wanted to be a community midwife. I was one of the older student midwives, having been a practising counsellor for 15 years when I started my midwifery training. I was a mother of 3 boys and galloping towards my middle years and I had a strong yearning within my very soul that I wanted to be a midwife. This yearning wasn't new. It is something I had wanted to do as a young child but had been distracted and found a different path. I love being a counsellor (I still practise) but this was a pull I couldn't ignore.

Realising I wanted to be a midwife was a birth in itself! I was applying for, and not getting, lots of counselling jobs. I had a busy private practice but needed the security of a regular income, so applying for jobs became an ongoing project. After one particularly difficult job rejection, my supervisor (all counsellors have psychological supervision every month from a trusted experience counsellor) advised me to sit with the discomfort, reflect, and meditate instead of reacting by applying for yet more jobs. By taking a step back and freeing up my subconscious to explore, I dreamt I was a midwife and I knew this was the pathway for me.

Applying for a midwifery degree and getting the 'within 5 years' qualification I needed to be accepted was another journey but I did it, started my training, and graduated with a first. I was elated.

And so I found myself with the difficult decision of head or heart when choosing the preceptorship programme for me. One to One Midwives was a big commitment not only for me but also for my family as I was on call a lot (5 out of 7 days) and the job was 30 miles away, whereas the other job was in a local hospital with no on-calls. However, my heart won and the opportunity to practise as a midwife within an autonomous, holistic, compassionate model of care was too much to pass up. I didn't know then that this was the last opportunity I would have to work within this model as I was in the last group of preceptors to be employed by One to One Midwives before they went into administration, so I am forever grateful my heart won.

This is how I found myself standing, on a Sunday afternoon, in a woman's conservatory, with a nervous dad taking a shower upstairs, a sausage dog running around the pool, and 2 children excitedly awaiting the arrival of their new sibling. No wonder I couldn't believe my luck!

There was an absolutely unique joy of seeing women in their own home for antenatal appointments without the pressure of task-focussed care as is common within the NHS. The holistic nature of relational care meant I knew the families' journey to this point; I knew their personalities, their fears, and their hopes for birth.

Birth is not just about the safe arrival of a baby into a family. It is the birthing of a mother and a parent. It is something that a woman will remember for the rest of her life. How a woman feels during birth will set the scene for the rest of her life. Not all women will have pool births in their conservatory with the sun streaming through the roof, but all women can feel powerful and empowered during birth if they are heard, supported, and respected during the entire pregnancy continuum, regardless of the birth they choose.

This particular day, I had already attended a birth … or more precisely a BBA (born before arrival) where the baby was in such a rush to arrive that she decided to make an appearance just 15 minutes after ringing me! I was back home enjoying a cup of tea and starting to think about my plans for the afternoon when I received the phone call to inform me the woman had felt her 'waters go' and she was experiencing regular surges.

When I arrived the woman was clearly in the active first stage of labour. We did not offer vaginal examinations as routine, a practice I have continued into my experiences as an NHS midwife. When offering vaginal examinations for cervical dilatation there must be a strong clinical reason to do so and offering them as routine felt arbitrary, intrusive, and unnecessary. As a very experienced midwife told me when I was a student midwife questioning how she possibly knew a woman was ready to push and was 'fully dilated' (I had only been present at very medicalised births at this point) she said 'she will push when she feels she needs to push and I will know her cervix is fully dilated when we see a head' ... I had held onto this!

I was encouraged as a Midwife to trust the process, trust women, and trust that the majority of women would birth their babies whether we were there or not! My role was supporter, 'reassurer', and birth space guardian. The birth space belonged to the family; I was merely an observer who had been invited in.

So when I say the woman was clearly in the active first stage what I mean is she was behaving in a way which informed me her labour was progressing. We had already discussed what she wanted from labour and birth and she had consented to intermittent auscultation of the fetal heart and requested a vaginal examination before entering the pool. The woman was worried about getting in the pool 'too early' and slowing labour down. Although I did not feel she required an examination it was her choice and upon examination I found her cervix to be 5 cm dilated.

When she entered the pool her labour was progressing quite quickly, and my colleague called to see if I needed her but I did not feel birth was imminent, so I advised her to finish her Sunday lunch and head over after (I am still rubbish at predicting birth – I was very wrong when I stated birth was not imminent ... babies arrive when they arrive!).

It had been a very rainy day but as the woman started to make noises like we were going to meet a baby soon, the clouds parted, the sun streamed in, and we readied ourselves. As the only adult present not birthing a baby, I was very fortunate that both the children were a little older and wanted to help! The baby's big sister wanted to be a midwife and had watched a lot of birthing programmes, so as the head was born, she clocked and announced the time! Dad made it downstairs just as the baby's head was crowning. Big brother was in charge of filming the birth, of which he did a remarkable job. By the time the second midwife arrived mother and baby were cuddling in the pool and the older children were beaming with pride at the part they had played in the birth.

We had a wonderful afternoon preparing the placenta for freezing (the woman had requested to eat the placenta as she had experienced postnatal depression following her previous birth and had read consuming the placenta could prevent a return of depression), reflecting on the birth, drinking tea, and basking in the oxytocin high which was always surprising to me but by now not an unfamiliar feeling. Following my first attendance at a homebirth I was so high when I came home that I spent a fortune on candles at a certain online shopping store, so now I was banned from shopping following a homebirth from fear of bankrupting us!

I always cry at births and I cried driving home from that particular birth. The power of the woman in the moment of birth as she brought her baby earthside and the connections made in that family as the children played an active role in supporting their mum overwhelmed me. I felt humbled that part of my job meant I was allowed to be present and witness one of the most absolutely private and intimate of human experiences.

This reflection is a thank you to One to One Midwives for allowing me the space and autonomy to midwife the way I knew I could, a thank you to my family for supporting me, and most of all a thank you to every single woman and family, who allow me into their space and continue to trust me to do so.

Thank you to the woman who birthed as we raved to MTV 90s classics.

Thank you to the woman who forgave me for flooding her kitchen!

Thank you to the woman who trusted me when I advised we transfer to hospital when my instinct told me something felt wrong (I was right but everyone was fine!)

Thank you to the couple who loved their baby out with such intimacy and mutual respect that I cried from start to finish!

Thank you to the couples with whom we have laughed, danced, cried, sung, eaten cake, drunk tea, eaten chef-standard food (who doesn't love it when a partner announces they're a chef when they offer you a snack!), watched films, and knitted quietly and who have welcomed me into their homes.

Thank you to the single parents, the same-sex parents, the IVF parents, and the surrogate parents. Thank you to the mothers who shout their babies out with power and primal energy and thank you to the women who slowly, quietly rock their babies earthside.

Thank you to every single person who has allowed me to be present as their baby was born whether that be a homebirth, a hospital birth, a midwife-led unit (MLU) birth, or a planned caesarean – you are all magic and full of power.

INDEX

Page numbers followed by *"b"* indicate boxes, *"f"* indicate figures, *"t"* indicate tables.